CASE FILES®
High-Risk Obstetrics

Eugene C. Toy, MD
The John S. Dunn Senior Academic Chair and Program Director
Obstetrics and Gynecology Residency Program
Vice Chair of Academic Affairs
Department of Obstetrics and Gynecology
The Methodist Hospital-Houston
Clerkship Director and Clinical Professor
Department of Obstetrics and Gynecology
University of Texas Medical School at Houston
Houston, Texas

Edward Yeomans, MD
Professor, Chairman, and Residency Program Director
Robert H. Messer, MD Endowed Chair
Texas Tech University Health Sciences Center
Department of Obstetrics and Gynecology
Lubbock, Texas

Linda Fonseca, MD
Assistant Professor of Maternal-Fetal Medicine
Northwestern University Feinberg School of Medicine
Chicago, Illinois

Joseph M. Ernest, MD
Chair, Department of Obstetrics and Gynecology
Carolinas Medical Center
Clinical Professor, University of North Carolina at Chapel Hill
Professor Emeritus, Wake Forest University School of Medicine
Charlotte, North Carolina

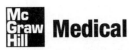

Mc Graw Hill Medical

New York   Chicago San Francisco   Lisbon   London Madrid Mexico City
Milan New Delhi San Juan Seoul   Singapore Sydney Toronto

Case Files®: High-Risk Obstetrics

1 2 3 4 5 6 7 8 9 0   DOC/DOC   14 13 12 11 10

ISBN 978-0-07-160543-4
MHID 0-07-160543-6

Notice

Medicine is an ever-changing science. As new research and clinical experience broaden our knowledge, changes in treatment and drug therapy are required. The authors and the publisher of this work have checked with sources believed to be reliable in their efforts to provide information that is complete and generally in accord with the standards accepted at the time of publication. However, in view of the possibility of human error or changes in medical sciences, neither the authors nor the publisher nor any other party who has been involved in the preparation or publication of this work warrants that the information contained herein is in every respect accurate or complete, and they disclaim all responsibility for any errors or omissions or for the results obtained from use of the information contained in this work. Readers are encouraged to confirm the information contained herein with other sources. For example and in particular, readers are advised to check the product information sheet included in the package of each drug they plan to administer to be certain that the information contained in this work is accurate and that changes have not been made in the recommended dose or in the contraindications for administration. This recommendation is of particular importance in connection with new or infrequently used drugs.

This book was set in Goudy by Glyph International.
The editors were Catherine A. Johnson and Cindy Yoo.
The production supervisor was Catherine Saggese.
Project management was provided by Rajni Pisharody, Glyph International.
The designer was Janice Bielawa.
RR Donnelly was printer and binder.

This book is printed on acid-free paper.

Library of Congress Cataloging-in-Publication Data

Case files. High-risk obstetrics / Eugene C. Toy ... [et al.].
  p. ; cm.
  Other title: High-risk obstetrics
  Includes bibliographical references and index.
  ISBN 978-0-07-160543-4 (pbk. : alk. paper)
  1. Pregnancy—Complications—Case studies.   2. Pregnancy—Complications—Problems, exercises, etc.   I. Toy, Eugene C. II. Title: High-risk obstetrics.
  [DNLM: 1. Pregnancy Complications—Case Reports.   2. Pregnancy Complications—Problems and Exercises.   3. Pregnancy, High-Risk—Case Reports.   4. Pregnancy, High-Risk—Problems and Exercises.   WQ 18.2 C3366 2010]
  RG571.C328 2010
  618.2—dc22   2010023056

McGraw-Hill books are available at special quantity discounts to use as premiums and sales promotions, or for use in corporate training programs. To contact a representative please e-mail us at bulksales@mcgraw-hill.com

To Terri, my lovely wife of 25 years, my best friend, my biggest encourager and supporter. It is her sacrifice and inspiration that allowed me to succeed in writing and teaching.

— ECT

To an entire generation of residents, medical students, and fellows who made teaching such a gratifying endeavor.

— ERY

To my parents and siblings, who together laid down the foundation for my future; to John, for his enduring support and encouragement; and my colleagues/friends, for their contributions to this textbook.

— LF

To all students, residents, fellows, and most importantly patients, who have taught me what is important about medicine, health, and life...

— JME

CONTENTS

CONTRIBUTORS

Irene E. Aga, MD
Assistant Professor
Department of Obstetrics, Gynecology, and Reproductive Sciences
University of Texas Health Science Center at Houston
Houston, Texas
Vaginal Breech Delivery

Leah W. Antoniewicz, MD
Assistant Professor
Department of Obstetrics, Gynecology, and Reproductive Medicine
University of Texas-Houston
Houston, Texas
Acute Kidney Injury

William H. Barth Jr, MD
Chief
Division of Maternal-Fetal Medicine
Massachusetts General Hospital
Associate Professor
Department of Obstetrics, Gynecology, and Reproductive Biology
Harvard Medical School
Boston, Massachusetts
VBAC—The "Approach to Counseling and Management"

Robert Casanova, MD
Associate Professor
Department of Obstetrics and Gynecology
Texas Tech University Health Sciences Center, School of Medicine
Lubbock, Texas
Shoulder Dystocia

Jude P. Crino, MD
Assistant Professor
Division of Maternal-Fetal Medicine
Department of Gynecology and Obstetrics
Johns Hopkins University School of Medicine
Baltimore, Maryland
Sickle Cell Disease

Christina M. Davidson, MD
Assistant Professor
Division of Maternal Fetal Medicine
Department of Obstetrics and Gynecology
Baylor College of Medicine
Houston, Texas
Asthma in Pregnancy
Abruption/Dead Fetus

Jeffrey Dungan, MD
Associate Professor
Division of Clinical Genetics
Department of Obstetrics and Gynecology
Northwestern University, Feinberg School of Medicine
Chicago, Illinois
First-Trimester Screening
Second-Trimester Serum Screening

Angela Earhart, MD
Division of Maternal Fetal Medicine
Department of Obstetrics and Gynecology
The Methodist Hospital-Houston
Houston, Texas
HELLP Syndrome
Breast Cancer in Pregnancy

Naghma Farooqi, MD, FACOG
Assistant Professor and Clerkship Director
Department of Obstetrics and Gynecology
Texas Tech University Health Sciences Center
Lubbock, Texas
Cesarean Section Leading to Cesarean Hysterectomy

Alfredo Gei, MD, FACOG
Director, Division of Maternal Fetal Medicine
Director, Division of Obstetrics
The Methodist Hospital-Houston
Houston, Texas
Preterm Premature Rupture of Membranes (PROM)
Peripartum Cardiomyopathy

R. Moss Hampton, MD
Associate Professor and Chairman
Department of Obstetrics and Gynecology
Texas Tech University Health Sciences Center of the Permian
 Basin
Odessa, Texas
Severe Preeclampsia

Andrew W. Helfgott, MD, MHA, CPE
Professor and Chief
Division of Maternal-Fetal Medicine
Department of Obstetrics and Gynecology
Medical College of Georgia
Augusta, Georgia
Postpartum Hemorrhage

Christopher Hobday, MD
Clinical Instructor
Department of Obstetrics and Gynecology
Weill Medical College of Cornell University
Houston, Texas
Preterm Premature Rupture of Membranes (PROM)

Marium G. Holland, MD, MPH
Fellow
Division of Maternal-Fetal Medicine
Department of Obstetrics, Gynecology, and Reproductive Sciences
University of Texas Health Sciences Center at Houston
Houston, Texas
Idiopathic Thrombocytopenic Purpura

Richard H. Lee, MD
Assistant Professor of Clinical Obstetrics and Gynecology
Department of Obstetrics and Gynecology.
Keck School of Medicine
University of Southern California
Los Angeles, California
Placenta Accreta

Alita Loveless, MD
Instructor
Department of Obstetrics and Gynecology
Texas Tech University Health Sciences Center
Lubbock, Texas
Septic Shock

Carla Ann Martinez, MD
Assistant Professor
Division of Maternal Fetal Medicine
Department of Obstetrics and Gynecology
Texas Tech University Health Science Center at Houston
El Paso, Texas
Stillbirth

Nathalie Dauphin McKenzie, MD, MSPH
Clinical Fellow
Division of Gynecologic Oncology
Department of Obstetrics and Gynecology
University of Miami, Miller School of Medicine
Miami, Florida
Adnexal Masses in Pregnancy

Hugh E. Mighty, MD, MBA
Associate Professor and Chair
Department of Obstetrics, Gynecology, and Reproductive Sciences
University of Maryland School of Medicine
Baltimore, Maryland
Ventilator Management

Manju Monga, MD
Professor
Department of Obstetrics, Gynecology, and Reproductive Sciences
University of Texas Health Science Center at Houston
Houston, Texas
Idiopathic Thrombocytopenic Purpura

LaTasha D. Nelson, MD, MSc
Assistant Professor
Department of Obstetrics and Gynecology
Division of Maternal-Fetal Medicine
Northwestern University, Feinberg School of Medicine
Chicago, Illinois
Pregestational Diabetes
Gestational Diabetes

J. Matt Pearson, MD
Assistant Professor
Department of Obstetrics and Gynecology
Division of Gynecologic Oncology
Sylvester Comprehensive Cancer Center
University of Miami, Miller School of Medicine
Miami, Florida
Adnexal Masses in Pregnancy

Kimberly A. Pilkinton, MD, MPH
Assistant Professor
Scott & White Memorial Hospital and Clinic
Texas A&M University System Health Science Center College
 of Medicine
Assistant Program Director, Obstetrics and Gynecology Residency
 Program
Director, Division of Education for Department of Obstetrics
 and Gynecology
Department of Obstetrics and Gynecology
Temple, Texas
Cesarean Section Leading to Cesarean Hysterectomy

Emily J. Su, MD, MS
Assistant Professor
Department of Obstetrics and Gynecology
Division of Maternal-Fetal Medicine
Northwestern University Feinberg School of Medicine
Chicago, Illinois
Thrombophilia

Alison C. Wortman, MD
Resident
Department of Obstetrics and Gynecology
Brian Allgood Community Hospital
United States Army
Seoul, South Korea
Puerperal Vulvovaginal Hematoma

Christopher M. Zahn, MD
Professor and Interim Chair
Department of Obstetrics and Gynecology
Professor
Department of Pathology
Uniformed Services University of the Health Sciences
Bethesda, Maryland
Puerperal Vulvovaginal Hematoma

ACKNOWLEDGMENTS

The curriculum that evolved into the ideas for this series was inspired by Larry C. Gilstrap III, MD when he was chairman of obstetrics and gynecology at the University of Texas Medical School at Houston. Dr. Gilstrap is a man of such a myriad of talents, and is my personal inspiration for much of the teaching that I do today. It has been a tremendous joy to work with my excellent coauthors: Ed Yeomans, who is a brilliant, talented clinician and never-tiring teacher; Dr. Linda Fonseca who set up the first case for this postgraduate series several years ago; and to my dear friend and colleague, Dr. Joseph "Mac" Ernest, whose leadership, vision, and practical approach are evident in all that he does. I am greatly indebted to my editor, Catherine Johnson, whose exuberance, experience, and vision helped to shape this series. I appreciate McGraw-Hill's believing in the concept of teaching through clinical cases, and I would like to especially acknowledge Cindy Yoo for her editing expertise and Catherine Saggese and Rajni Pisharody for the excellent production. I appreciate Linda Bergstrom for her sage advice and support. At Methodist, I appreciate Drs. Judy Paukert, Dirk Sostman, Marc Boom, Karin Larson-Pollock, Ayse McCracken, and Alan Kaplan for their leadership; and David Campbell and Tyler Kinney, who hold the department together. Without my dear colleagues, Drs. Konrad Harms, Jeane Holmes, and Priti Schachel, this book could not have been written. Most of all, I appreciate my ever-loving wife Terri, and our four wonderful children, Andy, Michael, Allison, and Christina, for their patience and understanding.

Eugene C. Toy

HOW TO USE THIS BOOK

Mastering the right diagnostic and therapeutic approaches within a field as broad as high risk obstetrics is a formidable task. It requires drawing on a knowledge base to procure and filter through the clinical and laboratory data, to develop a differential diagnosis, and finally to make a rational treatment plan. To gain these skills, the clinician is best guided and instructed by experienced teachers and accomplished surgeons, and inspired toward self-directed, diligent reading and practicing one's craft. Clearly, there is no replacement for experience at the bedside, delivery room, or operating room. Unfortunately, younger physicians will not have encountered the diversity of clinical situations, or dealt with the more unusual maternal-fetal complications. Perhaps the best alternative is a carefully crafted patient case designed to stimulate the clinical and surgical approach and decision making. In an attempt to achieve that goal, we have constructed a collection of clinical vignettes to teach diagnostic, therapeutic, and surgical approaches relevant to obstetrics and gynecology. Most importantly, the explanations for the cases emphasize the underlying principles, rather than merely rote questions and answers.

This book is organized for versatility: It allows the physician "in a rush" to go quickly through the scenarios and check the corresponding answers, and it provides more detailed information for the clinician who wants thought-provoking explanations. The answers are arranged from simple to complex: a summary of the pertinent points, the bare answers, an analysis of the case, an approach to the topic, a comprehension test at the end for reinforcement and emphasis, and a list of resources for further reading. The clinical vignettes are purposely placed in random order to simulate the way that real patients present to the practitioner. A listing of cases is included in Section III. The information is presented with the degree of evidence of support. Several multiple-choice questions are included at the end of each case discussion (comprehension questions) to reinforce concepts or introduce related topics.

Each case is designed to simulate a patient encounter with open-ended questions. At times, the patient's complaint is different from the most concerning issue, and sometimes extraneous information is given. The answers are organized into four different parts:

PART I
1. **Summary:** The salient aspects of the case are identified, filtering out the extraneous information to identify the key issues(s).
2. A straightforward answer is given to each open-ended question, often with a differential diagnosis.
3. The analysis of the case is comprised of two parts:
   a. **Objectives of the case:** A listing of the two or three main principles that are crucial for a practitioner to manage the patient. Again, the students are challenged to make educated "guesses" about the objectives of the case upon initial review of the case scenario, which helps to sharpen their clinical and analytical skills.
   b. **Considerations:** A discussion of the relevant points and brief approach to the specific patient.

PART II
Approach to the disease process: It consists of two distinct parts:

   a. **Definitions:** Terminology pertinent to the disease process.
   b. **Clinical approach:** A discussion of the approach to the clinical problem in general, including tables, figures, and algorithms.

PART III
Comprehension questions: Each case contains several multiple-choice questions, which reinforce the material, or which introduce new and related concepts. Questions about material not found in the text will have explanations in the answers.

PART IV
Clinical pearls: Several clinically important points are reiterated as a summation of the text. This allows for easy review, such as before an examination.

SECTION I

How to Approach Clinical Problems

Part 1. Approach to the Patient

As delineated in nearly every clinical book and guide, the first step in the approach to the patient is gathering information and establishing the database. This includes taking the history; performing the physical examination; and obtaining selective laboratory examinations or special evaluations, such as umbilical Doppler studies and/or imaging tests. Of these, the historical examination is the most important and useful. The obstetrician should be unbiased and balanced in the approach to the patient; discipline should be exercised to refrain from being influenced by preconceived ideas of the patient's findings or best therapy. An appropriate balance of open-ended and directive questioning is prudent to efficiently determine the diagnosis, yet not ignore other patient concerns. Additionally, because patients may be anxious due to possible serious fetal malformations or genetic disorders, the obstetrician must be nondirective in counseling the patient, and refrain from "coloring" the discussion with excessive preconceived beliefs or notions, but allow the patient and her family to receive the information in an unbiased fashion.

Clinical Pearl

> ➤ The history is usually the single most important tool in obtaining a diagnosis. The art of seeking the information in a nonjudgmental, sensitive, and thorough manner cannot be overemphasized.

HISTORY

1. Basic information:
   a. Age: Must be recorded because some conditions are more common at certain ages; for instance, women younger than 17 or those older than age 35 are at increased risk for hypertensive disease of pregnancy; pregnant women older than 35 years are at increased risk for fetal karyotypic abnormalities.
   b. Gravidity: Number of pregnancies including current pregnancy (includes miscarriages, ectopic pregnancies, and stillbirths).
   c. Parity: Number of pregnancies that have ended at gestational age(s) greater than 20 weeks, including any complications with the gestations.
   d. Abortuses: Number of pregnancies that have ended at gestational age(s) less than 20 weeks (includes ectopic pregnancies, induced abortions, and spontaneous abortions).
2. Last menstrual period (LMP): The first day of the last menstrual period. In obstetric patients, the certainty of the LMP is important in determining the gestational age in pregnancy. Because of delay in ovulation in some cycles, this is not always accurate. Use of hormonal contraception and regularity or irregularity of menses are important to document.

3. Chief complaint: What is it that brought the patient into the hospital or office? Is it a scheduled appointment, or an unexpected symptom, such as abdominal pain or vaginal bleeding in pregnancy? The duration and character of the complaint, associated symptoms, and exacerbating and relieving factors should be recorded. The chief complaint engenders a differential diagnosis, and the possible etiologies should be explored by further inquiry. The chief complaint should be explored with respect to how the pregnancy may affect a disease condition, and also how the disease condition may affect the pregnancy.

Clinical Pearl

> The chief complaint, as voiced by the patient or identified by the physician as most urgent, is probed through the clinical database, which yields a differential diagnosis.

4. Past gynecologic history:
   a. Menstrual history
      i. Age of menarche (should normally be older than 9 years and younger than 16 years).
      ii. Character of menstrual cycles: Interval from the first day of one menses to the first day of the next menses (normal is 28, +/− 7 days; or between 21 and 35 days).
      iii. Quantity of menses: Menstrual flow should last less than 7 days (or be less than 80 mL in total volume). Menstrual flow that is excessive, menorrhagia, should be further characterized as associated with clots, pain, or pressure.
      iv. Menometrorrhagia, which involves both excessive bleeding and irregular bleeding should be distinguished from menorrhagia, and usually involves anovulatory cycles or genital lesions such as endometrial or cervical cancer.
   b. Contraceptive history: Duration, type, and last use of contraception, and any side effects. Some agents such as the intrauterine contraceptive device may be associated with ectopic pregnancy in a pregnant woman, or pelvic inflammatory disease.
   c. Sexually transmitted diseases: A positive or negative history of herpes simplex virus, syphilis, gonorrhea, *Chlamydia*, human immunodeficiency virus (HIV), pelvic inflammatory disease, or human papilloma virus. Number of sexual partners, whether a recent change in partners, and use of barrier contraception.
5. Obstetric history: Date and gestational age of each pregnancy at termination, and outcome; if induced abortion, then gestational age and method. If delivered, then whether the delivery was vaginal or cesarean; if applicable, vacuum or forceps delivery, or type of cesarean (low-transverse vs classical). All complications of pregnancies should be listed.

6. Past medical history: Any illnesses, such as hypertension, hepatitis, diabetes mellitus, cancer, heart disease, pulmonary disease, and thyroid disease, should be elicited. Duration, severity, and therapies should be included. Any hospitalizations should be listed with reason for admission, intervention, and location of hospital.

7. Past surgical history: Year and type of surgery should be elucidated and any complications documented. Type of incision (laparoscopy vs laparotomy) should be recorded. The operative report is useful particularly with attention to the intra-abdominal findings, surgery performed, and possible complications.

8. Allergies: Reactions to medications should be recorded, including severity and temporal relationship to medication. Non-medicine allergies such as to latex or iodine are also important to note. Immediate hypersensitivity should be distinguished from an adverse reaction.

9. Medications: A list of medications, dosage, route of administration and frequency, and duration of use should be obtained. Prescription, over-the-counter, and herbal remedies are all relevant. The patient's symptoms and whether there is improvement or change with the use of medications is important to record. Use or abuse of illicit drugs, tobacco, or alcohol should also be recorded.

10. Review of systems: A systematic review should be performed but focused on the more common diseases. For example, in pregnant women, the presence of symptoms referable to preeclampsia should be queried, such as headache, visual disturbances, epigastric pain, or facial swelling. In an elderly woman, symptoms suggestive of cardiac disease should be elicited, such as chest pain, shortness of breath, fatigue, weakness, or palpitations.

PHYSICAL EXAMINATION

1. General appearance: Cachectic versus well-nourished, anxious versus calm, alert versus obtunded.

2. Vital signs: Temperature, blood pressure, heart rate, and respiratory rate. Height and weight are often placed here including body mass index (weight in kg/height in m^2).

3. Head and neck examination: Evidence of trauma, tumors, facial edema, goiter, and carotid bruits should be sought. Cervical and supraclavicular nodes should be palpated.

4. Breast examination: Inspection for symmetry, skin or nipple retraction with the patient's hands on her hips (to accentuate the pectoral muscles), and with arms raised. With the patient supine, the breasts should then be palpated systematically to assess for masses. The nipple should be assessed for discharge, and the axillary and supraclavicular regions should be examined for adenopathy.

5. Cardiac examination: The point of maximal impulse (PMI) should be ascertained, and the heart auscultated at the apex of the heart as well as base. Heart sounds, murmurs, and clicks should be characterized. Systolic flow murmurs are fairly common due to the increased cardiac output, but prolonged or louder systolic, or significant diastolic murmurs are unusual.

6. Pulmonary examination: The lung fields should be examined systematically and thoroughly. Wheezes, rales, rhonchi, and bronchial breath sounds should be recorded.

7. Abdominal examination: The abdomen should be inspected for scars, distension, masses or organomegaly (ie, spleen or liver), and discoloration. For instance, the Grey-Turner sign of discoloration at the flank areas may indicate intra-abdominal or retroperitoneal hemorrhage. Auscultation of bowel sounds should be accomplished to identify normal versus high-pitched, and hyperactive versus hypoactive sounds. The abdomen should be percussed for the presence of shifting dullness (indicating ascites). Careful palpation should begin initially away from the area of pain, involving one hand on top of the other, to assess for masses, tenderness, and peritoneal signs. Tenderness should be recorded on a scale (eg, 1-4, where 4 is the most severe pain). Guarding, whether it is voluntary or involuntary, should be noted.

8. Back and spine examination: The back should be assessed for symmetry, tenderness, or masses. In particular, the flank regions are important to assess for pain on percussion since that may indicate renal disease.

9. Pelvic examination (adequate preparation of the patient is crucial including counseling about what to expect, adequate lubrication, and sensitivity to pain and discomfort):

   a. The external genitalia should be observed for masses or lesions, discoloration, redness, or tenderness. Ulcers in this area may indicate herpes simplex virus, vulvar carcinoma, or syphilis; a vulvar mass at the 5-o'clock or 7-o'clock positions can suggest a Bartholin gland cyst or abscess. Pigmented lesions may require biopsy since malignant melanoma is not uncommon in the vulvar region. The level of estrogen effect should also be characterized, such as vaginal rugae and vaginal pH.

   b. Speculum examination: The vagina should be inspected for lesions, discharge, estrogen effect (well-rugated vs atrophic), and presence of a cystocele or a rectocele. The appearance of the cervix should be described, and masses, vesicles, or other lesions should be noted.

   c. Bimanual examination: Initially, the index and middle finger of the one gloved hand should be inserted into the patient's vagina underneath the cervix, while the clinician's other hand is placed on the abdomen at the uterine fundus. With the uterus trapped between the two hands, the examiner should identify whether there is cervical motion tenderness, and evaluate the size, shape, and directional axis of the uterus. The adnexa should then be assessed with the vaginal hand in the lateral vaginal fornices. The normal ovary is approximately the size of a walnut.

   d. Rectal examination: A rectal examination will reveal masses in the posterior pelvis, and may identify occult blood in the stool. Nodularity and tenderness in the uterosacral ligament can be signs of endometriosis. The posterior uterus and palpable masses in the cul-de-sac can be identified by rectal examination. Occult blood should not be assessed through digital examination, since false positives may occur.

10. Extremities and skin: The presence of joint effusions, tenderness, skin edema, and cyanosis should be recorded.

11. Neurologic examination: Patients who present with neurologic complaints usually require a thorough assessment including evaluation of the cranial nerves, strength, sensation, and reflexes.

Clinical Pearl

➤ Significant diastolic murmurs in the pregnant woman is usually abnormal.

12. Laboratory assessment for obstetric patients:
   a. Screening laboratory tests usually include:
     i. Complete blood count to assess for anemia and thrombocytopenia.
     ii. Basic or comprehensive metabolic panel to assess for electrolytes, renal and liver function tests.
     iii. Hepatitis B surface antigen: Indicates that the patient is infectious. Further testing will determine whether this is a chronic carrier status (normal liver function tests), or active hepatitis (elevated liver function tests).
     iv. Syphilis nontreponemal test (RPR or VDRL): A positive test necessitates confirmation with a treponemal test, such as MHA-TP or FTA-ABS.
     v. Human immunodeficiency virus test: The screening test is usually the ELISA and, when positive, will necessitate the Western blot or other confirmatory test.
     vi. Urine culture or urinalysis: To assess for asymptomatic bacteriuria.
     vii. Cytologic examination: To assess for cervical dysplasia or cervical cancer; involves both ectocervical component and endocervical sampling. Evidence is pointing toward the liquid-based media as being superior cellular sampling and allows for HPV subtyping.
     viii. Endocervical assays for gonorrhea and/or *Chlamydia trachomatis* for high-risk patients.
     ix. Pregnancy test: Urine pregnancy assays are both sensitive and specific, and quantitative serum hCG assays can be used to follow the progress of a pregnancy.
   b. Other tests are dependent on age, presence of coexisting disease, and chief complaint.

13. Common scenarios:
    a. Threatened abortion: Quantitative hCG and/or progesterone levels may help to establish the viability of a pregnancy and risk of ectopic pregnancy.
    b. Indirect Coombs: Antibody identification and titer are assessed when the antibody screen (indirect Coombs) is positive.
14. Imaging procedures:
    a. Ultrasound: Can be used for establishing gestational age (biometry), estimated fetal weight, fetal presentation, amniotic fluid volume, cervical length.
    b. Doppler flow: Can be used as an adjunct in assessing possible fetal anemia, or in IUGR.
    c. MRI: Can be used to assess for uterine malformations, possible cervical pregnancies, or more recently fetal assessment.

Clinical Pearl

> ➤ Umbilical artery Doppler flow can be helpful in assessing possible IUGR, especially when the end-diastolic velocity is absent or there is reverse flow. In these circumstances, the risk of perinatal death within 48 hours is high.

Part 2. Approach to Clinical Diagnosis and Staging

There are typically six distinct steps that a clinician undertakes to solve most clinical problems systematically:
1. Identifying the most important condition
2. Developing a differential diagnosis
3. Making a diagnosis
4. Assessing the severity and/or stage of the disease
5. Rendering a treatment based on the stage of the disease
6. Following the patient's response to the treatment

IDENTIFYING THE MOST IMPORTANT CONDITION

The patient's chief complaint is generally the problem to be evaluated and worked up; however, at times, the physician may identify an issue that is more concerning than the patient's reason for seeking care. Whatever the key clinical problem is, that issue should be clearly defined and communicated to the patient. If the clinical problem is different from the patient's chief complaint, then the reason for its priority should also be explained so as not to alienate the patient. Other clinical problems should likewise be listed and noted, but the primary condition should be highlighted.

DEVELOPING A DIFFERENTIAL DIAGNOSIS

After the key issue or issues have been identified and prioritized, then the next step is to develop a differential diagnosis. The differential diagnosis is usually between three to five disease processes based on clinical presentation, risk factors, disease prevalence, and potential danger of the disease. A seasoned clinician will "key in" on the most important possibilities. A good clinician also knows how to ask the same question in several different ways, and use different terminology. For example, patients at times may deny having been treated for "pelvic inflammatory disease," but will answer affirmatively to being hospitalized for "a tubal infection." Reaching a diagnosis may be achieved by systematically reading about each possible cause and disease. The patient's presentation is then matched up against each of these possibilities, and each is either placed high up on the list as a potential etiology, or moved lower down because of disease prevalence, the patient's presentation, or other clues. A patient's risk factors may influence the probability of a diagnosis.

Usually, a long list of possible diagnoses can be pared down to two to three most likely ones, based on selective laboratory or imaging tests. For example, a woman who complains of lower abdominal pain and has a history of a prior sexually transmitted disease may have salpingitis; another patient who has abdominal pain, amenorrhea, and a history of prior tubal surgery may have an ectopic pregnancy. Furthermore, yet another woman with a 1-day history of periumbilical pain localizing to the right lower quadrant may have acute appendicitis.

MAKING THE DIAGNOSIS

The diagnosis is made by a careful evaluation strategy. An efficient, cost-effective, and evidence-based approach is best. The clinician should be careful not to have "blinders" to only focus on one diagnosis, such as a 25-year-old woman with a pelvic mass has uterine fibroids, but rather keep an "open mind" to various diagnosis and be on the alert for "red flags" that may indicate inconsistencies with the primary diagnosis. Patients are conscious of the time, convenience, and number of visits required to reach a diagnosis, and these factors should also be taken into account in formulating the diagnostic plan. Finally, the diagnostic plan should be individualized for the particular patient, since a preconceived algorithm is rarely "one size fits all." Surgery is sometimes performed for diagnostic purposes to establish the diagnosis. In general, surgery should be reserved after noninvasive methods are unrevealing, or when an urgent condition exists.

Clinical Pearl

➤ The first three steps in clinical problem solving include identifying the key issue(s), developing a differential diagnosis, and making the diagnosis.

ASSESSING THE SEVERITY AND/OR STAGE OF THE DISEASE

After ascertaining the diagnosis, the next step is to characterize the severity of the disease process; in other words, describe "how bad" a disease is. With malignancy, this is done formally by staging the cancer. Most cancers are categorized from stage I (least severe) to stage IV (most severe). Some diseases, such as preeclampsia, may be designated as mild or severe. With other ailments, there is a moderate category. With some infections, such as syphilis, the staging depends on the duration and extent of the infection, and follows along the natural history of the infection (ie, primary syphilis, secondary, latent period, and tertiary/neurosyphilis).

Clinical Pearl

➤ The fourth step is to establish the severity or stage of disease. There is usually prognostic or treatment significance based on the stage.

RENDERING A TREATMENT BASED ON THE STAGE OF THE DISEASE

Many illnesses are stratified according to severity because prognosis and treatment often vary based on the severity. If neither the prognosis nor the treatment was influenced by the stage of the disease process, there would not be a reason to subcategorize a disease as mild or severe. As another example, urinary tract infections may be subdivided into lower tract infections (cystitis) that are treated by oral antibiotics on an outpatient basis, versus upper tract infections (pyelonephritis) that generally require hospitalization and intravenous antibiotics.

Bacterial vaginosis (BV), which has been associated with preterm delivery, endometritis, and vaginal cuff cellulitis (following hysterectomy), does not have a severe or mild substaging. The presence of BV may slightly increase the risk of problems, but neither the prognosis nor the treatment is affected by "more" BV or "less" BV. Hence, the student should approach a new disease by learning the mechanism, clinical presentation, staging, and the treatment based on stage.

Treatment is broadly divided into medical therapy and surgical therapy. The astute clinician will be aware of the various types of medical therapy available, and the indications for surgery. Often, there will be various types of surgical approaches, and possible associated or prophylactic procedures are considered with the primary operation. For instance in a 44-year-old woman undergoing a hysterectomy for symptomatic uterine fibroids that have failed medical management, should the ovaries be removed? Current review of the literature, assessing the risks and benefits of each alternative, and a careful discussion with the patient and her family is paramount.

Clinical Pearl

➤ The treatment, whether medical or surgical, is tailored to the extent or "stage" of the disease.

FOLLOWING THE PATIENT'S RESPONSE TO THE TREATMENT

The final step in the approach to disease is to follow the patient's response to the therapy. The "measure" of response should be recorded and monitored. Some responses are clinical, such as improvement (or lack of improvement) in a patient's abdominal pain, temperature, or pulmonary examination. Obviously, the physician must work on being more skilled in eliciting the data in an unbiased and standardized manner. Subjective complaints such as uterine pain may be followed by an analogue pain scale and by having the patient point to the location of the pain. Other responses such as amniotic fluid volume or estimated fetal weight are followed by intermittent monitoring. When the patient's symptoms do not respond (pain, fever, anemia), then the practitioner should reconsider the diagnosis, or reevaluate with another approach.

Clinical Pearl

➤ The final step is to monitor treatment response or efficacy, which may be measured in different ways. It may be symptomatic (patient feels better), or based on physical examination (fever), a laboratory test (hemoglobin level after iron supplementation), or an imaging test (ultrasound size of ovarian cyst).

REFERENCES

1. Cunninham FG, Leveno KJ, Bloom SL, Hauth JC, Rouse DJ, Spong CY. *Williams Obstetrics*, 23 rd ed., New York, McGraw-Hill, 2009.
2. Queenan JT, Hobbins JC, Spong CY. *Protocols for High-Risk Pregnancies*. Wiley-Blackwell, 5th ed, Hoboken, NJ, 2010.

Clinical Cases

Case 1

A 22-year-old primigravida is seen in your office at 28 weeks' gestation for a routine prenatal visit. Her pregnancy has been uneventful to date. She expresses her concern about several moles on her back, which have been enlarging over the past several weeks and for increasing difficulty with constipation. She also relates less energy to complete her job-related responsibilities at work and feels it may be related to the 18-lb weight gain she has experienced since becoming pregnant. She also has noted some gradual shortness of breath over the past 4 to 6 weeks especially when she climbs the three flights of stairs to her office at work. She wears contact lenses and relates that her visual acuity is not as good as before she became pregnant.

Physical examination reveals her height to be 5 ft 8 in, her weight to be 158 lb, and her blood pressure to be 90/60 mm Hg. She has several pigmented nevi over her shoulders and back. She has a darkened line on her skin from her xiphoid process to her symphysis. Examination of her heart reveals a 2/6 systolic ejection murmur heard best over the second left intercostal space. Her lungs are clear to auscultation and percussion. Abdominal examination reveals a 28 cm fundal height with normal bowel sounds, and she has trace pretibial pitting edema.

Laboratory values reveal a hemoglobin level of 12.0 g/dL and a platelet count of 125,000/mm^3. Urinalysis reveals no nitrites or leukocyte esterase, 2+ glucose, and no albuminuria. Fasting metabolic package reveals a sodium of 138 mEq/L (normal 135-145), potassium of 4.6 mEq/L (normal 3.5-5.0), calcium level of 9.2 mg/dL (normal 9.3-10.1), and albumin level of 3.1 g/dL (normal 3.3-4.0). Fasting glucose level was 65 mg%.

➤ Does this patient have any metabolic or physiologic changes not associated with a normal pregnancy?

➤ What is your next step in her evaluation?

ANSWERS TO CASE 1:
Physiologic Adaptation to Pregnancy

Summary: This is a 22-year-old primigravida who is 28 weeks' pregnant. She has the following complaints: enlarging skin moles, lack of energy, weight gain, mild dyspnea on exertion, and blurred vision. Your significant clinical findings are BP 90/60 mm Hg, several pigmented nevi, a grade 2/6 systolic ejection murmur, a fundal height 28 cm, and trace pretibial pitting edema. The significant lab results are platelet count of 125,000/mm^3, 2+ glucosuria and negative albuminuria on urinalysis, and a fasting serum glucose of 65 mg/dL.

> **Metabolic or physiologic changes not associated with a normal pregnancy:** No, all the symptoms, signs, and laboratory values are consistent with the physiologic adaptations of pregnancy.

> **Next step in evaluation:** The following are indicated in this patient: (1) Careful dermatological evaluation of her pigmented nevi to rule out the presence of malignant melanoma. (2) Thyroid function studies should be drawn to evaluate her "lack of energy," and (3) This patient should be advised to report any worsening of her shortness of breath.

ANALYSIS

Objectives

1. Be familiar with the physiologic adaptations associated with a normal pregnancy.
2. Be able to differentiate between certain signs and symptoms that can be common to both disease processes and to physiologic adaptations of pregnancy.
3. Learn to counsel patients of signs and symptoms to expect during a normal pregnancy.

US Preventive Services Task Force Study Quality

Level I.   Evidence obtained from at least one properly designed randomized controlled trial.

Level II-1. Evidence obtained from well-designed controlled trials without randomization.

Level II-2. Evidence obtained from well-designed cohort or case-control analytic studies, preferably from more than one center or research group.

Level II-3. Evidence obtained from multiple time series with or without the intervention. Dramatic results in uncontrolled experiments could also be regarded as this type of evidence.

Level III.   Opinions of respected authorities, based on clinical experience, descriptive studies, or reports of expert committees.

Considerations

This 22-year-old primigravida has presented to your office at 28 weeks' gestation with signs and symptoms that commonly occur in pregnancy but that may be the evidence of disease. Initial evaluation includes differentiating normal from pathologic processes, reassuring the gravida about those which are normal, and educating her to discern the difference. Thus, an awareness of the physiologic changes of pregnancy such as the increase in cardiac output, intravascular volume, glomerular filtration rate are essential in the interpretation of the history, physical, and lab findings in pregnancy.

APPROACH TO
Physiologic Adaptation to Pregnancy

Skin Changes

Pregnancy produces many changes in the skin that are commonly noted by patients. Increased pigmentation in the skin occurs in over 90% of pregnant women. Areas noted to be commonly involved include the face, the areola of the breast, the linea alba, the axilla, and the genital skin. Melasma gravidarum (the mask of pregnancy) involves the forehead, the cheeks, and the bridge of the nose. Pigmented nevi are also commonly affected.

Melanocyte-stimulating hormone (MSH) is increased in pregnancy. This and other sex steroids may be responsible for the generalized hyperpigmentation seen in pregnancy. This hyperpigmentation seems to be more pronounced in dark-skinned women than in those with fair complexions.

Other changes occur in the skin as a result of vascular engorgement and vessel proliferation. Spider angiomata are particularly common in Caucasian women. These are most commonly seen in the sun-exposed areas of the body. Blushing of the palms and the soles of the feet can be seen. This is transient and resolves postpartum.

Changes are also seen in hair growth. In the immediate postpartum period the percentage of hair follicles in the telogen phase (resting phase) reaches 30% to 40%. This results in hair loss. This loss is transient and resolves spontaneously in around 6 to 12 months.

Striae gravidarum (stretch marks of pregnancy) occur in 50% of all pregnancies. Involving the abdomen, the breast, the buttocks, and the thighs, these are thought to represent linear tears in dermal skin under the influence of estrogen. Striae appear red in the present pregnancy, pale slowly after delivery, and there is no known method of prevention.

Weight Gain

Weight gain in pregnancy has been the subject of great debate for many years. Current recommendations for weight gain in pregnancy should be based on the Institute of Medicine guidelines. These guidelines suggest for the normal woman a weight gain of 25 to 35 lb. For overweight women a weight gain of 15 to 25 lb is more appropriate and for the obese woman a weight gain of 15 lb is suggested. Normal weight is defined by the World Health Organization and the National Institutes of Health as a body mass index (BMI) of 18.9 to 24.9, overweight as a BMI of 25 to 29.9, and obesity as a BMI of 30 or greater.

Cardiovascular Changes

Significant cardiovascular changes occur in the pregnant woman beginning as early as the fifth week of gestation. While most are easily recognizable, many can be mistaken for cardiac disease.

During pregnancy, the heart is displaced upward and to the left from changes in the shape of the rib cage and from superior displacement of the diaphragm. It also rotates on its long axis. This moving of the apex of the heart in a lateral fashion can be misperceived on chest x-ray as representing cardiomegaly. Other changes in the structure of the heart resemble those found as a result of physical training. Physiologic myocardial hypertrophy is a result of expanded blood volume, peaks at 30 to 34 weeks' gestation, and reverses itself after the pregnancy is over.

Cardiac output (CO) is the product of stroke volume (SV) and heart rate (HR). During pregnancy CO is increased tremendously. By 5 weeks gestation it rises to 10 % over prepregnancy levels and by 34 weeks peaks at some 50% above those levels seen prior to pregnancy. Heart rate begins to rise in the first trimester and continues to rise until it peaks at 15 to 20 beats above normal at 34 weeks. Cardiac output varies greatly with maternal position. It is highest in the knee-chest and lateral recumbent positions and lowest in the supine position (some 30% lower). Late in pregnancy because of the development of a dilated paravertebral collateral circulation, venous return from the lower extremities is maintained in the supine position even when the vena cava is completely occluded by the pregnant uterus. In spite of this, 5% to 10% of pregnant women show signs of "supine hypotension," and experience dizziness, nausea, and even syncope when supine. This may represent a failure of those women to develop an adequate paravertebral collateral system.

Systemic vascular resistance (SVR) diminishes in early pregnancy. Reaching its nadir at mid-pregnancy, it gradually rises until term but even then remains approximately 20% lower than prior to pregnancy. This phenomenon is thought to be a direct effect of progesterone on the smooth muscle in the capillary beds, and increased levels of circulating nitric oxide and cyclic adenosine monophosphate also play a role. Since the pregnant woman's blood pressure is a product of her cardiac output and SVR, we see a similar change in blood pressure throughout pregnancy.

Venous blood pressure rises in the lower extremities gradually during pregnancy. Femoral venous pressure rises from 10 cm H_2O to 25 cm H_2O at term. Consequently edema, hemorrhoids, varicose veins, and an increased risk of deep vein thrombosis are common.

It is often difficult to distinguish between signs and symptoms caused by physiologic adaptations to pregnancy and those of true cardiac disease. S1 becomes louder by the end of the first trimester, and 90% of pregnant women will develop an S3. Systolic ejection murmurs along the left sternal border develop in more than 90% of pregnant women, thought to be caused by increased blood flow across the pulmonic and aortic valves.

Dyspnea can be seen in both pregnancy and with cardiac disease. The dyspnea associated with pregnancy usually arises gradually prior to 20 weeks gestation and by the third trimester is present in 75% of pregnancies. While fatigue, orthopnea, syncope, and chest discomfort can be experienced in normal pregnancy, the presence of hemoptysis, angina, increasing orthopnea, or nocturnal dyspnea should be evaluated promptly.

Respiratory System

Because of increased hyperemia and increased estrogen levels the nasopharyngeal mucosa becomes edematous and irritated. Nasal stuffiness, epistaxis, and nasal polyps occur frequently during pregnancy, and resolve spontaneously postpartum.

Due primarily to change in the size and shape of the chest cavity, the following alterations in lung capacities are seen:

1. Respiratory rate—Unchanged
2. Vital capacity—Unchanged
3. Inspiratory capacity—Increased 5% to 10%
4. Tidal volume—Increased 30% to 50%
5. Inspiratory reserve volume—Unchanged
6. Functional residual capacity—Decreased 20%

During pregnancy, increased levels of progesterone cause a state of relative hyperventilation resulting in a chronic respiratory alkalosis. This relatively low pCO_2 in the pregnant mother is beneficial in clearing CO_2 from the fetal circulation.

Hematologic Changes

Maternal blood volume is comprised of the plasma volume plus the red blood cell mass. This total blood volume begins increasing as early as 6 weeks gestation and plateaus at 30 to 34 weeks of pregnancy, increasing by some 40% to 50% in most gravidas. Plasma volume begins to increase at 10 weeks gestation and plateaus at 30 weeks' gestation while the red blood cell mass begins increasing at 10 weeks and continues its rise until term. The reasons for these expansions remain unknown. The use of iron supplementation has been shown to enhance the increase in RBC mass from 18% to 30% by term. Since at mid-pregnancy the plasma volume increases more than that of red blood cell mass, there appears a transient physiologic anemia of pregnancy.

A gradual decline in platelets has been observed throughout pregnancy, but 98% of pregnant women will have platelet counts of greater than 116,000/mm^3. Values below this should be evaluated for causes of thrombocytopenia.

Renal Changes

Renal plasma flow begins to rise early in pregnancy becoming 75% higher than prior to pregnancy by 16 weeks gestation. Glomerular filtration rate rises as early as 5 to 7 weeks and reaches a level 50% greater than in the nonpregnant female.

The altered mechanism of handling glucose in the proximal tubules during pregnancy remains to be completely understood. Glucose excretion into the urine occurs in most pregnant women. While the nonpregnant female excretes less than 100 mg/d, in pregnancy this can reach 1 to 10 g of glucose per day.

The Eye

Pregnancy affects the eye in two ways. Corneal thickening develops as early as the first trimester and lasts until several weeks postpartum. Pregnant women can perceive this as loss of visual acuity especially those who wear glasses or contact lenses. Intraocular pressure drops by as much as 10% during pregnancy. There appears to be little to no change in visual fields in pregnancy.

Comprehension Questions

1.1   A 25-year-old G3P2A0 patient presents complaining of chest discomfort with usual daily activities. This patient is at 26 weeks' gestation and as part of your workup a chest x-ray is read as consistent with cardiomegaly. Which of the following is the best diagnostic test to rule out congestive heart failure?
        A. ECG with rhythm strip
        B. MRI of the chest cavity
        C. Echocardiography evaluation
        D. Arterial blood gases

1.2   A 36-year-old woman at 34 weeks' gestation presents for her routine pre-
        natal visit. Her urine dip for glucose is noted to be 4+. Of note an
        O'Sullivan test (1-h GTT) done at 28 weeks was returned as 110 mg/dL.
        Which of the following is the most appropriate course of action?
        A. Reassure patient that this is a normal occurrence in pregnancy and
            no further evaluation is necessary.
        B. Random finger stick blood sugar to assure euglycemic state.
        C. Repeat O'Sullivan.
        D. Proceed to a 3-hour GTT.

1.3   A 36-year-old G4P3A0 patient presents at 30 weeks' gestation for her
        routine prenatal visit. Her prenatal course has been unremarkable up
        to the present. Her BP is 110/65 mm Hg, and her urine is negative for
        both protein and glucose. She mentions that she has noticed blurred
        vision for the past few weeks. She has worn contact lenses for several
        years and has an appointment to have her eyes checked. On gross
        evaluation of her visual fields they appear intact and symmetrical.
        Which of the following is the most appropriate advice for this patient?
        A. Proceed with ophthalmologic evaluation and have her prescrip-
            tions updated on her contact lenses.
        B. Proceed with ophthalmologic evaluation to assure that visual
            fields are intact but delay changes in her lenses until after the
            puerperium.
        C. Ignore all changes in visual acuity or visual field changes as these
            are normal for pregnancy.
        D. In the absence of headaches visual change can be ignored.

ANSWERS

1.1   **C.** In pregnancy the heart is displaced up and to the left. It also
        rotates on its long axis to the left. On x-ray this can be confused with
        cardiomegaly. This should be evaluated with an echocardiogram,
        especially if the patient is complaining of dyspnea or orthopnea.

1.2   **B.** Although the alteration in glucose handling in the proximal
        tubules remains to be accurately understood, glucosuria is common
        in the gravid female. The nonpregnant female excretes less than
        100 mg/d. In pregnancy 90% of women with normal blood sugars
        will excrete up to 10 g per day.

1.3   **B.** Because of thickening of the cornea in pregnancy decreased visual
        acuity can occur. Eye testing is best done in the nonpregnant state.
        The presence of decreased visual fields, however, deserves evaluation.

Clinical Pearls

See US Preventative Services Task Force Study Quality levels of evidence on page 4

➤ Cardiac output increases by almost 50% during pregnancy. It is position dependent and actually falls in the supine and standing positions (Level II-3).

➤ Pregnancy causes a chronic respiratory alkalosis. The resulting decrease in maternal pCO_2 promotes the clearing of CO_2 from the fetal circulation (Level II-3).

➤ Though not completely understood, glucosuria is common in pregnant women even with normal blood sugars (Level II-3).

➤ Two common effects of pregnancy on the eye are corneal thickening and decreased intraocular pressure (Level II-3).

REFERENCES

1. Bernstein I, Zeigler W, Badger G. Plasma volume expansion in early pregnancy. *Obstet gynecol*. 2001;97:669.
2. Bhagwat A, Engel P. Heart disease and pregnancy. *Cardiol Clin*. 1995;13:163.
3. Davison J, Hytten F. The effect of pregnancy on the renal handling of glucose. *Br J Obstet Gynaecol*. 1975;82:374.
4. Davison J, Noble F. Glomerular filtration during and after pregnancy. *J Obstet Gynaecol Br Commonw*. 1974;81:588.
5. Dinn R, Harris A, Marcus P. Ocular changes in pregnancy. *Graefes Arch Clin Exp Ophthalmol*. 2003;58:137.
6. Duvekot J, Peeters L. Maternal cardiovascular hemodynamic adaptation to pregnancy. *Obstet Gynecol surv*. 1994;49:S1.
7. MacGillivray I, Rose G, Rowe B. Blood pressure survey in pregnancy. *Clin Sci*. 1969;37:395.
8. O'Brien JR. Platelet count in normal pregnancy. *J Clin Patho*. 1976;29:174.
9. O'Rourke R, Ewy G, Marcus F, et al. Cardiac auscultation in pregnancy. *Med Ann D C*. 1970;39:92.
10. Parmley T, O'Brien T. Skin changes during pregnancy. *Clin Obstet Gynecol*. 1990;33:713.
11. Schatz M, Zeiger R. Diagnosis and management of rhinitis during pregnancy. *Allergy Proc*. 1988;9:545.
    A clinical approach to the cold symptoms of pregnancy
12. Theunissen I, Parer J. Fluid and electrolytes in pregnancy. *Clin Obstet Gynecol*. 1994;37:3.
    This is a good review of how pregnancy alters fluid and electrolyte handling.

Case 2

A 36-year-old G2P1001 woman presents as a transfer of care at 10 weeks' gestation. She was previously receiving care with another obstetrician until her insurance changed. She has no significant medical or family history. Her last pregnancy 4 years ago ended in a term delivery of a healthy female infant. She is aware of the increased likelihood of fetal chromosome disorders associated with maternal age over 35. She was advised by her previous doctor to undergo amniocentesis later in pregnancy. She is uneasy about waiting until after 16 weeks to get any information on the fetal chromosome status. Conversely, she is also uneasy about putting this pregnancy at risk by undergoing an invasive prenatal diagnostic procedure.

➤ What first-trimester screening/testing options does this patient have to address her risk for fetal aneuploidy?

➤ Would your recommendations for screening versus testing be any different if she was 26 years old instead of 36 years old?

ANSWERS TO CASE 2:
First-Trimester Screening

Summary: A G2P1001 at 10 weeks' gestation with advanced maternal age seeks information regarding aneuploidy testing.

> **First-trimester screening/testing options to address risk for fetal aneuploidy:** This patient has the option of aneuploidy screening with serum biochemical markers in combination with nuchal translucency or invasive testing with chorionic villus sampling (CVS) if available.

> **Recommendations for screening versus testing if patient was 26 years old instead of 36 years old:** Obviously the difference for these two patients would be the *a priori* risk for fetal chromosome abnormalities each of these patients has. If patients truly understand the nuances and limitations of screening versus testing, there should be no important differences in the type of counseling each of these age groups should receive. All patients should be offered invasive testing for prenatal diagnosis of fetal chromosome abnormalities, and all patients should be offered noninvasive screening, if they choose to do so, before deciding about invasive testing.

ANALYSIS

Objectives

1. Become familiar with first-trimester screening and diagnostic testing options for aneuploidy.
2. Understand the biochemical and ultrasound components for aneuploidy screening in the first trimester.
3. Understand combination first- and second-trimester screening modalities and their detection rates.

Considerations

This patient should first decide about any further testing from two broad options: noninvasive screening or diagnostic invasive testing. This patient is of a maternal age that has historically been called "advanced." There is a long-recognized increase in the risk for fetal aneuploidy with advancing maternal age, and the increased risk takes a dramatic turn upward after the mid-thirties. Historically, women who would be age 35 or older on the estimated delivery date were automatically offered invasive testing. With improvement in screening algorithms, detection rates, and improved safety profiles of invasive testing, the rationale for limiting invasive testing to this age group is no longer valid.

Currently there are no noninvasive tests commercially available that will *diagnose* fetal chromosome abnormalities. Available noninvasive tests can only provide refinement of a patient's risk for carrying a fetus with a chromosome abnormality beyond that based on her age alone. This is because a series of serum analytes are found to be discrepant from the average to an extent enough to serve as a screening tool. None performs spectacularly alone, but in combination, such as the 4-marker quad test performed in the second trimester, the detection rates for fetal trisomies 21 or 18 reach suitable levels for screening purposes (see Table 2–1).

The availability of earlier first-trimester invasive testing in the form of chorionic villus sampling (CVS) allows for implementation of earlier *screening* modalities as well. In modern practice, first-trimester screening is typically accomplished by combining results of *biochemical* testing and *sonographic* information that includes the **nuchal translucency** (fluid-filled space in the posterior fetal neck) between 11 and 14 weeks gestational age. Either component can be performed independently, but overall detection rates are improved when used in combination.

Patients found to have an abnormal or positive screening test are subsequently offered invasive testing. Accordingly, there is no reason to exclude consideration of noninvasive screening for a woman who has an elevated age-related risk. Many of these women will have their risks lowered by the

Table 2–1 MEDIAN (MOM) VALUES OF SERUM MARKERS IN PREGNANCIES AFFECTED WITH FETAL TRISOMY 21

MARKER	FIRST TRIMESTER[a]	SECOND TRIMESTER
AFP	0.86[b]	0.74
uE3	0.99[b]	0.66
Free beta-hCG	1.70	2.66[b]
Total hCG	0.96[b]	1.93
Inhibin A	0.94[b]	2.28
PAPP-A	0.40	1.11[b]

Data derived from FASTER and SURUSS results.
[a]For data from FASTER trial, median levels at 12 weeks gestation were used in calculating the medians for this table.
[b]Data from SURUSS only.

screening algorithm, to a point where they may choose to forego invasive testing. As such, this particular patient who will be 35 years or more at delivery can benefit from aneuploidy screening. All patients regardless of age should be offered the opportunity to have either noninvasive screening or invasive testing for prenatal diagnosis of fetal chromosomal abnormalities.

APPROACH TO
First-Trimester Screening

1. Obtain nuchal translucency measurement (NT) by sonography.
2. Obtain maternal serum for PAPP-A and beta-hCG (free or total).

These data are then combined with the mother's *a priori* age-related risk to calculate a new risk for fetal DS (and trisomy 18). If the level reaches a predetermined cutoff, the lab interprets this as "screen positive." Alternatively, the patient may opt to proceed with invasive testing based on her impression of the degree of fetal aneuploidy risk determined by the screening process.

Measurement of Nuchal Translucency

In order to obtain reliable and reproducible screening performance, strict adherence to careful measurement of the nuchal translucency is paramount. Sonography units/practitioners adhere to the standards set forth by various certifying bodies to maintain high-quality images and measurements (eg, the Nuchal Translucency Quality Review or NTQR program). The fetus must be of sufficient size to perform NT measurement, and this can generally be accomplished when the **crown to rump length (CRL) is between 45 and 84 mm (approximately 11 wk-14 wk).** Other criteria for proper NT measurement are as follows: margins of NT edges need to be clearly defined; fetus needs to be in mid-sagittal plane; fetus occupies majority of image; fetal head must be in neutral position; fetus must be away from amnion; measurement should be at widest NT space; proper caliper alignment. Figure 2–1 depicts proper alignment of fetus and location of calipers when measuring NT. This fetus has an increased NT measurement and was found to have trisomy 21 by CVS.

There is no single NT measurement that serves as the cut off between normal and abnormal. All NT measurements obtained for screening purposes are considered in the context of the patients' gestational age. However, NT greater than 3.5 mm is not only a risk factor for fetal trisomy 21 or trisomy 18, but may also indicate presence of congenital heart disease. Such patients should be offered later assessment of fetal heart anatomy, such as can be accomplished with fetal echocardiography even in those with negative aneuploidy screen results or normal chromosomes by invasive testing (1; level II-3).

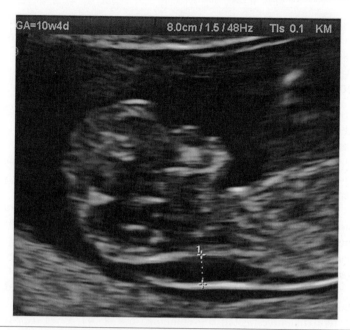

GA=10w4d   8.0cm / 1.5 / 48Hz   TIs 0.1   KM

Figure 2–1. Nuchal translucency as demonstrated by the clear area between the two cursors. (*Courtesy of Dr. Jeff Dungan*).

Biochemical Screening in First Trimester

Levels of **PAPP-A** (pregnancy-associated plasma protein A produced by trophoblasts) in fetal trisomy 21 tend to be significantly lower than from pregnancies with chromosomally normal fetuses. Additionally, hCG levels are typically elevated. See Table 2–2 for PAPP-A and hCG values in pregnancy. Analogous to the use of serum analytes in second trimester screening algorithms, these first trimester analytes are converted into multiples of the median (MoM), and used to calculate relative likelihood ratios for fetal trisomy 21. When multiplied by the patients existing age-related risk, a new risk is then calculated.

Table 2–2 PAPP-A AND hCG VALUES IN PREGNANCY		
	PAPP-A (MoM)	FREE BETA-hCG (MoM)
Median value in euploid	1.0	1.0
Median value in fetal trisomy 21	0.47 ↓	1.94 ↑
Median value in fetal trisomy 18	0.24	0.19

(Gestational age 12 weeks—Data from FASTER trial)

If NT screening is not available at one's center, biochemical screening is still valid with detection rates of fetal aneuploidy comparable to that obtainable with traditional second-trimester serum screening.

Detection Rates

The combined use of NT measurement with levels of PAPP-A and hCG are reported to be able to detect about 85% of fetuses with trisomy 21 with a 5% false-positive rate (FPR) when all maternal ages are screened. Given the underlying higher prevalence of trisomy 21 in women of advanced maternal age, the positive predictive value of any abnormal screen in women over age 35 will be higher than in women under age 35.

The Serum, Urine, and Ultrasound Screening Study (SURUSS) trial was designed to compare screening performance of first trimester, second trimester, and integrated screening algorithms. This trial contained over 40,000 women from multiple centers. Use of maternal age, NT assessment, and levels of free beta-hCG plus PAPP-A resulted in 83% detection rate with a FPR of 5% (2; level II-2). In the United States, the results of the Biochemistry, Urine, Nuchal Translucency (BUN) study were reported in 2003. This multicenter, prospective trial investigated the combined use of NT, PAPP-A, and free beta-hCG collected during first trimester (74-97 days, gestation) from over 8500 patients. When using a risk cutoff of 1 in 270 for trisomy 21, they identified 85.2% of trisomy 21 fetuses, with a FPR of 9.4%. If the FPR had been fixed at 5%, then 78.7% of trisomy 21 fetuses were detected. When stratified by maternal age, screening performance was not quite as favorable for those women under age 35, as expected. When maternal age was less than 35 years, then this screening regimen detected 66.7%, and in those more than 35 years, detection rate was 89.8% (3; level II-3). The First- and Second-Trimester Evaluation of Risk (FASTER) trial also examined screening performance in the first trimester. The first-trimester algorithm utilized by this multicenter trial was able to detect 86% of trisomy 21 fetuses at a false positive rate of 5.6% (utilized risk cut off of 1 in 300) (4; level II-2). When considering women of all ages, 90% of trisomy 18 cases are detected with first trimester screening with a FPR of 2% (3; level II-3). Risk assessment for trisomy 21 with serum analytes in multiple gestations is less accurate than in singleton gestations.

First-trimester screening performance, however, is maintained only by a rigorous training and QA implementation. The NT measurement is best performed between 11 and $13^6/_7$ weeks; however, the highest detection rates occur with scans done at 12 to 13 weeks as shown by Wald et al. in the SURUSS trial. Visualization at earlier gestational age can be technically difficult. On the other hand, performance of PAPP-A as a serum marker is highest at the earlier end of the screening window (10 wk), and so overall, earlier screening results improve detection rates at lowest false-positive rates. Resolution of the increased NT over time is not a contraindication to invasive testing, as the NT is known to resolve in many aneuploid fetuses.

Combination First- and Second-Trimester Screening

Screening tests performed in both the first and second trimester should not be evaluated independently, but rather as part of an established integrated or sequential screening algorithm. The false-positive rate using independently calculated second-trimester quad screening is unacceptably high for women who have already undergone a first-trimester evaluation. (This is because the majority of the true positives will not be rescreened in the second trimester, and thus the underlying prevalence of trisomy 21 will be much lower in this "prescreened" group than that used by the risk calculation software.) On the other hand, additional fetuses with trisomy 21 missed by the first-trimester screen will be detected by means of a second-trimester risk assessment, and therefore the highest detection rates are found with screening algorithms that incorporate information from the first and the second trimester.

In the large FASTER trial, the researchers sought to determine the optimal combination of first- and second-trimester serum screening with first-trimester NT assessment. Optimal test performance was achieved by the so-called "**integrated**" approach. In this method, the screening results from the first-trimester assessment are withheld until the second-trimester serum analysis is performed. In other words, there is no option for invasive testing if the first-trimester screen shows an elevated risk for fetal trisomy 21. After the second-trimester screen is performed, the two calculated risks are "integrated" into a single calculated risk. By using this approach, these investigators were able to identify 96% (87/92) of the fetuses with trisomy 21 from the group of over 33,000 women who underwent both first and second-trimester assessments. Several authorities have voiced concern over the withholding of first-trimester screening information from women found to have elevated risks. A compromise approach is **sequential screening**, in which women are informed of the first-trimester screening results, and offered invasive testing if the calculated risk is deemed "sufficiently" elevated. Those women who have a normal, or negative, first-trimester screen then go on to have serum screening drawn at 16 to 18 weeks, with a final risk calculation provided that incorporates information from both serum specimens and the first-trimester ultrasound. If the second (final) risk calculation is elevated, the patient is offered amniocentesis. Sequential screening was shown in the FASTER trial to have comparable test performance to integrated screening, that is, 95% detection of Down syndrome with an overall false-positive rate of about 5%.

With so many different options for aneuploidy testing, a patient can easily feel confused and overwhelmed. The differences between screening and diagnostic testing should be discussed with the patient. The patient who presents early enough in the first trimester should be offered combined first and second-trimester screening or diagnostic testing (either CVS or amniocentesis). Sequential screening provides a high detection rate with low false-positive rates. It also provides the patient the option of knowing her first-trimester screening results and the option of waiting until the second trimester for an adjusted risk assessment that combines the results of the second-trimester screen. If there is a lack of personnel to perform nuchal translucency, serum integrated screening (combined first- and second-trimester serum biochemical markers) can be a reasonable approach. If CVS is not available, either sequential or integrated screening can be performed depending on the patient's desire. If a patient desires diagnostic testing and CVS is not available, then a second-trimester amniocentesis is a reasonable alternative.

Comprehension Questions

2.1   A 29-year-old G1 at 8 weeks' gestation with triplet gestation presents for prenatal care. She is sure she does not desire to have invasive testing as a first step but desires "to have some information" regarding her risk for fetal Down syndrome. What option do you recommend?

A. Integrated screen
B. Sequential screen
C. Quad screen
D. Nuchal translucency only

2.2   A 22-year-old woman is being seen at 11 weeks' gestation for an ultrasound examination. Besides the nuchal translucency, which other sonographic finding is associated with fetal aneuploidy?

A. Fetal biparietal diameter
B. Fetal cerebellar diameter
C. Fetal nasal bone
D. Fetal crown rump length

ANSWERS

2.1   **D.** Serum screening tests are less sensitive in multiple gestations compared to singletons given that analytes from both fetuses (normal and abnormal) enter maternal circulation and are averaged together. Although data is limited, it is reasonable to offer nuchal translucency measurement to those with triplets as long as the patient is informed that the sensitivity is lower compared to first-trimester screening in singleton gestations.

2.2   **C.** The fetal nasal bone should be visualized by 11 weeks' gestation, and should be noted in the fetus in mid sagittal plane. An absent or shortened nasal bone is associated with fetal Down syndrome.

Clinical Pearls

See US Preventive Services Task Force Study Quality levels of evidence in Case 1

➤ All women, regardless of age, should be counseled regarding screening and diagnostic testing options for aneuploidy (Level III).

➤ Integrated or sequential first- and second-trimester screening have the highest detection rates for Down syndrome with lower false-positive rates than first-trimester screening alone (Level II-2).

➤ Nuchal translucency measurement ≥ 3.5 mm is associated with an increased risk of congenital heart defect (Level II-2).

REFERENCES

1. Bahado-Singh RO, Wapner R, Thom E, et al. Elevated first-trimester nuchal translucency increases the risk of congenital heart defects. First Trimester Maternal Serum Biochemistry and Fetal Nuchal Translucency Screening Study. *Am J Obstet Gynecol.* 2005;192:1357-1361.
   Increased nuchal translucency was associated with a higher risk of major congenital hearing defects in chromosomally normal pregnancies. At ≥ 3.5 mm, the incidence was 1 in 43 pregnancies (level II-3).
2. Malone F, Vonick JA, Ball RH, et al. First-trimester or second-trimester screening, or both, for Down's syndrome. First- and Second-Trimester Evaluation of Risk (FASTER) Research Consortium. *N Eng J Med.* 2005;353:2001-2011.
   This multicenter prospective study of over 38,000 participants showed that stepwise sequential screening and integrated screening had the highest detection rates (95% and 96%, respectively) with low FPR (level II-2).
3. Wald NJ, Rodeck C, Hackshaw AK, Walters J, Chitty L, Mackinson AM. First and second trimester antenatal screening for Down's syndrome: the results of the Serum, Urine and Ultrasound Screening Study (SURUSS) [published erratum appears in J Med Screening Study. 2006;13:51-21]. *J Med Screen.* 2003;10:56-104.
   A prospective multicenter European trial of approximately 47,000 participants that showed the use of maternal age, NT assessment, and levels of free beta-hCG plus PAPP-A resulted in 83% detection rate with a FPR of 5% (level II-2).
4. Wapner R, Thome E, Simpson JL, et al. First trimester screening for trisomies 21 and 18. First Trimester Maternal Serum Biochemistry and Fetal Nuchal Translucency Screening (BUN) Study Group. *N Eng J Med.* 2003;349:1405-1413.
   A large multicenter prospective study of 8872 participants in whom serum beta-hCG, PAPP-A, and nuchal translucency was measured. The detection rate for trisomy 21 was 85% with a 9% FPR (1:270 risk cutoff rate). For trisomy 18, the detection rate was 91% with a 2% FPR. This study provided data supporting that first-trimester screening is superior to maternal age alone, maternal age and biochemistry, and maternal age and nuchal translucency (level II-3).

Case 3

A 31-year-old G1 Caucasian female at $17^2/_7$ weeks' gestation undergoes a second-trimester maternal serum quad screen. Her medical history is unremarkable. Her weight is 235 lb, however, and she reports having somewhat irregular menstrual periods. At her 16-week visit, she was counseled about maternal serum screening for fetal abnormalities and opted to undergo the blood draw for this. Her values are as follows:

AFP	uE3	hCG	Inhibin A
3.1 MoM	1.4 MoM	0.9 MoM	0.8 MoM

Based on these results, she is referred for genetic counseling and targeted sonography.

➤ What are some possible explanations for her elevated maternal serum alpha-fetoprotein (MSAFP)?

➤ Should this screening test be repeated?

ANSWERS TO CASE 3:

Second-Trimester Serum Screening

Summary: A 31-year-old G1 at $17^2/_7$ weeks' gestation has an elevated MSAFP of 3.1 MoM.

➤ **Some possible explanations for elevated MSAFP:** Fetal open spina bifida, multiple gestations, anencephaly, erroneous gestational age, encephalocele, fetal death, ventral wall defect, miscellaneous metabolic/structural abnormalities.

➤ **Repetition of screening test:** No, because of the markedly elevated value.

ANALYSIS

Objectives

1. Describe the types of second-trimester serum testing for fetal aneuploidy.
2. Describe the role of serum testing for fetal neural tube defects.
3. Understand the diagnostic approach to abnormal second-trimester screening.

Considerations

In this patient, the MSAFP is 3.1 multiple of the median (MoM). Repeat testing of MSAFP levels will result in a reduction of the false-positive rate by nearly half. This is a result of regression toward the mean, a statistical property that states the more often a test is repeated, the more likely the result will represent the "true" value—meaning at or near "normal," (assuming the fetus is structurally intact). From a practical standpoint, however, most centers do not advocate repeat testing if the initial value exceeds 3.0 MoM. This is because the repeat level is not likely to reach normal limits when the initial value is this elevated. Additionally, the likelihood of some type of pregnancy abnormality is inherently higher with increasing values of MSAFP (open spina bifida, ventral wall defect, twins). At the time of her ultrasound examination, the patient is found to be carrying a 17-week size fetus with open neural tube defect or **myelomeningocele** of the lumbosacral spine.

APPROACH TO
Second-Trimester Serum Screening

Elevated MSAFP

Is amniocentesis warranted if open spina bifida (OSB) is identified on sono?

Rarely, spina bifida is associated with fetal aneuploidy. Some series report the incidence as high as around 15%, especially if additional anomalies are present. When isolated, the actual risk is probably around 1% to 2%. For this reason, karyotyping of the fetus is indicated. An abnormal karyotype would have significant impact on prognosis, and for this reason, patients may wish to know this information for decision making about continuing or terminating the pregnancy. Recurrence risk for this condition would be different if the fetal karyotype is normal, and the recommended tests in subsequent pregnancies would also be affected. Additionally, since an option of in utero treatment in the form of fetal surgery is being studied, a normal fetal karyotype should be confirmed. Measurement of amniotic fluid AFP has no correlation with degree of severity, size of lesion, or anticipated neurologic complications.

How should a couple found to have a fetus with an open spina bifida (OSB) be counseled about outcomes?

The long-term management of spina bifida in children (and adults) continues to evolve. At our center, consultation with a pediatric neurosurgeon is performed to give the prospective parents the latest information. Most newborns (80%-90%) will require ventriculoperitoneal shunting. The need for shunt revisions is based on development of shunt infection (around 5% in most institutions) or obstruction (0-6 per 10 patients-years) [1; level III]. Frequent shunt revision is associated with worse prognosis for neurologic function. For newborns with lumbosacral open spina bifida, most will require some combination of wheelchair assistance and/or crutches with braces. Mobility tends to deteriorate with age. Cognitive impairment is seen frequently, with reports of 15% incidence of mild mental retardation and 70% incidence of learning disability in children with low lesions (below L3). Higher lesions and larger lesions are associated with higher rates of these types of disabilities.

Is route of delivery important in prognosis for newborn?

There are conflicting and scant data about whether route of delivery impacts prognosis for the newborn with open spina bifida. There is no clear evidence that elective cesarean delivery has a direct benefit on outcome (2; level II-2). If the fetus is in a breech presentation, most would advocate for elective cesarean. Some centers report lower infection rates in the newborn's CNS if delivered by elective C-section, but the long-term implications from this are unclear (1; level III). Others recommend C-section based on the following fetal criteria: (1) lesion protrudes more than 1 cm from surface of the back; (2) intact knee movement; and (3) absence of other severe, untreatable anomalies. With respect to timing and coordination of ancillary medical teams, a scheduled cesarean offers advantages, as these newborns typically need surgical closure relatively soon after delivery.

What risk factors for fetal neural tube defects does she have that are modifiable? (3; level III)

Weight (obese women about 2× higher risk)

Use of folate supplements (400 µg/d is recommended in low-risk women)

Teratogenic drugs and alcohol

Maternal diabetes (optimal glucose control preconceptionally)

Maternal fever

Genetic susceptibility (personal history or previous affected fetus) is not modifiable.

What form of prenatal testing is warranted in subsequent pregnancies?

Should the fetus in this current affected pregnancy have a normal chromosome complement, subsequent pregnancies need to be evaluated for recurrence of neural tube defects (NTD). Prior to conception, she should receive daily folic acid supplementation in the dose of 4 mg, typically given as 1 mg 4× each day (4; Level I). Early sonography is reasonable to exclude anencephaly. Amniocentesis would be indicated in subsequent pregnancies in the early second trimester, when visualization of a small spinal defect may not be readily accomplished. Testing for amniotic fluid acetylcholinesterase in subsequent pregnancies is routinely performed as well as AFP measurement.

What obstetrical implications are associated with an unexplained MSAFP?

Numerous retrospective series have delineated a relationship between unexplained elevated MSAFP and a variety of adverse outcomes. Higher rates of stillbirth, preterm labor, preeclampsia, and intrauterine growth restriction (IUGR) have all been reported from series of women with high MSAFP values (typically ≥ 2.5 MoM). However, use of midtrimester MSAFP to accurately predict complications is not feasible, given the poor sensitivity and specificity of this biomarker. Accordingly, no large-scale prospective trial of increased antepartum surveillance for these patients has demonstrated any added benefit in the early identification or prevention of such complications. Nonetheless, most clinicians choose to evaluate growth and fetal well-being in the third trimester as they would other high-risk pregnancies (5; Level III).

What does the evaluation consist of with an unexplained elevated MSAFP?

Once wrong dates, twins, and fetal anomalies that can be associated with an elevated MSAFP have been excluded by ultrasound, the option of amniocentesis should be presented. Measurements of amniotic fluid AFP (AFAFP) together with acetylcholinesterase (AChE) improve the accuracy of detecting an open neural tube defect. AChE is derived predominantly from fetal neural tissue and is therefore more specific for central nervous lesions. However, targeted ultrasound *in experienced hands* can also be as sensitive and specific as AFAFP plus AChE and this information may be helpful to a patient when deciding on whether to proceed with invasive testing. The higher the MSAFP level the greater the risk of fetal abnormalities. Exceedingly high levels of MSAFP (> 5 or 6 MoM and AFAFP > 10 MoM) are associated with **congenital nephrosis**. This is an autosomal recessive disorder that leads to nephrotic syndrome. It is more common in the Finnish population, however, it can also occur in those of non-Finnish decent. Nephrotic syndrome in infancy can be lethal without treatment which may involve dialysis or renal transplant. Antenatal diagnosis can be strongly suspected in those with a very high MSAFP level, however, additional genetic testing for the most common mutations involving the nephrin (*NPHS*) gene may also be offered to improve the accuracy of antenatal diagnosis.

Comprehension Questions

3.1   A 25-year-old G1P0 at 19-weeks' singleton by last menstrual period (LMP) consistent with 7-week crown to rump length (CRL) gestation is found to have an elevated MSAFP 3.1 MoM. An ultrasound is done confirming a singleton fetus without apparent anatomical abnormalities. What is the next step in management?
A. Offer amniocentesis for measurement of AFAFP and AChE.
B. Offer chorionic villus sampling.
C. Offer repeat serum alpha-fetoprotein in 2 weeks.
D. Explain to the patient that with a normal ultrasound, there are unlikely to be any complications to the pregnancy.

3.2   A 27-year-old woman G2P1 at 16 weeks' gestation is noted to have a decreased MSAFP, with an increased risk of trisomy 18. Which of the following statements is most accurate?
A. A fetal ultrasound showing wrong dates is unlikely to show a change in the trisomy 18 risk.
B. The serum hCG level is likely higher than expected.
C. The serum unconjugated estriol level is likely higher than expected.
D. The serum PAPP-A level is part of the calculation of the aneuploidy risk.

ANSWERS

3.1 **A.** Although amniocentesis should be offered in anyone with an unexplained elevated MSAFP, a targeted ultrasound in experienced hands can be just as sensitive and specific as AFAFP plus AChE in detecting open neural tube defects, thus avoiding the need to perform amniocentesis. Ultimately the decision to pursue invasive testing can be left to each individual patient and recommendation for further testing can be based on whether additional genetic testing for other conditions is warranted. Although there is no standard way of managing patients with an unexplained MSAFP level, it is not unreasonable to monitor fetal growth with periodic ultrasounds in the third trimester given the association with IUGR.

3.2 **A.** An increase in the fetal trisomy 18 risk is associated with a decrease in the serum analytes of hCG, AFP, and unconjugated estriol. Unlike Down syndrome, where the gestational age correction can alter the Down syndrome risk, with trisomy 18, wrong gestational age rarely leads to a normalization of the trisomy 18 risk. This difference is principally due to the direction of the hCG level with gestational age, which falls from 10 weeks gestation through 20 weeks gestation, and the fact that Down syndrome is associated with an elevated hCG.

Clinical Pearls

See US Preventive Services Task Force Study Quality levels of evidence in Case 1

➤ All women of reproductive age should consume healthy diets, including foods rich in folic acid. Because dietary sources are rarely adequate, periconceptional use of folic acid supplementation (400 μg daily in low-risk women) is recommended (Level I).

➤ Maternal serum screening for fetal neural tube defects (and other anomalies) should be offered to all pregnant women in the early second trimester (Level I).

➤ Further evaluation must be offered to all women found to have elevated levels of maternal serum alpha-fetoprotein (Level II-3).

➤ Women found to be carrying a fetus with a neural tube defect should receive appropriate counseling from specialists knowledgeable about treatment and prognosis for these conditions as part of the decision-making process about pregnancy management (Level III).

➤ Delivery options for fetuses with neural tube defects should be individualized depending on expected prognosis and specific characteristics of the lesion (Level III).

REFERENCES

1. Doherty D, Shurtleff DB. Pediatric perspective on prenatal counseling for myelomeningocele. *Birth Defects Res (Pt A)*. 2006;76:645-653.
   Overview of key features of this malformation, focusing on prognosis and typical postnatal course (Level III).
2. Lewis D, Tolosa JE, Kaufmann M, et al. Elective cesarean delivery and long-term motor function or ambulation status in infants with meningomyelocele. *Obstet Gynecol*. 2004;103:469-473.
   In this retrospective review of one center's experience with long-term assessment of motor function in children born with spina bifida, there was no advantage to elective cesarean delivery in terms of preserving motor function or ambulation status (Level II-2).
3. Mitchell LA. Epidemiology of neural tube defects. *Amer J Med Genet (Pt C)*. 2005;135C:88-94.
   Review of risk factors and known etiologies of common neural tube defects, emphasizing preventable causes amenable to preconceptional and periconceptional interventions (Level III).
4. MRC Vitamin Study Research Group. Prevention of neural tube defects: results of the Medical Research Council Vitamin study. *Lancet*. 1991;338:131-137.
   This large multicenter randomized controlled trial demonstrated a 72% reduction in recurrence of NTD when 4 mg folic acid are consumed daily prior to and during subsequent pregnancies (level I).
5. Wilkins-Haug L. Unexplained elevated maternal serum alpha-fetoprotein: what is appropriate follow-up? *Curr Opin Obstet Gynecol*. 1998;10:469-474.
   In this review of studies examining outcomes of pregnancies associated with unexplained elevated MSAFP, it is clear that while these women are at higher risk, current means of antepartum surveillance fall short of achieving reductions in adverse outcomes (level III).

Case 4

A 36-year-old G3P2002 at 38 weeks' gestation presents to labor and delivery (L&D) with uterine contractions, and is found to be in active labor with the fetus in breech presentation. She has had an uncomplicated antepartum course with good prenatal care including a normal anatomy scan in the second trimester. Her prior infants, each weighing approximately 3000 g, were delivered vaginally without complications. Ultrasound evaluation upon presentation to L&D confirms that the infant is in frank breech presentation and the head is flexed; the estimated fetal weight (EFW) is 3200 g. Clinical assessment of the maternal pelvis is determined to be adequate for a fetus of this estimated weight. The cervix is 5 cm dilated, 100% effaced and the fetal sacrum is at zero station, frank breech, left sacrum transverse. After being counseled on delivery options, the patient states that she would like to avoid a cesarean section if at all possible.

➤ What are the prerequisites for offering women at term with breech presentation an attempt at vaginal breech delivery?

➤ With careful selection criteria, how do the perinatal outcomes of vaginal breech delivery compare to those of infants delivered via cesarean?

➤ What technical principles are important to optimize perinatal outcome?

ANSWERS TO CASE 4:
Vaginal Breech Delivery

Summary: A multiparous woman with a frank breech presentation at term, with a clinically adequate pelvis, desires to avoid cesarean delivery. Following the steps outlined in the subsequent discussion will assist caregivers in achieving satisfactory results.

➤ **Prerequisites:** Frank or complete breech presentation, estimated fetal weight between 2500 and 4000 g, flexed fetal head, adequate maternal pelvis, patient counseling and consent, and an experienced operator present at delivery are all important prerequisites.

➤ **Perinatal outcomes comparing vaginal delivery to cesarean:** The largest randomized trial conducted by Hannah and colleagues found an increased neonatal morbidity and mortality for infants delivered vaginally compared to those delivered by cesarean.[1] A follow-up report of surviving infants from that trial at 2 years of life revealed no significant differences between groups.[2] Since the publication of that large trial, several smaller nonrandomized reports have documented better outcomes than those obtained in the large trial.[3]

➤ **Important technical principles:** These include conscientious labor management, delivery in a setting with immediate cesarean capability, avoidance of early operator interference, adequate episiotomy if indicated, gentle manipulation of the infant, and the use of forceps for the aftercoming head.

ANALYSIS

Objectives

1. Identify an appropriate candidate for vaginal breech delivery.
2. Effectively counsel a woman regarding risks, benefits, and alternatives related to vaginal breech delivery.
3. Become familiar with the technical principles involved in achieving satisfactory neonatal outcomes.

Considerations

Ideally, the fetus in breech presentation should be diagnosed between 36 and 39 weeks gestation in the prenatal clinic where the option of external cephalic version can be discussed. Many women who present at term in labor with a fetus in breech presentation are not candidates for vaginal breech delivery.

The first step in management is therefore to identify appropriate cases for attempted vaginal breech delivery[4,5] and delivery by cesarean for the women who do not meet strict selection criteria. The next section will outline in detail these selection criteria. The second step is to counsel potential candidates regarding risks, benefits, and alternatives to vaginal breech delivery. This counseling step is critically important and should reflect institutional and individual operator experience in the context of the available evidence, and should take into account their local results. A variable portion of women who satisfy the first two steps will require cesarean delivery in labor, for either abnormal progress or nonreassuring fetal status. At most institutions less than 50%, and at some centers only 10%, of carefully selected women will achieve successful vaginal breech delivery. To optimize outcomes for those who do, the final step in management consists of proper technique in the performance of the delivery itself.

APPROACH TO
Vaginal Breech Delivery

DEFINITIONS

TYPES OF BREECH: A frank breech has hips flexed and knees extended. A complete breech has both hips and knees flexed. An incomplete breech has one or both hips extended, such that part of a lower extremity is palpable in the birth canal below the buttocks. Planned vaginal breech delivery should only apply to fetuses in frank or complete breech presentation.

CLINICAL PELVIMETRY: Some authors prefer to call this clinical pelvic assessment rather than measuring (-metry) the pelvis, but the end result is the same. The aftercoming head of the fetus will not have time to mold as it passes through the birth canal. Thus, the operator must determine that the pelvis is sufficiently large to accommodate the unmolded head using only physical examination skills and not radiographic pelvimetry.

LOVSET MANEUVER: There are many eponyms associated with the various maneuvers used in vaginal breech delivery. Lovset of Norway is credited with describing rotational movement of the fetal trunk once the lower third of the scapula has become visible to allow for delivery of the anterior fetal arm and shoulder first, followed by a 180 degree rotation to deliver the remaining shoulder anteriorly as well. In difficult cases the posterior shoulder of the fetus may need to be delivered first and this maneuver is not associated with Lovset.

CLINICAL APPROACH

Unfortunately, selection criteria for candidates for planned vaginal breech delivery vary throughout the literature. For this chapter four important requirements are recommended: frank or complete breech presentation, adequate maternal pelvis, estimated fetal weight 2500 to 4000 g, and a flexed fetal head.[6] Ultrasound is an important tool for assessing each criterion except pelvic adequacy, which depends on physical examination by an experienced clinician, supplemented at some centers by radiographic pelvimetry. Confirmation of fetal head flexion is difficult using only clinical examination; the use of either ultrasound or a flat-plate radiograph is recommended. Hyperextension of the fetal head is associated with an unacceptable risk of cervical spine injury and possible head entrapment. Restricting planned vaginal breech delivery to frank or complete breech presentation is designed to reduce the risk of umbilical cord prolapse associated with incomplete breech presentation. The lower estimated-weight limit of 2500 g should eliminate both premature and growth restricted fetuses. The upper limit of 4000 g should reduce the possibility of attempting to deliver a macrosomic infant vaginally.

Counseling a well-selected candidate for vaginal breech delivery may be the key to her decision regarding the options of planned vaginal versus planned cesarean delivery (assuming that the option of external cephalic version has been previously addressed). If the counselor begins the session with a statement like "the baby's head may get trapped and that could cause brain damage or even death," the woman will most likely choose cesarean delivery. In contrast, a statement like "our careful selection process has minimized many of the risks of vaginal breech delivery and we have a proven track record of good outcomes" may persuade more women to carefully weigh the risks to themselves of cesarean delivery. If an obstetrician experienced in vaginal breech delivery is not available, cesarean delivery is a safer option.

If residents in training are not taught the technical skills of vaginal breech delivery, they will be unable to offer this option to their patients. Simulation training[7] and vaginal breech delivery of second twins can help to enhance the resident's understanding of many of the technical aspects of breech delivery. The same techniques that facilitate safe vaginal breech delivery are also applicable to cesarean breech delivery.

In order to arrive at the moment where vaginal delivery techniques can be employed, one must first manage the woman's labor adroitly (Figures 4–1 to 4–4). Careful attention to fetal heart rate monitoring and judicious, infrequent use of oxytocin are recommended. Delivery should occur in a

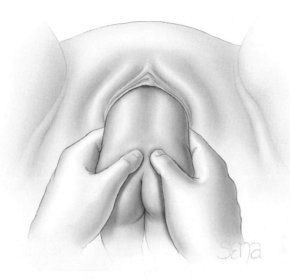

Figure 4–1. Delivery of the body. The hands are applied, but not above the pelvic girdle. Gentle downward rotational traction is accomplished until the scapulas are clearly visible. (*Reproduced, with permission, from Cunningham FG, Leveno KJ, Bloom SL, et al. Williams Obstetrics. 23rd ed. New York, NY: McGraw-Hill; 2010.*)

fully equipped operating room with the capability of proceeding immediately with cesarean delivery if necessary. The operator should grasp the fetal pelvis over bony prominences (sacrum and iliac crests) and should apply pressure parallel to, and not transverse to, long bones. Either Piper or Laufe-Piper forceps should be used routinely to deliver the aftercoming head (Figure 4–5). Laufe-Piper forceps can be easily applied to the aftercoming head at cesarean delivery, whereas Piper forceps are a bit unwieldy when used at cesarean section. In certain circumstances, an assistant may apply suprapubic pressure to facilitate engagement and flexion of the fetal head, but frequently this step is not necessary.

The patient presented in the case scenario is an ideal candidate for vaginal breech delivery. Astute labor management coupled with the presence of an experienced obstetrician at delivery should produce excellent maternal and perinatal outcomes.

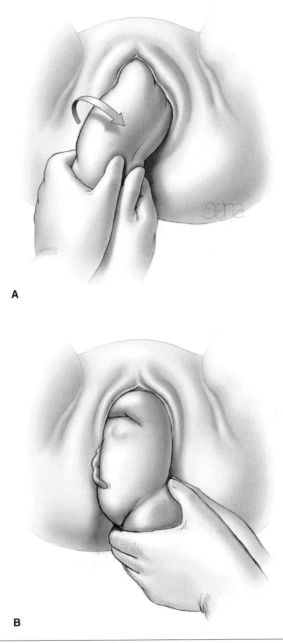

Figure 4–2.   Delivery of body is accomplished using clockwise rotation of the fetal pelvis to bring the sacrum to left sacrum transverse, which gentle downward traction, and gently splinting the arm against the body delivers the arm. (*Reproduced, with permission, from Cunningham FG, Leveno KJ, Bloom SL, et al.* Williams Obstetrics. *23rd ed. New York, NY: McGraw-Hill; 2010.*)

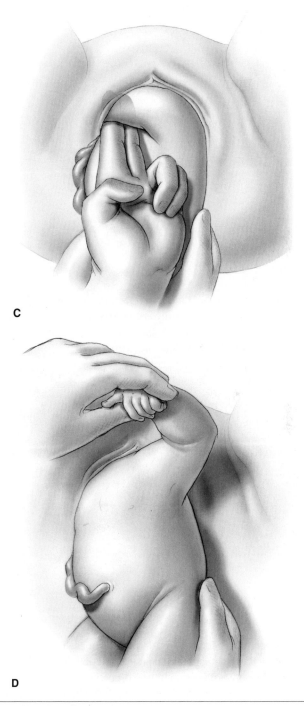

C

D

Figure 4–2. (*Continued*)

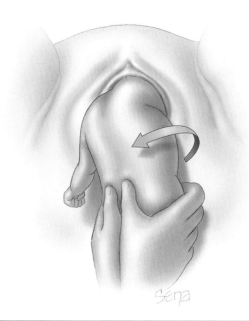

Figure 4–3. Counterclockwise rotation from sacrum anterior to right sacrum transverse along with gentle traction downward effects delivery of the right scapula. (*Reproduced, with permission, from Cunningham FG, Leveno KJ, Bloom SL, et al. Williams Obstetrics. 23rd ed. New York, NY: McGraw-Hill; 2010.*)

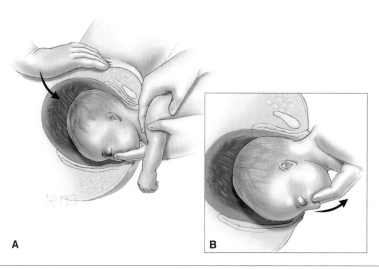

A   **B**

Figure 4–4. Delivery of the fetal head using the Mauriceau maneuver, and flexion of the fetal head by the assistant maintaining suprapubic pressure (A). Pressure on the maxilla as careful outward traction is used (B). (*Reproduced, with permission, from Cunningham FG, Leveno KJ, Bloom SL, et al. Williams Obstetrics. 23rd ed. New York, NY: McGraw-Hill; 2010.*)

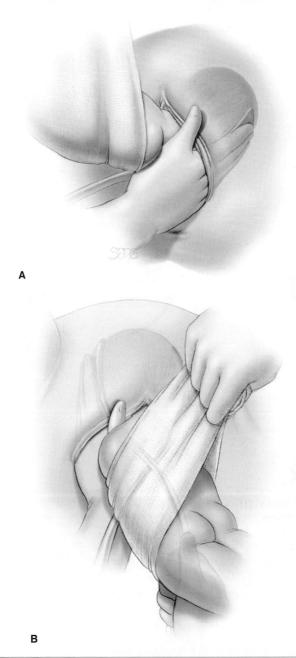

A

B

Figure 4–5.   Piper forceps are used for the delivery of the aftercoming head. The fetal body is elevated using a warm towel and the left blade of the forceps is applied to the aftercoming head (A). The right blade is applied with the body still elevated (B). Forceps delivery of the aftercoming head, with the movement of the forceps is shown by the arrow (C). (*Reproduced, with permission, from Cunningham FG, Leveno KJ, Bloom SL, et al. Williams Obstetrics. 23rd ed. New York, NY: McGraw-Hill; 2010.*)

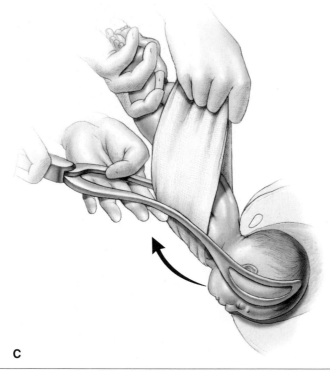

C

Figure 4–5. (*Continued*)

Comprehension Questions

4.1   Which of the following ultrasound findings would be a contraindication to planned vaginal delivery of a term breech?
      A. EFW of 3600 g
      B. Fetal pyelectasis
      C. Extension (> 90 degrees) of the fetal head
      D. Complete breech presentation

4.2   Which of the following named maneuvers are used to deliver the fetal arms during vaginal breech delivery?
      A. Pinard maneuver
      B. Lovset maneuver
      C. Mauriceau-Smellie-Veit maneuver
      D. Prague maneuver

4.3 Which of the following types of obstetrical forceps has been shown to be useful for delivery of the aftercoming head at either abdominal or vaginal delivery?
A. Simpson
B. Kielland
C. Laufe-Piper
D. Piper

ANSWERS

4.1 **C.** Extension of the fetal head increases the risk of C-spine injury. The weight of 3600 g is within the suggested weight range of 2500 to 4000 g. Fetal pyelectasis (dilation of the fetal renal pelvis of > 7 mm at term) is a relative common ultrasound finding which has no bearing on route of delivery. Vaginal delivery is reasonable for either frank or complete breech presentation.

4.2 **B.** Lovset was a Norwegian obstetrician who advocated rotation of the fetal trunk to facilitate freeing the anterior fetal arm. Pinard was a French obstetrician whose maneuver is used to deliver one or both fetal legs. Mauriceau (French), Smellie (English), and Veit (German) have their names attached to a manual method of delivering the aftercoming head (although forceps are preferable). Finally, the Prague maneuver should be used when the fetus, whose body is delivered, cannot be rotated to dorsum anterior.

4.3 **C.** Laufe modified the Piper forceps by considerably shortening the length and changing the lock from English to pivot. The short length of the Laufe-Piper facilitates their use at abdominal breech delivery. Simpson forceps have a pelvic curve which is a disadvantage. Kielland forceps are seldom used for either abdominal or vaginal breech delivery. Piper forceps are useful for vaginal breech delivery, but unwieldy for use at cesarean delivery.

Clinical Pearls

See US Preventive Services Task Force Study Quality levels of evidence in Case 1

➤ In order for a practitioner to feel confident in deciding that a pelvis is adequate for attempted vaginal breech delivery, pelvic assessment should be a routine element for all laboring women (Level II-3).

➤ Long bone fractures complicate both vaginal and abdominal breech deliveries. In their handling of fetal extremities, operators should ensure that pressure is applied parallel to, and not perpendicular to long bones (Level II-3).

➤ Strong consideration should be given to conducting vaginal breech delivery in an operating room with personnel and equipment to proceed with immediate cesarean delivery should that be necessary (Level III).

➤ An experienced operator should be present for all breech deliveries, vaginal or abdominal (Level III).

➤ A woman's choice of delivery mode once she has been appropriately counseled should be respected (Level III).

REFERENCES

1. Hannah ME, Hannah WJ, Hewson SA, Hodnett ED, Saigal S, Willan AR. Planned caesarean section versus planned vaginal birth for breech presentation at term: a randomized multicentre trial. *Lancet.* 2000;356:1375-1383.
2. Whyte H, Hannah ME, Saigal S, et al. Outcomes of children at 2 years after planned cesarean birth versus planned vaginal birth for breech presentation at term: the International Randomized Term Breech Trial. *Am J Obstet Gynecol.* 2004;191:864-871.
3. American College of Obstetricians and Gynecologists. ACOG Committee Opinion No. 340, Mode of term singleton breech delivery. *Obstet Gynecol.* 2006;108:235-237.
4. Alarab M, Regan C, O'Connel MP, Keane DP, Herlihy C, Foley ME. Singleton vaginal breech delivery at term: still a safe option. *Obstet Gynecol.* 2004;103:407-412.
5. Albrechtsen S, Rasmussen S, Reigstad H, Markestad T, Irgens LM, Dalaker K. Evaluation of a protocol for selecting fetuses in breech presentation for vaginal delivery or cesarean section. *Am J Obstet Gynecol.* 1997;177:586-592.
6. SOGC Clinical Practice Guideline: Vaginal delivery of breech presentation, Guideline no. 226. JOGC. June 2009.
7. Yamamura Y, Ramin KD, Ramin, SM. Trial of vaginal breech delivery: current role. *Clin Obstet Gynecol.* 2007;50:526-536.

Case 5

A 32-year-old G4P3003 Hispanic female with no prenatal care presents to the hospital at 40 weeks stating that her membranes ruptured the day before and her contractions began about 8 hours prior to this admission. For the past 4 hours she has noted progressively severe pain and decreased fetal movement. A recent immigrant from El Salvador, her primary language is Spanish. She is a single mother with three children, ages 12, 10, and 1 year old. She states that her first delivery was by cesarean section because she never went into labor, second was a normal vaginal delivery, and third was a cesarean section at a public hospital in San Antonio, Texas when she "...went into labor early and the baby was in the wrong position." She states that she did not want second cesarean because her first one had been complicated by a wound infection that required 2 months of packing and cleaning.

She tells you that she is very worried about having another cesarean section, but also wants to do whatever is the safest for her fetus. She denies diabetes, hypertension, or any chronic medical illnesses. She does not smoke, drink, or use illicit drugs. Both of her parents are obese with diabetes and hypertension.

On physical examination she is in moderate distress with frequent contractions and complains that her right shoulder hurts. The maternal heart rate is 140 beats per minute (bpm). Her blood pressure is 80/40 mm Hg. Her temperature is normal. She is obese with a BMI of 35 kg/m^2. Her fundal height is difficult to measure, but appears near term. Her abdomen is mildly tender in all quadrants. The nurse reports that fetal heart tones by external Doppler are 140 bpm with absent variability and no accelerations. On pelvic examination she is 8 cm dilated, 90% effaced, and the fetal vertex is floating above the pelvic inlet.

➤ What is the differential diagnosis?

➤ What is the most likely diagnosis?

➤ What are your next steps in caring for this patient?

ANSWERS TO CASE 5:

VBAC—The "Approach to Counseling and Management"

Summary: This is a patient with two prior cesareans, one prior vaginal delivery, nonrepetitive indications for the prior cesareans, an unknown scar(s), an inter-pregnancy interval of only 30 weeks and current risk factors for macrosomia. Her presentation suggests hemodynamic instability and possible fetal compromise.

> **Differential diagnosis:** Uterine rupture, abruptio placenta, chorioamnionitis with sepsis, pyelonephritis, appendicitis, cholecystitis or other intra-abdominal acute processes.

> **Most likely diagnosis:** Uterine rupture.

> **Next steps:** This is a life-threatening emergency for both, the mother and the fetus. Quickly notify essential personnel such as anesthesia, operating room staff, blood bank, and laboratory services. Immediately obtain large bore IV access. Simultaneously obtain blood for cross match and coagulation studies with one red-top tube taped to a wall to observe for clotting. Resuscitation with volume repletion is important while assessing the mother and determining fetal status. As the fetal heart rate is the same as the mother's, a quick ultrasound to assess fetal viability should be obtained but should not delay the next steps. While continuing to resuscitate the mother, the patient should be immediately moved to the operating room as surgical management is imperative at this point even if the fetus is already dead. Usually, a general anesthetic is indicated, as this clinical situation does not permit the time required for a regional anesthetic.

ANALYSIS

Objectives

1. Be familiar with historical, antenatal, and intrapartum factors that influence the **likelihood of success** if attempting a trial of labor.
2. Be familiar with historical, antenatal, and intrapartum factors that influence one's **risk of uterine rupture** during a trial of labor.
3. Be able to counsel patients regarding the **maternal and newborn outcomes** associated with (1) trial of labor, (2) elective repeat cesarean, and (3) uterine rupture in labor.
4. Describe the **most common signs** of intrapartum uterine rupture.
5. Describe the intrapartum and operative **management of uterine rupture.**

Considerations

The most recent report of births from the National Center for Health Statistics shows that the VBAC (vaginal birth after cesarean) rate in the United States continues to decline and is now less than 10%.[1] While the reasons for this are multiple, an unavoidable effect is that women who plan larger families will increasingly face the specter of multiple cesarean sections over a reproductive lifetime. In light of the individual and societal consequences, appropriate counseling about primary and repeat cesarean delivery is essential.

The counseling and management for vaginal birth after a previous cesarean section presents a number of opportunities and challenges. As much as possible, the counseling should be specific for the individual patient. Information gained from a thorough review of the events surrounding the previous cesarean section(s) may inform a particular patient's likelihood of successful VBAC as well as her risk of uterine rupture. Similarly, characteristics of the current pregnancy and labor may also modify the chances of success or the likelihood of uterine rupture. Consequently, VBAC counseling is not necessarily a one-time event and may need to be readdressed as circumstances of the current pregnancy change. In addition to an objective description of the maternal and newborn outcomes associated with a successful or failed trial of labor, patients should also be informed of the maternal and fetal consequences of uterine rupture. Finally, if uterine rupture does occur, prompt recognition and management are vital to optimize outcomes for both the mother and her fetus.

APPROACH TO

Vaginal Birth After Cesarean: The "Approach to Counseling and Management"

FACTORS AFFECTING THE LIKELIHOOD OF SUCCESS OF A TRIAL OF LABOR

Large observational studies from a wide range of practice environments suggest that the overall likelihood of success with an attempted VBAC is between 60% and 80%.[2,3] Studies with more selective criteria for VBAC candidates usually report success rates of about 75%, while studies with more liberal inclusion criteria report success rates closer to 60%. The two most important factors in determining a particular patient's chances of success are a history of a prior vaginal birth and the indication for the previous cesarean delivery.[4-6] The chance of a successful VBAC with a prior vaginal birth is generally reported as 85% compared to 60% without such a history. Similarly, the chance of success if the prior cesarean was performed for a nonrepetitive indication such as malpresentation or a nonreassuring fetal heart rate tracing also approaches 80% to 85%. Women whose previous cesarean section was performed for dystocia generally have a success rate closer 50% to 60%. Other factors associated with a lower likelihood of success include an unfavorable cervix, need for induction of labor, maternal obesity (BMI > 30), fetal weight greater than 4000 g, fetal weight more than 500 g greater than the previous newborn, maternal diabetes, and a maternal age greater than 35 years. Several investigators have tried to combine these and other predictive factors by creating sophisticated prediction models to identify an individual patient's likelihood of success. Unfortunately, none of these models has proven clinically useful when applied prospectively. With the possible exception of the negative prognostic effect of a previous cesarean for second-stage arrest, none of the previously mentioned factors, alone or in combination, will reliably predict a success rate below 50%.

Factors Affecting the Risk of Uterine Rupture

The likelihood of a successful VBAC may influence an individual patient's decision to undergo a trial of labor, but the risk of uterine rupture usually weighs more significantly in that decision. Large prospective cohort studies and a large meta-analysis suggest that the overall risk of uterine rupture during a trial of labor is about 0.6% to 0.7%.[2,7] When counseling an individual patient about the risk of uterine rupture, it is important to identify factors that may predict a higher risk of uterine rupture. These include the conduct and circumstances of the prior cesarean(s), antenatal factors, and intrapartum factors.

First among these is a careful review of the operation reports from prior cesarean sections or other uterine surgeries. Prior classical uterine incisions, "T-shaped" incisions, or large resections of intramural fibroids may be associated with rupture rates as high as 6% or 8% and should be considered contraindications to a trial of labor.

Other historical factors influencing the risk of uterine rupture include a prior vaginal delivery, the number of previous cesareans, the technique of the previous uterine closure, endometritis following the prior cesarean, and the inter-pregnancy interval.[8,9] A prior vaginal delivery reduces the likelihood of uterine rupture in a subsequent trial of labor by as much as 60%.[5,10] Although the number of previous cesarean sections is important, it may not have as much of an effect on the risk of rupture as early studies had indicated. Early small retrospective cohort studies suggested that the risk of uterine rupture with two prior low-transverse cesarean sections was between 2.3% and 3.7% or about four times that of a patient with only one prior cesarean.[11] On the basis of studies that were available at that time, the American College of Obstetricians and Gynecologists published a practice bulletin suggesting that women with two prior cesarean deliveries were not appropriate candidates for a trial of labor unless they had had a previous vaginal delivery. However, more recent data from a larger prospective cohort study suggest that the risk of uterine rupture with two prior cesareans is not that different than with only one

(0.9% vs 0.7%).[12] Several retrospective cohort studies and one secondary analysis of a clinical trial have examined the relationship between technique of single- versus double-layer and the subsequent risk of uterine rupture during a trial of labor.[13-15] Although not all of the studies are consistent, on balance the results suggest an increased risk of rupture with a single-layer closure. While these reports do not preclude a trial of labor after a single-layer closure, the information may support two-layer closure at the time of cesarean section for women who might consider a trial of labor in the future. Finally, a review of prior inpatient records may also be informative. The authors of a retrospective cohort study reported that post-cesarean fever was associated with a fourfold increase in the risk of uterine rupture in a subsequent trial of labor.[16]

In addition to the conduct and circumstances surrounding the prior cesarean delivery, clinicians should also consider factors associated with the current pregnancy when counseling patients regarding the risks and benefits of a trial of labor. Maternal age greater than 30 years has been suggested as a risk factor for uterine rupture, but this has not been observed in large studies using statistical modalities to control for other factors. Several authors have reported that a short inter-pregnancy interval is associated with an increased risk of rupture, but there is no uniform agreement as to the critical time. One of the larger studies demonstrated odds ratios for uterine rupture of 2.6 and 4.8 for inter-delivery intervals of less than 24 months and less than 12 months, respectively.[17] Prematurity in the current pregnancy appears to be associated with a decreased risk of uterine rupture. Surprisingly, while fetal macrosomia may decrease the chance of a successful VBAC, it is not associated with an increased risk of uterine rupture.[18]

Lastly, the relationships between intrapartum factors and the risk of uterine rupture are complex. Most, but not all, large observational studies demonstrate an increase in the risk of uterine rupture with induction of labor with an absolute risk of 1% to 3% regardless of the method of induction.[2] Reports of studies examining the relationship between methods of induction of labor and the risk of uterine rupture have produced conflicting results. One large observational study suggested a significant risk of rupture with any use of prostaglandins compared to induction with oxytocin alone while two larger studies showed either no similar risk or only a very small incremental risk in uterine rupture.[2,19,20] Nonetheless, at this time the American College of Obstetricians and Gynecologists recommends against the use of prostaglandins for the induction of labor in third-trimester patients with a previous cesarean delivery.

Maternal and Newborn Outcomes With Trial of Labor Versus Elective Repeat Cesarean

When counseling patients about VBAC, it is also important to inform them of the maternal and newborn outcomes associated with the different options. At this time, the best estimates of maternal and newborn outcomes are those

Table 5–1 MATERNAL OUTCOMES WITH TRIAL OF LABOR VERSUS ELECTIVE REPEAT CESAREAN SECTION

OUTCOME	TRIAL OF LABOR (%)	REPEAT CESAREAN (%)	ODDS RATIO	P VALUE
Hysterectomy	0.20	0.30	0.77	.22
Thromboembolic disease	0.04	0.10	0.62	.32
Transfusion	1.7	1.0	1.71	<.001
Endometritis	2.9	1.8	1.62	<.001
Maternal death	0.02	0.04	0.38	.21
Other morbidity	0.4	0.3	1.09	.66
Any of the above	5.5	3.6	1.56	<.001

Reproduced, with permission, from Landon MB, Hauth JC, Leveno KJ, et al. Maternal and perinatal outcomes associated with a trial of labor after prior cesarean delivery. *N Eng J Med.* 2004;351:2581-2589. Copyright © 2004 Massachusetts Medical Society. All rights reserved.

reported from the large, multicenter prospective cohort study conducted by the NICHD Maternal-Fetal Medicine Units (MFMU) research network.[2] This was a prospective cohort study with 17,898 trials of labor and 15,801 elective repeat cesarean sections all reported with strict ascertainment rules. Maternal outcomes are shown in Table 5–1 and fetal outcomes are shown in Table 5–2. It is important to discuss both the absolute and the relative risks of these adverse outcomes in order to avoid bias. Often, patients will ask, "What happens if the uterus does rupture?" Here again, the results of the MFMU report are helpful. Rounding to numbers that are easier for counseling, if the uterus ruptures one can expect 1/50 infants to die, 1/20 to have hypoxic ischemic encephalopathy, 1/3 to have a pH less than 7.0, and about half to be admitted to the neonatal intensive care unit. At this point, it is often helpful to return to the previous estimates of absolute risks associated with either a trial of labor or elective repeat cesarean. Conversations concerning these discussions with the patient should be documented in the medical record and at the time of informed consent.

Signs of Uterine Rupture

A number of studies have reported the signs and symptoms of uterine rupture during a trial of labor. The most common sign is an abnormal fetal heart rate tracing, usually prolonged, persistent fetal bradycardia. Less common signs

Table 5–2 PERINATAL OUTCOMES WITH TRIAL OF LABOR VERSUS ELECTIVE REPEAT CESAREAN DELIVERY

OUTCOME	TRIAL OF LABOR (%)	REPEAT CESAREAN (%)	ODDS RATIO	P VALUE
Stillbirth 37-38	0.40	0.10	2.93	.008
Stillbirth ≥ 39	0.20	0.10	2.7	.07
Intrapartum 37-38	0.02	0	—	.43
Intrapartum ≥ 39	0.01	0	—	1.00
HIE	0.08	0	—	<.001
Neonatal death	0.08	0.05	1.82	.19
Any of above	0.38	0.13	2.9	<.001

Reproduced, with permission, from Landon MB, Hauth JC, Leveno KJ, et al. Maternal and perinatal outcomes associated with a trial of labor after prior cesarean delivery. *N Eng J Med.* 2004;351:2581-2589. Copyright © 2004 Massachusetts Medical Society. All rights reserved.

include abdominal pain, loss of fetal station, gross hematuria, cessation of uterine contractions, vaginal bleeding, or signs of massive intra-abdominal bleeding with shock as in the current case scenario.

Management of Uterine Rupture

Suspected intrapartum uterine rupture is a true surgical emergency with two patients at risk. In the present scenario, the mother needs volume; initially two large-bore intravenous lines should be placed and isotonic crystalloids infused, but given her degree of shock she will almost certainly require blood transfusion. With severe maternal tachycardia and this degree of systolic hypotension, the patient has probably lost at least 30% to 40% of her blood volume. In this situation, O-negative or type specific non–cross-matched blood should be released for possible use until cross-matched blood is available. The risks of a hemolytic transfusion reaction from O-negative or type specific, non–cross-matched blood are small and greatly outweighed by the need for red cells in this situation. Importantly, vasopressors play a limited role in the management of massive hemorrhage. Recent evidence from a large, multicenter, prospective cohort study of patients with hemorrhagic shock from blunt trauma shows that when compared to early crystalloid resuscitation, the use of vasopressors of any type is associated with a twofold increased risk of mortality at both 12 and 24 hours.[21] The use of vasopressors in the setting of massive hemorrhage should be limited to those patients who are not responding despite aggressive volume resuscitation while moving toward definitive surgical control.

Surgical management of suspected uterine rupture requires immediate laparotomy, delivery of the fetus, and exploration of the extent of injury to the uterus and surrounding organs. However, even with heroic efforts at emergency cesarean, fetal deaths or injuries cannot always be prevented even with delivery times of less than 10 minutes. The location and extent of the uterine injury will dictate the appropriate surgical management, but hysterectomy is not necessarily required. Because uterine ruptures are often irregular and do not always involve the previous uterine scar, it is important to thoroughly explore the posterior and lateral aspects of the uterus, the uterine vasculature, and the bladder and surrounding organs.

Comprehension Questions

5.1   Which of the following is associated with the greatest likelihood of a successful vaginal birth after a previous cesarean section?
A. Prior cesarean performed due to arrest of dilation at 6 cm
B. Prior cesarean performed for arrest of descent in the second stage
C. Prior cesarean section for an unknown reason
D. Prior cesarean section for breech presentation

5.2   Which of the following is least likely to be associated with an increased risk of uterine rupture during a trial of labor?
A. An inter-delivery interval of greater than 2 years
B. A history of prolonged fever following the prior cesarean section
C. A single-layer closure of the prior cesarean hysterotomy
D. Two prior cesarean sections with no prior vaginal delivery

5.3   Which of the following is the most common sign of an intrapartum uterine rupture?
A. Loss of fetal station
B. Maternal pain
C. Loss of contractions
D. Maternal shock
E. Sudden onset, prolonged fetal bradycardia

5.4   The overall risk of a serious complication defined by hysterectomy, neonatal death, or hypoxic ischemic encephalopathy from an attempted vaginal delivery is closest to which of the following?
A. 1/10
B. 1/100
C. 1/1000
D. 1/10,000

ANSWERS

5.1 **D.** Estimates of the likelihood of successful VBAC based on the indication for the prior cesarean are as follows: (1) prior cesarean for breech—80% to 85%, (2) prior cesarean for nonreassuring fetal heart rate tracing—80% to 85%, and (3) prior cesarean for dystocia in the active phase—50% to 65%.

5.2 **A.** Although various authors have defined a short inter-pregnancy or inter-delivery differently, most of the literature suggests that an inter-delivery interval greater than 18 or 24 months is associated with a decreased risk of uterine rupture.

5.3 **E.** Although all of the choices should be of concern and raise the concern for uterine rupture during a trial of labor, multiple authors have demonstrated that the most common sign is an abnormal fetal heart rate tracing, usually prolonged bradycardia. Serious variables and late decelerations have also been described and are of particular concern when followed by the onset of prolonged bradycardia.

5.4 **C.** The authors writing for the NICHD MFMU research network prospective cohort study group suggested a risk of neonatal death or hypoxic ischemic encephalopathy of 1 in 2000 trials of labor. An analysis from the Agency for Healthcare Research and Quality (AHRQ) suggests a risk of maternal hysterectomy or newborn hypoxic ischemic encephalopathy of 1 in 1250 trials of labor.

Clinical Pearls

See US Preventive Services Task Force Study Quality levels of evidence in Case 1

➤ The best numeric risks for the maternal and fetal outcomes associated with a trial of labor or repeat cesarean section are those from the NICHD MFMU research network prospective cohort study of women with a prior cesarean delivery as depicted in Tables 5–1 and 5–2 (Level II-2).

➤ The best predictor of a successful VBAC is a prior vaginal delivery (Level II-2).

➤ To avoid biased counseling, both absolute and relative risks of a trial of labor versus an elective repeat cesarean should be presented (Level III).

➤ The use of prostaglandins for cervical ripening or induction of labor for women with a prior cesarean section is generally proscribed by current guidance from the American College of Obstetricians and Gynecologists (Level II-B).

REFERENCES

1. National Institutes of Health Consensus Development Conference Statement, Vaginal birth after cesarean: New insights, March 8-10, 2010. *Obstet Gynecol* 2010;115:1279-1295.
2. Landon MB, Hauth JC, Leveno KJ, et al. For the National Institute of Child Health and Development Maternal-Fetal Medicine Units Research Network. Maternal and perinatal outcomes associated with a trial of labor after prior cesarean delivery. *N Engl J Med.* 2004;351:2581-2589. (Level II-2)
3. Harper LM, Macones GA. Predicting success and reducing the risks when attempting vaginal birth after cesarean. *Obstet Gynecol Surv.* 2008;63:538-545. (Systematic Review)
4. Landon MB, Leindecker S, Spong CY, et al. for the National Institute of Child Health and Human Development Maternal-Fetal Medicine Units Network. The MFMU Cesarean Registry: factors affecting the success of trial of labor after previous cesarean delivery. *Am J Obstet Gynecol.* 2005;193:1016-1023. (Level II-2)
5. Mercer BM, Gilbert S, Landon MB, et al. for the National Institute of Child Health and Human Development Maternal-Fetal Medicine Units Network. Labor outcomes with increasing number of prior vaginal births after cesarean delivery. *Obstet Gynecol.* 2008;111:285-291. (Level II-2)
6. Brill Y, Windrim R. Vaginal birth after caesarean section: review of antenatal predictors of success. *J Obstet Gynaecol Can.* 2003;25:275-286. (Level II-2)
7. Chauhan SP, Martin JN, Henricks CE, Morrison JC, Magann EF. Maternal and perinatal complications with uterine rupture in 142,075 patients who attempted vaginal birth after cesarean delivery: a review of the literature. *Am J Obstet Gynecol.* 2003;189:408-417. (Systematic Review)
8. Smith JG, Mertz HL, Merrill DC. Identifying risk factors for uterine rupture. *Clin Perinatol.* 2008;35:85-89. (Review)
9. Cahill AG, Macones GA. Vaginal birth after cesarean delivery: evidence-based practice. *Clin Obstet Gynecol.* 2007;50:518-525. (Review)
10. Zelop CM, Shipp TD, Repke JT, Cohen A, Lieberman E. Effect of previous vaginal delivery on the risk of uterine rupture during a subsequent trail of labor. *Am J Obstet Gynecol.* 2000;183:1184-1186. (Level II-2)
11. Caughey AB, Shipp TD, Repke JJ, et al. Rate of uterine rupture during a trial of labor in women with one or two prior cesarean deliveries. *Am J Obstet Gynecol* 1999;181:872-876.
12. Landon MB, Spong CY, Thom E, et al. Risk of uterine rupture with a trial of labor with multiple and single prior cesarean deliveries. *Obstet Gynecol* 2006;108:12-20.
13. Bujold E, Bujold C, Hamilton EF, et al. The impact of a single-layer or double-layer closure on uterine rupture. *Am J Obstet Gynecol.* 2002;186:1326-1330. (level II-2)
14. Durnwald C, Mercer B. Uterine rupture, perioperative and perinatal morbidity after single-layer and double-layer closure at cesarean delivery. *Am J Obstet Gynecol.* 2003;189:925-929.
15. Gyamfi C, Juhasz G, Gyamfi P, Blumenfeld Y, Stone JL. Single- versus double-layer uterine incision closure and uterine rupture. *J Matern Fetal Neonatal Med.* 2006;19:639-643.
16. Shipp TD, Zelop C, Cohen A, Repke JT, Lieberman E. Post-cesarean delivery fever and uterine rupture in a subsequent trial of labor. *Obstet Gynecol.* 2003;101:136-139. (Level II-2)

17. Bujold E, Mehta SH, Bujold C, Gauthier RJ. Interdelivery interval and uterine rupture. *Am J Obstet Gynecol.* 2002;187:1199-1202. (Level II-2)
18. Zelop CM, Shipp TD, Repke JT, et al. Outcomes of trial of labor following previous cesarean delivery among women with fetuses weighing > 4000 g. *Am J Obstet Gynecol.* 2001;185:903-905. (Level II-2)
19. Lydon-Rochelle M, Holt VL, Easterling TR, Martin DP. Risk of uterine rupture during labor among women with a prior cesarean delivery. *New Engl J Med* 2001; 345:3-8.
20. Macones GA, Peipert J, Nelson DB, et al. Maternal complications with vaginal birth after cesarean delivery: a multicenter study. *Am J Obstet Gynecol* 2005; 193:1656-62.
21. Sperry JL, Minei JP, Frankel HL, et al. Early use of vasopressors after injury: caution before constriction. *J Trauma.* 2008;64:9-14. (Level II-1)

Case 6

A 38-year-old African American woman, G7P6006, presents to triage at 40 weeks of gestation by last menstrual period because of painful contractions. She denies bleeding or leakage of amniotic fluid. All six of her previous pregnancies resulted in term vaginal deliveries. Vital signs are normal, height is 5 ft 4 in and weight is 190 lb (86 kg). Her fundal height is 47 cm, fetal heart tones are detected at 160 beats per minute and presentation cannot be ascertained on abdominal examination. Cervical examination reveals a bulging bag of water, dilation of 6 cm, complete effacement, and no presenting part in the pelvis. A bedside ultrasound is performed which indicates excessive amniotic fluid and a cephalic presentation. During the ultrasound examination the patient's membranes rupture spontaneously followed by vaginal passage of copious amounts of amniotic fluid and a prolapsed umbilical cord. An emergency cesarean delivery under general anesthesia results in the birth of a 4500 g male infant. After the placenta is removed, the uterus is flaccid and bleeding is brisk. There is no response to massage, bimanual uterine compression, and a variety of uterotonic agents. Blood loss is estimated at 2000 cc and bilateral uterine artery ligation produces no improvement. Blood pressure is now 80/40 mm Hg, pulse is 120 per minute, and type-specific blood has been requested.

➤ What is the most likely diagnosis?

➤ What is your next step?

➤ What are the complications of the next step?

ANSWERS TO CASE 6:

Cesarean Section Leading to Cesarean Hysterectomy

Summary: A 38-year-old G7P6006 at term, with polyhydramnios, who underwent an emergency cesarean delivery for cord prolapse after spontaneous rupture of membranes in labor. She experienced severe intraoperative blood loss leading to hemodynamic instability. Conservative treatment measures did not resolve the problem.

➤ **Most likely diagnosis:** Uterine atony refractory to conservative management.

➤ **Next step:** Proceed with cesarean hysterectomy.

➤ **Potential complications:** Urinary tract injury, high likelihood of transfusion, loss of fertility, admission to intensive care, death.

ANALYSIS

Objectives

1. Appreciate that both primary and repeat cesarean delivery are strong risk factors for cesarean hysterectomy.
2. Be familiar with the leading indications for cesarean hysterectomy.
3. Consider the ways in which proper performance of cesarean hysterectomy may enable the operator to avoid the known complications of the procedure.

Considerations

A **38-year-old grand multipara** with **polyhydramnios** undergoes spontaneous rupture of membranes and cord prolapse necessitating an emergent cesarean delivery under **general anesthesia** with delivery of a **macrosomic infant**. Each entry in bold in the previous sentence is a risk factor for uterine atony and combining such factors, as in the case presented, markedly increases the risk. Intraoperatively, when the expected uterine atony and hemorrhage is encountered, conservative management fails to reduce the bleeding. To prevent further morbidity or mortality a cesarean hysterectomy is performed.

APPROACH TO

Cesarean Section Leading to Cesarean Hysterectomy

DEFINITIONS

CESAREAN DELIVERY: A surgical incision through the abdominal wall (laparotomy) and uterus (hysterotomy) performed to deliver a fetus.

CESAREAN HYSTERECTOMY: An abdominal hysterectomy performed at the time of a cesarean delivery.

PERIPARTUM HYSTERECTOMY: A more inclusive term encompassing hysterectomy performed at the time of either cesarean or vaginal delivery or in the immediate postpartum period.

UTERINE ATONY: Inadequate contractility of the postpartum uterus leading to hemorrhage from the placental implantation site. Blood flow to this site averages 600 mL/min at term.

POLYHYDRAMNIOS: A term that is used to describe excessive amniotic fluid volume. Quantitatively, an amniotic fluid index above 24 cm, or above the 95th percentile for gestational age, or a maximum vertical pocket greater than 8 cm have each been used to define excessive fluid; sometimes only a qualitative assessment of too much fluid is used.

CLINICAL APPROACH

Safe cesarean childbirth is one of the greatest medical advances of the 20th century. Advances in anesthesia, broad-spectrum antibiotics, safe blood transfusion, and improved operative technique have resulted in incredibly low maternal mortality related to cesarean delivery. Ironically, it is the safety of the procedure that has contributed to unprecedented high rates in the United States and around the world.

The incidence of cesarean has increased in the United States from 5.5% in 1970 to its present rate of almost 32%. There are a myriad of "reasons" for this increased rate including lower tolerance for risks, high false-positive rate for detection of fetal hypoxia, increased use of electronic fetal monitoring, increased use of epidural anesthesia, decrease in VBACs, fear of litigation, patient choice, and physician convenience.[1]

Overall maternal mortality is extremely uncommon (< 10 deaths/100,000 live births) in the United States, but even here cesarean birth carries two to four times the risk for mortality compared to vaginal delivery. This risk notwithstanding, cesarean deliveries have been credited with saving the lives of some mothers and many infants. The case of cord prolapse presented in this case exemplifies the lifesaving nature of an emergency cesarean delivery for the infant. The indication for cesarean in our case is inarguable, but too often the indications are flimsy, and the serious risks of the procedure including hysterectomy and death are underemphasized. Of note, cesarean delivery is associated with a fivefold increase in pulmonary embolism compared to vaginal delivery. For a detailed discussion of cesarean delivery indications and technical considerations the reader is referred to standard texts on obstetrics. The remainder of this section outlines the clinical approach to cesarean hysterectomy.

The incidence of cesarean hysterectomy is 4 to 8/10,000 births; if peripartum hysterectomies are considered (see under "Definitions"), then the frequency will be slightly higher. Two recent reports examined the relationship of cesarean delivery to cesarean hysterectomy.[2,3] Compared with controls, women who had a peripartum hysterectomy were three times more likely to have had a previous cesarean section and the risk increased to 18 times for two or more prior cesareans. Even if one considers only cesarean delivery in the current gestation, the risk of hysterectomy is still seven times higher than after vaginal delivery.

Most peripartum hysterectomies are performed because of life-threatening hemorrhage. A smaller number are performed for concurrent gynecologic conditions such as leiomyomata or cervical dysplasia; these are classified as indicated nonemergency procedures. Relatively few are performed electively. In one series, hemorrhagic complications leading to cesarean hysterectomy included uterine atony 53%, abnormally adherent placenta 39%, uterine rupture 8%, and irreparable extension of the uterine incision 6%.[2] However, the majority of recent reports cite placenta accreta and its variants as the most frequent condition requiring hysterectomy.[4] If, as in our case, the indication is uterine atony, the initial management is aimed at preserving the uterus with medical measures, surgical measures, or both. In our case uterine artery ligation was the only surgical method attempted. Hypogastric artery ligation is not used often and is of uncertain value. Uterine suturing methods like the B-Lynch stitch may be useful in primiparous women or those of low parity, but choosing hysterectomy without such measures in a grand multipara is defensible. When placenta accreta is the indication, for example, in women with three or more prior cesareans and a placenta previa in the current gestation, proceeding with planned cesarean hysterectomy may be advisable and results in less blood loss.[5]

Peripartum hysterectomy is associated with considerable morbidity and mortality. Average blood loss in an emergency hysterectomy is 2500 +/-1300 mL. An adequately trained operator, experienced anesthesia personnel, and immediate availability of blood products are all essential to optimize outcomes. Technically, good exposure, extensive mobilization of the urinary bladder, careful attention to vascular pedicles, and constant traction on the uterus will minimize blood loss and avoid damage to adnexal structures and adjacent organs. If brisk bleeding is occurring then rapidly clamping and dividing the vessels supplying the uterus down to and including the uterine arteries has merit.[6] The surgeon can later return to suture ligate all the pedicles once the uterus has been devascularized.[6] Occasionally, the cervix is not safely approachable due to previous scarring and a supracervical hysterectomy may be chosen; significant blood loss may dictate this choice. Often, the cervix can be isolated and removed without adding substantially to the risk of the operation. Once the specimen has been removed, the instillation of sterile milk (infant formula is useful) into the maternal bladder through an indwelling Foley catheter may be advisable to confirm bladder integrity. Some surgeons would opt for cystoscopy to inspect the ureteral orifices and examine the bladder. Cesarean hysterectomy is almost always performed on relatively young women, so particular attention must be paid to preserving the ovaries.

Cesarean hysterectomy is a formidable surgical procedure, especially in the setting of massive hemorrhage. Some of the complications of cesarean hysterectomy and their approximate frequencies are presented in Table 6–1.[7] It is highly desirable for residency training programs to provide young physicians with the opportunity to participate in a few of these cases under controlled circumstances to avoid having them encounter their first emergency after training is completed. In those cases where hemorrhage is anticipated, calling in experienced assistance or transfer of the woman to a tertiary center are both prudent options.

Surgical Technique

The surgical technique for a hysterectomy performed after delivery (cesarean hysterectomy) is similar to that of an abdominal hysterectomy performed unrelated to recent delivery. One of the hardest components of performing a

Table 6–1 COMPLICATIONS OF CESAREAN HYSTERECTOMY

COMPLICATION	FREQUENCY (%)
RBC transfusion	84
Transfusion of other blood products	34
Admission to ICU	25-30
Postoperative fever	11
Unplanned removal of one ovary	5-15
Bladder injury	5-8
Subsequent laparotomy	4-8
Ureteral injury	3-7
Maternal death	2

hysterectomy after delivery is making the decision to perform the procedure if it was not planned previously. Delay in decision can lead to increased risk of additional hemorrhage and use of blood products in some cases.

As for all surgical procedures, exposure is crucial. The uterus should be elevated from the abdominal cavity to allow for exploration posteriorly, laterally, and caudally to review the anatomy and clear the gutters of blood and debris. Also, in keeping the uterus elevated on traction, this can decrease blood loss. If the placenta is still intact and there is suspicion of placenta accreta, one should evaluate the entire external uterine serosa to ensure that there is no evidence of percreta into surrounding organs, such as posteriorly to the bowel, caudally into the bladder, or laterally into the uterine vessels or otherwise. If so, additional consultation with a specialist in general surgery, urology, or vascular surgery, respectively may be beneficial. Some would advocate conservative surgery, leaving the placenta in place to avoid causing excessive bleeding from the placental site or myometrium if it is still in place at the time of investigation. The body of evidence that supports such an approach is limited.

If visualization of the ureters is difficult, then palpation is essential to ensure safety of placement of clamps to try to decrease the risk of ureteral injury. Due to the relatively young age of women undergoing hysterectomy after delivery, it is advisable to retain ovaries if possible.

The uterine incision can be quickly reapproximated. The round ligament is identified, doubly clamped, and ligated allowing for separation of the broad ligament in order to skeletonize the uterine arteries and their branches as quickly as possible. The ligation of the round ligament should be performed close to the uterus (Figure 6–1). The anterior leaf of the broad ligament should be extended to the vesicouterine serosa. The uterine arteries and associated veins can be tortuous and dilated at the time of a postpartum hysterectomy. One must ensure that the bladder has been dissected far enough away from the lower portion of the uterus to allow for the clamping, suturing, and ligation of the uterine artery. (Figures 6–2 and 6–3). Some advocate placing a clamp on the uterus itself to control back-bleeding.

Once hemostasis is obtained, attention can then be turned back to the utero-ovarian area (Figures 6–4 and 6–5).

The ovary needs to be elevated to allow for evaluation of the utero-ovarian area which often involves congested vessels during pregnancy. The posterior leaf of the broad ligament is perforated inferior to the fallopian tube, utero-ovarian ligaments, and their associated vessels which can be dilated significantly. Double clamping is advisable using first a free tie followed by suture ligation of the utero-ovarian pedicle. Attention can then be turned back to the area of the uterine cervix and bladder. In some cases it is safer and medically indicated to excise the uterus at the level of the internal cervical os; however, in other cases, a total abdominal hysterectomy is feasible. If a supracervical hysterectomy is performed, a series of interrupted figure-of-eight sutures on the cervical stump can decrease bleeding and help with healing. If the cervix is removed, then the cuff should be reapproximated to the

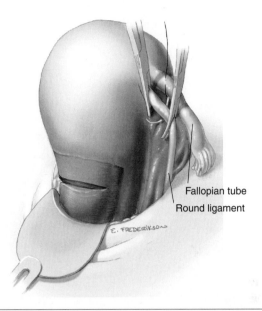

Fallopian tube

Round ligament

Figure 6–1. The round ligaments are clamped, ligated, and transected bilaterally. *(Reproduced, with permission, from Cunningham FG, Leveno KJ, Bloom SL, et al. Williams Obstetrics. 23rd ed. New York, NY: McGraw-Hill; 2010.)*

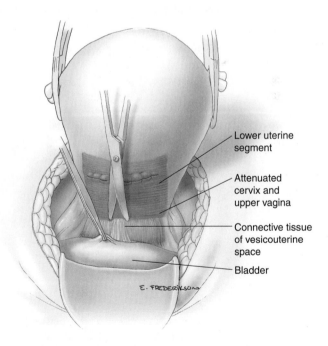

Lower uterine segment

Attenuated cervix and upper vagina

Connective tissue of vesicouterine space

Bladder

Figure 6–2. The bladder is dissected sharply from the lower uterine segment. *(Reproduced, with permission, from Cunningham FG, Leveno KJ, Bloom SL, et al. Williams Obstetrics. 23rd ed. New York, NY: McGraw-Hill; 2010.)*

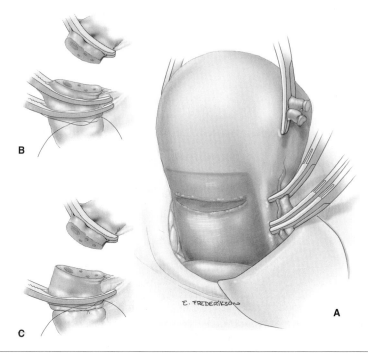

Figure 6–3. The uterine artery and veins on either side are doubly clamped immediately adjacent to the uterus and divided. *(Reproduced, with permission, from Cunningham FG, Leveno KJ, Bloom SL, et al. Williams Obstetrics. 23rd ed. New York, NY: McGraw-Hill; 2010.)*

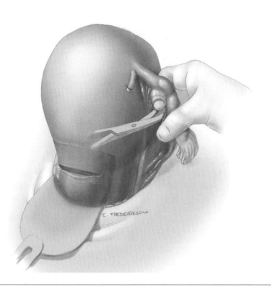

Figure 6–4. The posterior leaf of the broad ligament adjacent to the uterus is perforated just beneath the fallopian tube, utero-ovarian ligament, and ovarian vessels. *(Reproduced, with permission, from Cunningham FG, Leveno KJ, Bloom SL, et al. Williams Obstetrics. 23rd ed. New York, NY: McGraw-Hill; 2010.)*

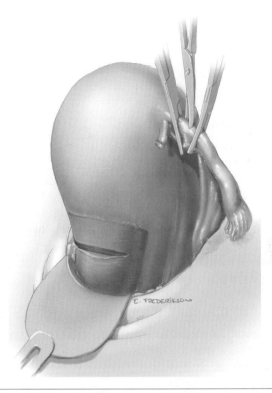

Figure 6–5. The utero-ovarian ligament and fallopian tube is clamped and cut bilaterally. (*Reproduced, with permission, from Cunningham FG, Leveno KJ, Bloom SL, et al. Williams Obstetrics. 23rd ed. New York, NY: McGraw-Hill; 2010.*)

uterosacral ligaments to reduce the risk of future vaginal vault prolapse. The uterosacral sutures should be held during continued progression of removal of the cervix so that the uterosacral ligaments can easily be identified at time of cuff closure. As in total abdominal hysterectomies unrelated to delivery, a curved clamp is placed across the lateral vaginal fornices immediately below the level of the cervix so that the tissue can be incised superiorly to the clamp to allow removal of the cervix and uterus. The angles of the lateral vagina are then reapproximated to the uterosacral ligaments that were previously held. The cuff is then closed in a series of interrupted figure-of-eight sutures or with a running-locked suture technique.

If there is any concern for bladder injury, the bladder can be filled with sterile milk (infant formula is suitable) via the Foley catheter. We recommend filling with at least 300 mL of fluid to ensure there is no leakage. If there is any question of ureteral injury, a small cystotomy can be performed in the dome of the bladder after IV infusion of indigo carmine to evaluate bilateral spill from both ureters or transurethral cystoscopy could be performed but would require some repositioning of the patient.

Irrigation of the abdominal cavity should be performed at the completion of the procedure prior to closure of the fascia and abdominal cavity.

Comprehension Questions

6.1 A 34-year-old woman at 35 weeks' gestation is being counseled about her condition and possible complications. Hemorrhage and the need for hysterectomy are explained. The patient asks what is the likelihood for hysterectomy. Which of the following causes of obstetrical hemorrhage is MOST likely to lead to cesarean hysterectomy?

    A. Placenta accreta
    B. Uterine atony
    C. Placental abruption
    D. Uterine rupture

6.2 A 32-year-old woman has just delivered vaginally, and profuse vaginal bleeding is encountered. The uterus is noted to be boggy. Which of the following is the best therapy for this patient?

    A. Intravenous misoprostol
    B. Bakri intrauterine balloon
    C. Oral ergot alkaloid
    D. Uterine curettage

6.3 Which of the following complications is most frequently encountered with a cesarean hysterectomy?

    A. Need for transfusion of blood products
    B. Urinary tract injury
    C. Endometritis
    D. Maternal death

ANSWERS

6.1   **A.** Placenta accreta complicates about 1 in 500 pregnancies and is increasing remarkably with the increase in cesarean delivery.

6.2   **B.** Uterine atony may be treated early on with uterine massage and pharmacological agents. Rectal or oral misoprostol can be used and intramuscular prostaglandin is an option. Oral ergot alkaloids are not absorbed quickly enough to be useful in the face of hemorrhage. An intrauterine balloon has been shown to be useful in postpartum hemorrhage due to uterine atony. When these conservative measures are not effective, then surgery is indicated.

6.3   **A.** Transfusion is the only logical choice and it is required in over 75% of emergency cases. Urinary tract injury occurs in up to 5% of cases. Death is uncommon and there is no endometrium remaining to get infected.

Clinical Pearls

See US Preventive Services Task Force Study Quality levels of evidence in Case 1

➤ Despite a careful examination of risk factors, a substantial number of women who undergo cesarean hysterectomy cannot be identified preoperatively (Level II).

➤ Women with a peripartum hysterectomy are 10 times more likely to have had one or more previous cesarean section (Level II).

➤ A diagnosis of hemorrhage is listed in the discharge of about 70% of peripartum hysterectomy patients (Level II).

➤ Cesarean hysterectomies are most often performed for uterine atony or abnormally adherent placenta. The latter is particularly concerning in light of the increasing cesarean delivery rate in contemporary obstetric practice (Level II).

➤ Hemorrhage, infections, and bladder injury are the most common complications of a peripartum hysterectomy. The integrity of the bladder should be evaluated, especially in patients with a previous cesarean section (Level II).

➤ After one previous cesarean section the risk of serious complications such as placenta previa, placenta accreta, uterine rupture increases in a subsequent pregnancy. Thus, every effort must be made to limit primary cesarean deliveries to those with a valid clinical indication (Level III).

REFERENCES

1. Sachs BP, Kobelin C, Castro MA, Frigoletto F. The risks of lowering the cesarean-delivery rate. *N Engl J Med.* 1999;340:54-57.
2. Knight M, Kurinczuk JJ, Spark P, Brocklehurst P. Cesarean delivery and peripartum hysterectomy. *Obstet Gynecol.* 2008;111:97-105.
3. Whiteman MK, Kuklina E, Hillis SD, et al. Incidence and determinants of peripartum hysterectomy. *Obstet Gynecol.* 2006;108:1486-1492.
4. Flood, KM, Said S, Geary M, et al. Changing trends in peripartum hysterectomy over the last 4 decades. *Am J Obstet Gynecol.* 2009;200:632.e1-632.e6.
5. Eller AG, Porter TF, Soisson P, Silver RM. Optimal management strategies for placenta accreta. *BJOG.* 2009;116:648-654.
6. Plauche WC. Cesarean Hysterectomy: Indications, technique, and complications. *Clin Obstet Gynecol.* 1986;29:318-328.
7. Shellhaas CS, Gilbert S, Landon MB, et al. The frequency and complication rates of hysterectomy accompanying cesarean delivery. *Obstet Gynecol.* 2009;114:224-229.

Case 7

A 26-year-old G1P0 at 34 $^3/_7$ weeks by last menstrual period (LMP) consistent with a first-trimester ultrasound (US) with singleton gestation presents to L&D because of mild contractions for the last 2 hours that are increasing in frequency and intensity. She also endorses decreased fetal movement since the onset of these contractions and had an episode of vaginal bleeding on arrival. She denies leakage of fluid or abdominal trauma. She has received scant prenatal care. She is Rh negative but has not received Rh immune globulin this pregnancy. She denies medical problems or surgeries.

Initial vital signs: T = 97.9°F, BP = 110/69 mm Hg, Pulse = 90 bpm, respiratory rate (RR) = 18 breaths/min. She appears uncomfortable due to contractions, lungs are clear, chest has regular rate and rhythm with grade 3/4 systolic ejection murmur, abdomen is tender in all quadrants and uterus feels hypertonic, extremities with 2+ edema bilaterally but without tenderness. The nurse is unable to detect fetal heart rate by external Doptones but contractions are detected by tocodynamometer every 2 to 3 minutes. A bedside US is performed and no fetal cardiac activity is detected. The placenta appears fundal and there is no evidence of retroplacental clot. Amniotic fluid is normal and fetal biometry is consistent with stated gestational age. On speculum examination, there is a golf-size clot in the vault and active bleeding noted. Her cervix is dilated to 2 cm, cervical length is 1 cm, and station is −2 on digital examination.

➤ What is the differential diagnosis?

➤ What is the most likely diagnosis?

➤ What should be involved in the management of this patient?

ANSWERS TO CASE 7:
Abruption/Dead Fetus

Summary: This is a primigravida at term with vaginal bleeding, fetal demise, preterm contractions, and hypertonic uterus.

➤ **Differential diagnosis of the patient's pain:** Placental abruption, placenta previa, and vasa previa are important consideration in any patient that presents with bleeding during pregnancy. Other conditions that should be considered but are less likely based on the clinical presentation are appendicitis, urinary tract infections, labor, fibroid degeneration, and ovarian pathology.

➤ **Most likely diagnosis:** The most likely diagnosis in this case is placental abruption severe enough to kill the fetus.

➤ **Next step in the management of this patient:** Maternal stabilization is the priority in this case involving fetal demise. Close monitoring of hemorrhage, vital signs, urine output, and laboratory results for assessment of anemia and coagulopathy will help to determine hemodynamic status.

ANALYSIS

Objectives

1. Describe the clinical presentation of placental abruption.
2. List the risk factors of placental abruption.
3. Describe the diagnostic strategy and therapy for abruption.
4. List the complications of placental abruption.

Considerations

This 26-year-old woman is noted to have significant vaginal bleeding and a dead fetus. The most likely diagnosis is placental abruption. The diagnosis is a clinical one, and also to rule out other causes of vaginal bleeding, such as an ultrasound to assess placental location. Meanwhile, the patient should have two large-bore IVs placed and receive fluid resuscitation. This individual very well could have a coagulopathy, and should have a clinical assessment for overt coagulopathy, as well as a red top for clot retraction testing. Delivery is important, and a vaginal delivery should be the plan.

   The diagnosis of placental abruption is a clinical one, however, presentation may vary. Most cases present with **vaginal bleeding (66%)** or **abdominal pain/back pain (78%)**. Other signs/symptoms include fetal heart rate abnormalities (60%), preterm labor (22%), high-frequency contractions (17%), uterine hypertonus (17%), and dead fetus (15%)[1] (Level II-2). The sensitivity of ultrasound in detecting placental abruption is poor (approximately 25%). As illustrated in this case, **the absence of a retroplacental clot should not exclude this diagnosis when it is clinically suspected**[2] (Level II-2). On the other hand, when a retroplacental clot is visualized by ultrasound the positive predictive value for an abruption at delivery is high.

Once the diagnosis is made, maternal resuscitation takes precedence in this patient of severe abruption with fetal demise. Regardless of gestational age, a vaginal delivery is recommended as long as the maternal hemodynamic status is stable. **When the abruption is severe enough to kill the fetus, maternal blood loss can be estimated as approximately 50% of her blood volume**[3] **(Level II-2).** Therefore, it is important to have blood crossed for at least 4 units of packed red blood cells (PRBCs) when considering this principle; however, each case should be individualized based on the severity of abruption. Abruption involving a dead fetus also has a high risk of causing disseminated intravascular coagulopathy (DIC). Critical laboratory tests that should be drawn at regular intervals are as follows: CBC with platelets, coagulations studies (PT/INR/aPTT, fibrinogen, fibrin degradation products), and a comprehensive metabolic panel. Correction of anemia and/or DIC should be undertaken according to the patient's hemodynamic status and/or laboratory results (see Table 7–1). Urine output should be closely monitored to ensure a minimum of 30 cc/h. Volume replacement with crystalloid or colloid applying the "3:1 rule" (3 mL of fluids for every 1 mL of blood loss) should be undertaken. Visual estimation of blood loss during an emergency is appropriate, however, weighing pads and chucks is a more accurate approach to the estimation of blood loss. This is done by subtracting the dry weight of disposable items (ie, pads) from the soiled material remembering that 1 g = 1 mL. If there is ongoing bleeding, a **multidisciplinary team approach** should be undertaken involving nursing staff, obstetricians, anesthesiologists, neonatologists (with viable fetus), specialists in gynecologic oncology, interventional radiologist, critical care as well as the laboratory, blood bank, and pharmacy personnel.

Preeclampsia labs should be drawn as well even in the absence of hypertension as elevated blood pressures may become apparent only after the maternal intravascular compartment has been refilled. Evaluation for fetal-maternal hemorrhage is important in this nonsensitized Rh-negative patient in order to determine the dose of Rh immune globulin to be administered. Toxicology screen should be considered if drug use such as cocaine is suspected. The placenta should be sent for pathologic examination.

Once maternal stabilization has been accomplished, induction or augmentation of labor should be initiated. The use of oxytocin, prostaglandins (E1 or E2), or mechanical dilators should be individualized. It is important to keep in mind that it is *not the interval of time to delivery* but rather maternal resuscitation

Table 7–1 BLOOD COMPONENT THERAPY

THERAPY	INDICATION	VOLUME PER UNIT	DOSE	RESULT
Packed red blood cells	Anemia; ↑O$_2$ carrying capacity	250 mL		↑Hgb 1 g/dL ↑Hct 3% per unit
Platelets	Bleeding/DIC or surgery with platelets < 50,000/mm³	50-75 mL	6 units (1 unit per 10 kg weight)	↑Platelets by 5,000/mm³ per unit
Fresh frozen plasma	Clotting factor deficiency[a]	200-250 mL	4-6 units (10-20 mL/kg)	↑Fibrinogen 10 mg/dL per unit
Cryoprecipitate	Fibrinogen < 100 mg/dL, concern for volume overload	~15 mL	1 unit per 10 kg weight	↑Fibrinogen 5-15 mg/dL per unit

[a]Prolonged PT/aPTT/INR, fibrinogen < 100 mg/dL.

with fluid and blood that predicts maternal outcome. Therefore, cesarean delivery should be considered only with special circumstances involving maternal hemodynamic instability or contraindications to vaginal delivery.

APPROACH TO
Abruption/Dead Fetus

Placental abruption is by definition premature separation of a normally implanted placenta. The frequency in which it occurs has been reported to be 1 in 200 deliveries. The incidence of placental abruption severe enough to kill a fetus has been reported as 1 in 1600 deliveries in recent years.[4]

Over half of all pregnancies complicated by placental abruption deliver preterm. Abruption is more common between 24 and 27 weeks gestational age[5] (level III). The perinatal mortality rate for placental abruption is *119 per 1000 births* compared with 8.2 per 1000 for all others. Although this high rate can be strongly associated with preterm delivery, the perinatal mortality was 25-fold higher with placental abruption at term.[6] The risk of neurologic injury depends on gestational age and severity of abruption.

Risk Factors

There are many known risk factors for placental abruption. The most significant risk factor is *hypertension* including preeclampsia, gestational or chronic. The risk of abruption with early onset severe preeclampsia is in the order of 4% to 30%. It is also important to note that approximately **50% of abruption cases severe enough to kill a fetus involve a hypertensive disorder that may not become apparent until the intravascular compartment has been adequately refilled**[7] (Level II-3).

The risk of abruption with *premature rupture of membranes* is 4% to 12%. *Abdominal trauma* also increases the risk of placental abruption as well as fetal hemorrhage. Clinically evident abruption occurs in up to 40% of severe abdominal trauma and in only 3% of minor direct abdominal trauma. *Uterine leiomyomas* may also be a risk factor for abruption especially when they are large and retroplacental in location. Other risk factors include increased parity, maternal age, multiple gestation, polyhydramnios, chorioamnionitis, thrombophilias, smoking, and cocaine use.

The recurrence rate of severe placental abruption is approximately 12%[8] (Level II-2) although up to 35% has been reported[9] (Level II-2). Recurrence has also been reported to occur 1 to 3 weeks prior to the gestational age of the previous abruption.

Pathophysiology

The precise pathophysiology that leads to abruption is unknown in many instances. Most would agree that the most important factor is hemorrhage at the decidual-placental interface. Acute vasospasm of small vessels may precede hemorrhage and placental separation. Progressive hemorrhage causes compression of the overlying intervillous space with subsequent destruction of placental tissue. Gross examination of the placenta often reveals an organized clot on a depressed area of maternal surface. The "age" of the clot is often difficult to determine. The placenta may also appear completely unremarkable if abruption occurs just before delivery not allowing enough time for clot formation. Data from the New Jersey–Placental Abruption Study showed that concordance between clinical and histologic criteria is poor. Of the clinically diagnosed cases of abruption, the sensitivity and specificity for a histologic confirmation of abruption were 30% and 100%, respectively. Retroplacental clots were the most common (77%) findings in clinically apparent cases. Acute lesions associated with abruption included chorioamnionitis and funisitis while placental infarction was the only chronic histologic lesion associated with abruption[10] (Level II-2).

A chronic placental disorder may be the underlying etiology of a placental abruption. Abnormal trophoblast invasion may lead to rupture of spiral arteries and premature separation of the placenta. There is also evidence suggesting that inflammatory cells which secrete cytokines and tumor necrosis factors (TNF) can lead to trophoblasts production of matrix metalloproteinase leading to premature placental detachment[11] (Level II-2). Intrauterine growth restriction, preeclampsia, and oligohydramnios are associated with placental abruption providing further evidence of placental insufficiency as a causative factor.

Clinical Presentation

In addition to the previously mentioned signs and symptoms of abruption (see case discussion) there are other important clinical consequences. *Abruption is the most common etiology in obstetrics of DIC.* **Consumptive coagulopathy is seen in approximately 30% of abruption cases severe enough to kill the fetus (fibrinogen <150 mg/dL in 38% and <100 mg/dL in 28%)[3] (Level II-2)**. Thromboplastin release from placental separation activates the *extrinsic* pathway of the coagulation cascade. This event, in combination with retroplacental fibrin deposition (although to a lesser extent), contributes to depletion of clotting factors. Fibrin degradation productions are elevated in 85% to 100% of patients with DIC and are formed from the degradation of fibrinogen and fibrin by plasmin. Placental separation associated with abruption contributes to an increase in higher than normal FDP levels after delivery. Data supports a **direct pathophysiologic relationship between high FDP (fibrin degradation products) levels (>300 mg/dL) and postpartum hemorrhage associated with abruption**. Elevated FDP levels interfere with myometrial contractility[12] (Level II-2). **Couvelaire uterus** is caused by extravasation of blood into the uterine musculature and serosa. This rarely interferes with myometrial contractility and is an unlikely reason for postpartum hemorrhage.

Acute renal failure secondary to under perfusion is common in untreated hemorrhage. Most cases are due to reversible acute tubular necrosis and less often due to irreversible cortical necrosis.

Concealed hemorrhage occurs when the placenta separates to some degree and the collection of blood behind the placenta is retained by the margins of the placenta or membranes that remain attached to the uterine wall or by the fetal head applied to the cervix. Concealed abruption is by far less common than external hemorrhage but just as clinically significant (Figure 7–1).

Management

The management of placental abruption depends on the presentation, gestational age, and the degree of maternal and fetal compromise.

A delay in recognizing hypovolemia due to hemorrhage can occur as a result of some of the normal physiologic changes that occur during pregnancy.

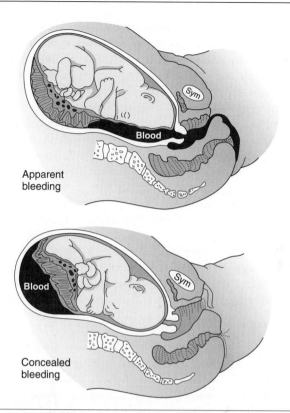

Apparent
bleeding

Concealed
bleeding

Figure 7–1.   Abruption/Dead fetus *(Reproduced, with permission, from DeCherney AH, Nathan L, Goodwin TM, et al.* Current Diagnosis & Treatment: Obstetrics & Gynecology, *10th ed. New York: McGraw-Hill 2007:332.)*

Pregnancy is normally a state of *hypervolemia* due to an approximate 50% increase in blood volume. With blood loss, vasoconstriction of vessels occurs to maintain perfusion of vital organs. This results in compensatory tachycardia and an increase in systemic vascular resistance. Blood pressures usually remain stable (normal to high) until blood loss exceeds 30% of the pregnancy blood volume. **It is therefore important to remember that the first vital sign to change is heart rate (tachycardia) and the last to change is blood pressure (hypotension).** Interventions to replace fluid and blood should not be delayed until hypotension develops. Preeclamptics are less tolerant of blood loss due to a constricted intravascular compartment. Normal blood pressures in a previously hypertensive patient should always be concerning for hemorrhage. Similarly, a normal hematocrit should *not* be considered reassuring in preeclamptics. Hemoconcentration is expected due to an underfilled intravascular compartment. It is therefore important to replace volume in these women in the early phase as they are more susceptible to renal failure compared to non-preeclamptics.

Although it is important to individualize each case according to severity of complications, the basic principles of resuscitation apply in all cases. Two large-bore infusion lines and Foley catheter should be inserted immediately. Type and cross, complete blood count, comprehensive metabolic panel, and coagulation studies should be sent stat. The decision on how much blood to cross should be individualized based on the severity of abruption. The **clot assay** is a useful and inexpensive bedside test for hypofibrinogenemia if laboratory results are not available within a reasonable time. A sample of blood is collected in a red-topped tube. If a clot does not form in 6 minutes or forms and lyses in 30 minutes, then the fibrinogen level is most likely less than 150 mg/dL.[13] Correction of anemia and/or coagulopathy should be undertaken. Vaginal delivery is preferable and usually proceeds quickly in the setting of abruption. This is because many patients are already experiencing signs of labor at presentation. Patients with any degree of placental abruption are at risk of postpartum hemorrhage and preparation in case of atony is critical. Uterotonic agents should be readily available. It is also important to be familiar with hospital resources in case there is a need for uterine artery embolization or peripartum hysterectomy.

Severe Abruption with Stillbirth   See Case Discussion.

Fetus is alive at or near term   When the fetus is alive at or near term, delivery should be expedited. If spontaneous labor is absent, induction or augmentation of labor may be necessary if the fetus is vertex and there is no contraindication for vaginal delivery. If delivery does not occur within a reasonable time and the patient has ongoing hemorrhage and is difficult to stabilize, then cesarean delivery is recommended. Cesarean delivery should also be performed at any time when the fetal heart rate tracing is concerning or for any contraindications to vaginal route of delivery. Surgery in a patient with DIC is life-threatening and must be corrected prior to surgery.

Fetus is alive at 24 to 34 weeks' gestation   If the maternal and fetal status is reassuring, conservative management is reasonable with close monitoring. Antenatal steroids can be administered during this period of observation given the high risk of preterm birth. Consultation with maternal-fetal medicine and neonatology specialists is important for counseling regarding maternal and neonatal outcomes. The patient needs to be counseled that abruption is unpredictable, that fetal death can occur at any time, and that normal fetal testing can occur before a catastrophic event. The risks to both mother and fetus associated with conservative management need to be balanced against the neonatal risks associated with preterm birth. Coexisting conditions such as preterm premature rupture of membranes (PPROM), preeclampsia, or intrauterine growth restriction should be factored into the decision on whether to recommend expectant management versus delivery. The use of tocolytics in the setting of abruption and contractions is controversial and not enough evidence exists to support or refute routine practice. Continued hospitalization until bleeding subsides is reasonable and outpatient management can be considered in well-selected cases, depending on the clinical circumstances.

Fetus is alive less than 24 weeks Antepartum bleeding in the second trimester is usually attributed to some degree of placental abruption. Exclusion of other causes such as previa, rupture of membranes or cervical causes should be undertaken before attributing bleeding to abruption. There is limited data to guide management of abruption prior to viability. Expectant management is reasonable as long as maternal hemodynamic status is stable. Intrauterine growth restriction, oligohydramnios, recurrent bleeding, previable and/or preterm birth, and cesarean delivery are potential risks of pregnancies complicated by early abruption. The goal of conservative management is to prolong the pregnancy in order to improve fetal/neonatal outcome. This must be balanced against the risks to the mother such as hemorrhage, anemia requiring blood transfusion or lifesaving procedure such as hysterectomy, and rarely maternal death. Consultation with maternal-fetal medicine specialists is recommended given that there are several factors to consider when determining the most reasonable management plan. One factor to consider is gestational age since counseling regarding prognosis may differ when the gestational age is 16 weeks versus 23 weeks, for example. The severity of abruption and coexisting maternal conditions (hypertension, cardiac disease, renal disease) are also important considerations as they affect pregnancy outcome. Most importantly, the patient's own wishes should be considered and the risks/benefits of both options, expectant management and termination of pregnancy, should be explained.

Abdominal Trauma If direct abdominal trauma has occurred and there is no evidence of maternal or fetal compromise, a period of observation to monitor for placental abruption is warranted. Delayed abruption is unlikely in the absence of frequent contractions (< 6 contractions per hour) with normal fetal heart rate tracing over a 4 to 6 hour period. The recommended monitoring period is a minimum of 4 hours from the trauma event. Further monitoring is also reasonable with other concerning signs or symptoms such as uterine tenderness, abdominal ecchymoses, vaginal bleeding, or frequent contractions[14] (Level III).

Hemorrhage from most cases of abruption is maternal in origin. **With blunt traumatic abruption, fetal bleeding is more common as a result of a tear or fracture in the placenta.** An evaluation of fetal-maternal hemorrhage with flow cytometry or Kleihauer-Betke test is useful in nonsensitized Rh-negative women with abruption, (traumatic or nontraumatic) as the information obtained guides in administering the appropriate dose of Rh immune globulin necessary to prevent alloimmunization. There is little evidence that tests of fetal-maternal hemorrhage (flow cytometry or Kleihauer-Betke test) in Rh-positive women predict adverse fetal or neonatal outcome due to fetal hemorrhage[15] (Level II-2). Significant fetal hemorrhage from abruption that would impact neonatal outcome usually results in fetal heart rate tracing abnormalities such as tachycardia, loss of variability, late decelerations, or sinusoidal pattern[14] (Level III). It is important to keep in mind that a negative test does not exclude the diagnosis of abruption and similarly a positive test does not confirm the diagnosis. A positive test for fetal-maternal hemorrhage simply guides the management of Rh-immune-globulin dose that needs to be administered in nonsensitized women.

Comprehension Questions

7.1   A 21-year-old G1P0 at 32 weeks' gestation presents to L&D after a fall involving direct abdominal trauma. She denies leakage of fluid, vaginal bleeding, contractions, or abdominal pain. On examination her vitals are normal and stable and her abdominal examination is nontender without evidence of trauma. Her cervix is closed and 2 cm in length. The fetal heart rate tracing is reassuring but irregular, infrequent contractions (every 25 min) are noted on external monitoring. She is Rh positive and has no medical problems. If her cervix is unchanged in 2 hours, how long will you observe her from the time of the traumatic event?

   A. 1 hour
   B. 2 hours
   C. 4 to 6 hours
   D. Until her contractions resolve

7.2   A 40-year-old woman G3P1010 at 39 weeks' gestation is being induced for preeclampsia. She has been on intravenous oxytocin, and is now at 5 cm dilation. Amniotomy is performed and bright red blood mixed with fluid is seen. Her BP is 143/89 mm Hg, pulse is 98, urine output is 55 cc/h, and abdomen is nontender although she has an epidural. The fetal heart rate tracing is reassuring with a baseline of 140, moderate variability, and no decelerations. Contractions are occurring every 2-4 minutes. Her obstetrical history is significant for one-term uncomplicated vaginal delivery. What is your next step in management?

   A. Place two large-bore IVs, repeat preeclampsia labs and coagulation studies.
   B. Recommend cesarean delivery at this time.
   C. Recommend amnioinfusion.
   D. Prepare for transfusion.

ANSWERS

7.1   **C.** The recommended time to observe a patient for abruption after direct abdominal trauma is 4 to 6 hours, however, reasonable judgment should be exercised. If this patient's contractions increase in frequency or if other worrisome signs/symptoms develop then she should be observed longer to evaluate for preterm labor and abruption.

7.2   **A.** This patient may continue to labor as long as the fetal heart rate tracing remains reassuring and she is progressing well in labor. At this time there is no need to prepare for transfusion given that her vitals signs are appropriate, however, close monitoring of vitals, urine output, and estimated blood loss is necessary. Preeclampsia labs should be repeated and coagulation studies should be ordered for suspected abruption.

Clinical Pearls

See US Preventive Services Task Force Study Quality levels of evidence in Case 1

➤ Over half of all pregnancies complicated by placental abruption deliver preterm.

➤ The sensitivity of ultrasound in detecting placental abruption is poor and therefore the absence of a retroplacental clot should not exclude this diagnosis when it is clinically suspected (Level II-2).

➤ When the abruption is severe enough to kill the fetus, maternal blood loss can be estimated as approximately 50% of her blood volume (Level II-2).

➤ Half of all cases of abruption cases severe enough to kill a fetus involve a hypertensive disorder that may only become apparent after the intravascular compartment has been adequately refilled (Level II-3).

➤ Consumptive coagulopathy is seen in approximately 30% of abruption cases severe enough to kill the fetus (Level II-2).

➤ Elevated FDP levels interfere with myometrial contractility and this increases the risk for postpartum hemorrhage (Level II-2).

➤ The first vital sign to change during hemorrhage is heart rate (tachycardia) and the last to change is blood pressure (hypotension). Volume replacement should not be delayed until there is hypotension since 30% of blood volume has been lost by this point.

➤ It is *not the interval of time to delivery* but rather maternal resuscitation with fluid and blood replacement that predicts maternal outcome in an abruption.

➤ In any case of antepartum or postpartum hemorrhage, a **multidisciplinary team approach** ensures both maternal and fetal/neonatal safety.

CONTROVERSIES

- Routine assessment of fetal-maternal hemorrhage in all cases of abruption involving Rh-positive women as there is little evidence that testing predicts fetal or neonatal outcome.

REFERENCES

1. Hurd WW, Miodovnik M, Hertzberg V, et al. Selective management of abruption placentae: a prospective study. *Obstet Gynecol.* 1993;61:467.
   A prospective study of 50 cases of placental abruption between 20 and 34 weeks' gestation. There was a significant increase in respiratory distress and low Apgar scores in study infants compared to controls but without a correlation with regard to mode of delivery or diagnosis to delivery interval (Level II-2).
2. Glantz C, Purnell L. Clinical utility of sonography in the diagnosis and treatment of placental abruption. *J Ultrasouund Med.* 2002;21:837. (Level II-2)
3. Pritchard JA, Brekken AL. Clinical and laboratory studies on severe abruptio placentae. *Am J Obstet Gynecol.* 1967;97:681. (Level II-2)
4. Cunningham FG, Leveno KJ, Bloom SL, et al. *Williams Obstetrics.* 23rd ed. New York, NY: McGraw-Hill; 2010.
5. Oyelese Y, Ananth CV. Placental Abruption. *Obstet Gynecol.* 2006;108:1005-1016. (Level III)
6. Ananth CV, Wilcox AJ. Placental abruption and perinatal mortality in the United States. *Am J Epidemiol.* 2001;153:332.
7. Pritchard JA, Cunningham FG, Pritchard SA, et al. On reducing the frequency severe abruption placentae. *Am J Obstet Gynecol.* 1991;165:345. (Level II-3)
8. Pritchard JA, Mason R, Corely M, et al. Genesis of severe placental abruption. *Am J Obstet Gynecol.* 1970;108:22. (Level II-2)
9. Matsaseng T, Bagratee JS, Moodley J. Pregnancy outcomes in patients with previous history of abruptio placentae. *Int J Gynecol Obstet.* 2006;92:253-254. (Level II-2)
10. Elsasser DA, Ananth CV, Prasad V, Vintzileos AM. Diagnosis of placental abruption: relationship between clinical and histopathological findings. *Eur J Obstet Gynecol Reprod Biology.* 2009;6762.
    A multicenter case-control study (New Jersey–Placental Abruption Study) which showed that the concordance between clinical and pathologic criteria for abruption is poor (Level II-2).
11. Ananth CV, Getahun D, Peltier MR, et al. Placental abruption in term and preterm gestations. Evidence for heterogeneity in clinical pathways. *Obstet Gynecol.* 2006;107:785-792. (Level II-2)
12. Basu HK. Fibrinolysis and abruption placenta. *J Obstet Gynaecol Br Commonw.* 1969; 76:481-496. (Level II-2)
13. Gabbe SG, Niebyl JR, Simpson JL. *Normal and Abnormal Pregnancy.* 4th ed. Philedelphia, PA: Churchill Livingstone; 2001.
14. Brown HL. Trauma in pregnancy. *Obstet Gynecol.* 2009;114:147-160. (Level III)
15. Boyle J, Kim J, Walerius H, Samuel P. The clinical use of the Kleihauer-Betke test in Rh positive patient. *Am J Obstet Gynecol.* 1996;174:343. (Level II-2)

Case 8

A 25-year-old G4P3003 at 19 weeks' gestation by LMP presents for ultra-sound appointment. The fetal anatomic survey is within normal limits but a complete anterior placenta previa is noted. In addition, there is a concern regarding thinning of the myometrium of the lower uterine seg-ment. Color Doppler shows a distance of approximately 1 mm between retroplacental vessels and the uterine serosa-bladder interface. In addi-tion, extensive intraplacental lakes are noted (see Figure 8–1). Given the concern for a placenta accreta, you are contacted by the sonologist performing the ultrasound. You review the patient's obstetrical and sur-gical history. Of note, the patient has a history of three prior lower trans-verse cesarean deliveries. The first one was performed for arrest of active phase after an elective induction of labor at 39 weeks and the next two were performed for a history of cesarean delivery. You have previously discussed with the patient contraception options and the patient has told you that she may want another child but is undecided. You call the patient to discuss the results of her ultrasound.

➤ What is your next step in evaluating the patient?

➤ What are the potential maternal/fetal complications associated with placenta previa/accreta?

ANSWERS TO CASE 8:
Placenta Accreta

Summary: A multipara with multiple prior cesarean deliveries now with ultra-sound confirming previa and findings suspicious for placenta accreta.

➤ **Next step in evaluating the patient:** After confirming the sonographic find-ings initially found by the sonologist, the next step would be to counsel the patient about placenta accreta and the increased morbidity and mortality it entails. The patient should be assessed for any treatable forms of anemia and also counseled on the possibility of blood transfusion with delivery. Furthermore, preparations should be made to have a planned cesarean delivery if the previa persists with the possibility of a hysterectomy.

➤ **Potential maternal/fetal complications associated with placenta previa/acc-reta:** Maternal complications include hemorrhage, infection, risks associated with blood transfusion, increased risk for injury to the bowel, ureters, blad-der; hysterectomy/sterilization, intensive care admission, and death. Fetal complications include malpresentation, intrauterine growth restriction (IUGR), and preterm birth.

ANALYSIS

Objectives

1. Describe the risk factors for placenta previa and accreta.
2. Describe the clinical presentation of these conditions.
3. Describe the diagnostic strategy and management of placenta previa and placenta accreta.

Considerations

Classically, **placenta previa** occurs when placental tissue overlies the internal cervical os; however, it can also occur when placental tissue is located next to or near the internal cervical os. The incidence of placenta previa is gesta-tional age-dependent. It is a common finding before 20 weeks' gestation, occurring in 1% to 6% of pregnant women during that time period. That said, nearly 90% of these cases demonstrate resolution of the placenta previa by the third trimester. The incidence of placenta previa after the second trimester is approximately 4 per 1000 pregnancies (0.4%). The recurrence rate of pla-centa previa is 4% to 8%[1] (Level III).

Risk factors for placenta previa include prior cesarean delivery, multiparity, advanced maternal age, prior uterine surgery, smoking, and multiple gestations.

This patient has two identifiable risk factors for placenta previa: multiparity and three prior cesarean deliveries. Multiple cesarean deliveries and ultrasound findings of complete previa also increase the risk for **placenta accreta**, or abnormal invasion of the placenta into the myometrium.

The diagnosis of placenta previa is made using ultrasound, either transvaginal or transabdominal. Transvaginal ultrasound has been shown to be superior to the transabdominal approach in detecting placenta previa. The advantage is that there are fewer false-positive diagnoses while being a safe approach in experienced hands. As with most cases, this patient was diagnosed with a placenta previa on routine ultrasound in the second trimester. In addition, ultrasound findings were suspicious for accreta. Although placenta accreta may not be definitely diagnosed by ultrasound imaging, the sensitivity and specificity of ultrasound is approximately 80% and 95%, respectively.

Management of a patient with a placenta previa and suspected accreta depends on whether or not the patient has active bleeding. This patient was diagnosed at her routine anatomy ultrasound and is without complaints of vaginal bleeding. Serial sonograms are recommended to assess placental location. This patient with a complete previa should be cautioned to seek emergency care if there is any vaginal bleeding. Although there are no data to support the efficacy of avoiding intercourse and excessive activity, it is reasonable to discuss with the patient that these should be avoided. Bedrest at home is not recommended as there is no evidence to support it is of any benefit.

Furthermore, if vaginal bleeding develops, the patient should ideally inform caregivers that she was diagnosed with a placenta previa and possible accreta so that the unbeknownst provider can avoid performing a digital cervical examination. This patient should also be evaluated for anemia periodically during pregnancy so that iron supplementation can be administered in preparation for delivery. The patient should also be counseled regarding the increased risk of antepartum and postpartum hemorrhage, possible blood transfusion, and risk of hysterectomy as a lifesaving procedure. It is important to discuss the patient's desire for future fertility in advance. She should be counseled that a reasonable effort will be made to preserve her fertility if she desires, as long as it does not comprise her health.

APPROACH TO
Placenta Previa/Accreta

There are four types of placenta previa. First, a **complete placenta previa** occurs when the placenta completely covers the internal os. Second, a **partial placenta previa** occurs when the placenta partially covers the internal os. Third, a **marginal placenta previa** happens when the placenta is located next to internal os. Finally, a **low-lying placenta** occurs when the placental margin is within 2 cm of the internal os but not next to the internal os.

Although the classic clinical presentation for placenta previa is painless vaginal bleeding, it is important to note that patients with placenta previa may also have painful bleeding due to marginal separation of the abnormally implanted placenta or secondary to contractions. Bleeding from a placenta previa can occur anytime throughout pregnancy; however, it usually does not occur until the late second trimester or beyond. During this time in pregnancy, bleeding may occur due to the formation of the lower uterine segment and dilation of the internal os resulting in tearing of the placental attachments. Moreover, muscle fibers comprising the lower uterine segment may be unable to constrict the bleeding vessels thus further intensifying vaginal bleeding.

Once the diagnosis of placenta previa has been made and in the absence of labor or vaginal bleeding, management would include repeat ultrasound at 32 to 34 weeks for placenta location. With advancing gestational age, the lower segment stretches allowing the placenta to localize away from the internal os. This "migration" occurs most often when the placenta does not completely cover the internal os. Persistence to term can be predicted based on the relationship between the placenta and the internal os in the second trimester. The majority of cases where the tip of the placenta does not touch or cover the internal os resolve[2] (Level II).

On the other hand, if there is active vaginal bleeding from a placenta previa, the patient should be stabilized, the fetus monitored, and both should be closely observed to assess for any signs of maternal and/or fetal compromise. Antenatal corticosteroids should be administered if vaginal bleeding occurs between 24 and 34 weeks. Two large-bore intravenous cannulas should be placed and blood should be sent for a blood count and type and screen (or cross) depending on the degree of bleeding. It is important to verify that the blood bank can provide 4 to 6 units of packed red blood cells and coagulation factors if necessary. Rh immunoglobulin should be administered to those who are Rh negative. Assessment for fetal-maternal hemorrhage with either Kleihauer-Betke test or flow cytometry should also be performed to determine if additional Rh immunoglobulin is necessary in these women. The use of tocolytics is controversial. The rationale for their use in those with bleeding and contractions is based on the logic that contractions may cause bleeding which in turn can lead to more contractions and bleeding. The benefit of tocolytic therapy has been demonstrated in two studies where prolongation of pregnancy and higher birth weights were noted; however, the data is limited and the results from these small studies should therefore be interpreted with caution[3,4] (Level II). Delivery may be necessary if there is a continued hemorrhage and/or nonreassuring fetal heart rate tracing at any gestational age. A lower threshold for delivery should also be considered for continued bleeding near term. Neonatology consultation to discuss the risks of prematurity is also of benefit to the patient and her family.

If bleeding has stopped and both fetal and maternal status is stable, the patient should be observed for any further bleeding. The decision to observe the patient as an inpatient or as an outpatient is dependent on the initial quantity of bleeding and the risk of recurrent bleeding. Outpatient management depends on the ability of the patient to return to the hospital in a timely fashion if bleeding recurs, her ability to rest at home and understand the risk of outpatient management, and the ability to call or come to the hospital if she has another bleeding episode. The only randomized trial of inpatient versus outpatient management of 53 women showed no significant difference in maternal or fetal outcomes[5] (Level II).

If the placenta previa persists into the third trimester, consideration should be given to timing of delivery. It is preferable to perform a cesarean delivery under controlled conditions rather than in an emergency. As gestational age increases, the risk of bleeding also increases. Testing fetal lung maturity via amniocentesis at 36 to 37 weeks' gestation is reasonable, although this approach is based primarily on expert opinion. The route of delivery for placenta previa is abdominal. This also includes low lying placentas that are within 2 cm of the internal os. Ideally the uterine incision should be made away from the placenta in order to avoid incising or lacerating fetal-placental vessels; however, even with knowledge of the placental location before delivery this cannot always be avoided. If such is the case, the fetus should be delivered as quickly as possible.

Placenta accreta occurs when there is an abnormally firm attachment of placental villi to the uterine wall with the absence of the normal intervening deciduous basalis and **Nitabuch layer**. There are three variants of this condition. In the most common form, accreta, the placenta is attached directly to the myometrium. When the placenta extends into the myometrium it is termed **placenta increta**. Last, when the placenta extends through the entire myometrial layer and uterine serosa it is termed **placenta percreta**. Over the past two decades, the reported incidence of placenta accreta ranged from 1 in 533 to 1 in 2510 deliveries[6,7] (Level II). However, as the national rate of cesarean deliveries continues to increase over time, the incidence of placenta accreta will likewise increase as well.

Several risk factors for placenta accreta have been identified. The two most important appear to be prior cesarean delivery and placenta previa. In women with placenta previa the incidence of placenta accreta appears to correlate with the number of previous cesarean sections. Clark et al reported a 5% incidence of placenta accreta among women with placenta previa and no previous cesarean sections[8] (Level II). The incidence increased to 24% with one previous cesarean section and to 45% with two or more. Among 723 women with prior cesarean delivery and previa, Silver et al reported the risk for accreta to be 3%, 11%, 40%, 61%, and 67% for one, two, three, four, and five or more cesarean deliveries, respectively. Among 29,409 women with cesarean delivery and no previa the risk for accreta was 0.03%, 0.2%, 0.1%, 0.8%, 0.8%, 4.7% for one, two, three, four, five, and six or more cesarean deliveries, respectively[9] (Level II). Advanced maternal age and placental location with respect to the previous uterine scar have also been reported to be independent risk factors for placenta accreta among women with placenta previa.

Miller reported a 2.1% incidence of accreta in women with placenta previa who were less than 35 years of age and had no previous cesareans. The incidence increased to 38.1% in women who were 35 years of age or older with two or more previous cesarean sections and a placenta previa overlying the uterine scar[6] (Level II).

Placenta accreta should be suspected in all women with placenta previa. A definitive diagnosis of accreta is not possible prior to delivery. That said, ultrasonography has yielded encouraging results in the prospective diagnosis of placenta accreta. The use of ultrasonography and color Doppler findings (diffuse intraparenchymal placental lacunar flow, bladder-uterine serosa hypervascularity, prominent subplacental venous complex, loss of subplacental Doppler vascular signals) has yielded sensitivities of approximately 80% and specificities of approximately 95% for the detection of accrete[10,11] (Level II). Using ultrasound color flow mapping, Twickler found if the myometrial thickness under the placenta was less than 1 mm, this was predictive of myometrial invasion with a sensitivity of 100%, specificity 72%, positive predictive value (PPV) 72%, and negative predictive value (NPV) 100% (Figure 8–1)[12] (Level II). MRI has been described to diagnose placenta accreta, although the sensitivity does not appear to be superior to sonography. Warshak et al evaluated the accuracy of

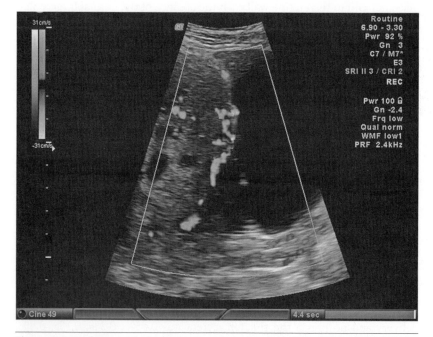

Figure 8–1. Ultrasound of a placenta accreta (increta). Note the hypervascularity at the bladder-lower segment interface as well as the inability to define a layer of myometrium between the placenta and the bladder. There is also lacunar lakes noted in the placenta. *(Courtesy of Dr. Richard H. Lee)*

sonography and MRI in the antenatal diagnosis of placenta accreta. Of 39 cases of confirmed placenta accreta, sonography had a sensitivity of 77% and specificity of 96% whereas gadolinium-enhanced MRI had a sensitivity of 88% and specificity of 100% and was able to exclude placenta accreta in 14/14 cases. The use of MRI must take into account cost, accessibility, and if gadolinium is used, the risks and benefits of fetal exposure to contrast agents[13] (Level II).

In women with placenta previa who are considered to be at high risk for placenta accreta, cesarean delivery should be performed electively. The timing of delivery differs among institutions. Delivery timing is based on several factors including patient stability, risk of future bleeding, and fetal maturity. That said, most experts generally agree that delivery should occur at approximately 35 to 37 weeks' gestation. The patient should be counseled preoperatively regarding the risks of hemorrhage, transfusion, and hysterectomy. The operating room should be staffed by experienced personnel, equipped with appropriate hysterectomy instruments, and blood products/blood salvage equipment should be available. The use of prophylactic intravascular balloon catheters for placenta accreta have failed to produce any substantial decrease in maternal morbidity[14] (Level II). Preoperative ureteral stents may be placed to avoid ureteral injury. It is important that other surgical specialties be available including gynecologic oncology and urology services.

At cesarean delivery the uterine incision is made vertically away from the suspected placental location. The fetus is delivered, spontaneous delivery of the placenta is awaited, or gentle traction is applied on the cord to await delivery of placenta. Attempts to manually deliver the placenta can cause massive hemorrhage if there is indeed a placenta accreta. However, it is important for the physician to be aware that focal placenta accreta may occur which may be treated with conservative approaches. If placental delivery is unsuccessful or if uncontrollable hemorrhage ensues, the surgeon should leave the placenta in place and proceed with hysterectomy. Hysterectomy remains the procedure of choice (Figures 8–2 and 8–3).

Control of potentially life-threatening hemorrhage is the first priority; however, the patient's desire for future fertility must be taken into consideration. If the patient is hemodynamically stable and strongly desires future fertility, conservative management may be cautiously considered—keeping in mind the literature regarding conservative management is based on case series or reports. The risks of **conservative management** include delayed hemorrhage (requiring reoperation) and infection. *If the patient is unstable, conservative management is not an option.*

Conservative techniques that have been described include curettage and/or over-sewing the placental bed, or wedge resection of the area of accreta with subsequent repair of the myometrium. In the vast majority of cases these techniques have been applied in the setting when a focal accreta is encountered after attempted removal of the placenta. **Planned conservative management** has been described in case reports when a placenta accreta is diagnosed before delivery and the patient strongly desires future fertility, this

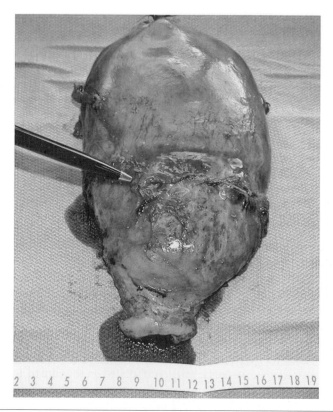

Figure 8–2. The cesarean hysterectomy specimen. Note the placenta can be visualized underneath the uterine serosa. *(Courtesy of Dr. Richard H. Lee)*

involves leaving the placenta in situ thereafter adjunctive therapy is administered either with uterine artery embolization, methotrexate, or delayed removal. These methods of management have not been subject to randomized control trials and should be considered investigational. This approach should only be considered in patients who strongly desire future fertility and who understand and accept the risks of delayed hemorrhage, infection, and death. The patient should be counseled that this approach cannot be used if she has profuse bleeding or is hemodynamically unstable. Timmermans et al. reviewed 60 pregnancies managed with the conservative management. The most common complication was that of vaginal bleeding (21/60). The timing of blood loss ranged from immediately postpartum up to 3 months after delivery. Treatment failure due to vaginal bleeding occurred in 15% of case (9/60). Fever occurred in 21/60 cases, 11/60 had endomyometritis, and 2/60 required hysterectomy for definitive treatment. Importantly, the authors caution that the number of complications may be falsely lowered due to publication bias of reported successful cases[15] (Level II).

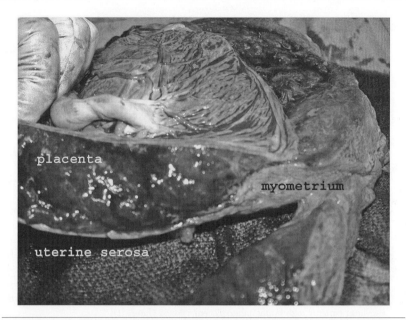

Figure 8–3. A macroscopic cross section of the specimen. Note the invasion of the placenta into the myometrium. The final pathologic diagnosis was placenta increta. *(Courtesy of Dr. Richard H. Lee)*

Clinical Pearls

See US Preventive Services Task Force Study Quality levels of evidence in Case 1

➤ Placenta previa is a common diagnosis before 20 weeks' gestation (1%-6%) (Level II-2).

➤ Approximately 90% of cases of placenta previa diagnosed before 20 weeks' resolve (Level II-2).

➤ The recurrence risk of placenta previa is 4% to 6% (Level II-3).

➤ Placenta accreta should be suspected in any patient with a prior cesarean delivery and a placenta previa (Level II-2).

➤ In an unstable, bleeding patient with a suspected placenta accreta, cesarean hysterectomy is the procedure of choice.

CONTROVERSIES

- The gestational age at which to electively deliver placenta previa.
- The gestational age at which to electively deliver a suspected placenta accreta.
- If MRI is of any added benefit to ultrasound in making the diagnosis of placenta accreta.

REFERENCES

1. Oyelese Y, Smulian JC. Placenta previa, placenta accreta, and vasa previa. *Obstet Gynecol.* 2006 Apr;107(4):927-941.
   The authors perform an in-depth review on the management of placenta previa, accreta, and vasa previa (Level III).
2. Taipale P, Hiilesmaa V, Ylostalo P. Transvaginal ultrasonography at 18-23 weeks in predicting placenta previa at delivery. *Ultrasound Obstet Gynecol.* 1998 Dec;12(6):422-425.
   The authors assess the persistence of placenta previa at the time of delivery (Level II).
3. Besinger RE, Moniak CW, Paskiewicz LS, Fisher SG, Tomich PG. The effect of tocolytic use in the management of symptomatic placenta previa. *Am J Obstet Gynecol.* 1995 Jun;172(6):1770-1775; discussion 5-8.
   The authors studied 112 preterm pregnancies with placenta previa and initial bleeding. They assessed outcomes after the administration of magnesium sulfate and/or beta-sympathomimetics. They found tocolytic therapy may prolong pregnancy and increase birthweight, but does not appear to alter the frequency or severity of bleeding (Level II).
4. Sharma A, Suri V, Gupta I. Tocolytic therapy in conservative management of symptomatic placenta previa. *Int J Gynaecol Obstet.* 2004 Feb;84(2):109-113.
   The authors found the use of ritodrine may prolong pregnancies and increase the birthweight in patients with symptomatic placenta previa (Level II).
5. Wing DA, Paul RH, Millar LK. Management of the symptomatic placenta previa: a randomized, controlled trial of inpatient versus outpatient expectant management. *Am J Obstet Gynecol.* 1996 Oct;175(4 Pt 1):806-811.
   The authors found that outpatient management may be used in a selected group of patients with symptomatic placenta previa (Level II).
6. Miller DA, Chollet JA, Goodwin TM. Clinical risk factors for placenta previa-placenta accreta. *Am J Obstet Gynecol.* 1997 Jul;177(1):210-214.
   The authors found among 155,670 deliveries, 1 in 2510 were complicated by a histologically confirmed placenta accreta. They found advanced maternal age and prior cesarean delivery to be independent risk factors for placenta accreta in women with placenta previa (Level II).
7. Wu S, Kocherginsky M, Hibbard JU. Abnormal placentation: twenty-year analysis. *Am J Obstet Gynecol.* 2005 May;192(5):1458-1461.
   An evalution on the incidence of placenta accreta between 1982 and 2002. The incidence of placenta accreta was found to be 1 in 533 (Level II).
8. Clark SL, Koonings PP, Phelan JP. Placenta previa/accreta and prior cesarean section. *Obstet Gynecol.* 1985 Jul;66(1):89-92.
   This retrospective cohort study evaluated 97,799 patients and found the risk of placenta previa in an unscarred uterus was 0.26%. The risk of plcenta accreta in the presence of placenta previa in an unscarred uterus was 5%. The risk of placenta previa/accreta was found to be increased with the number of prior cesarean births (Level II).
9. Silver RM, Landon MB, Rouse DJ, et al. Maternal morbidity associated with multiple repeat cesarean deliveries. *Obstet Gynecol.* 2006 Jun;107(6):1226-1232.
   The authors found increased morbidity as well as increased risk for accreta with increasing number of cesarean deliveries (Level II).
10. Chou MM, Ho ES, Lee YH. Prenatal diagnosis of placenta previa accreta by transabdominal color Doppler ultrasound. *Ultrasound Obstet Gynecol.* 2000 Jan;15(1):28-35.

The authors evaluated the sensitivity (82.4%) and specificity (96.8%) of various color Doppler parameters to diagnose placenta previa/accreta during pregnancy (Level II).

11. Comstock CH, Love JJ, Jr., Bronsteen RA, et al. Sonographic detection of placenta accreta in the second and third trimesters of pregnancy. *Am J Obstet Gynecol.* 2004 Apr;190(4):1135-1140.

   The authors conclude the ultrasonographic appearance of vascular spaces within the placenta (lacunae) has the highest positive predictive value for placenta accreta (Level II).

12. Twickler DM, Lucas MJ, Balis AB, et al. Color flow mapping for myometrial invasion in women with a prior cesarean delivery. *J Matern Fetal Med.* 2000 Nov-Dec;9(6):330-335.

   The authors found that a measurement of < 1 mm for the smallest myometrial thickness or presence of large intraplacental lakes was predictive of myometrial invasion with 100% sensitivity and 72% specficity (Level II).

13. Warshak CR, Eskander R, Hull AD, et al. Accuracy of ultrasonography and magnetic resonance imaging in the diagnosis of placenta accreta. *Obstet Gynecol.* 2006 Sep;108(3 Pt 1):573-581.

   The authors of this cohort study concluded that the combination of ultrasound and MRI would optimize diagnostic accuracy for placenta accreta (Level II).

14. Shrivastava V, Nageotte M, Major C, Haydon M, Wing D. Case-control comparison of cesarean hysterectomy with and without prophylactic placement of intravascular balloon catheters for placenta accreta. *Am J Obstet Gynecol.* 2007 Oct;197(4):402 e1-5.

   This case-control study did not find any significant difference with prophylactic placement of intravascular balloon catheters in patients undergoing cesarean hysterectomy for placenta accreta (Level II).

15. Timmermans S, van Hof AC, Duvekot JJ. Conservative management of abnormally invasive placentation. *Obstet Gynecol Surv.* 2007 Aug;62(8):529-539.

   A review of published literature between 1985 and 2006 that involved conservative management of abnormally invasive placentation (Level II).

Case 9

A 28-year-old G1P0 Caucasian female at 38 weeks' gestation presented in active labor. She progressed to complete dilation and began to push; after $3^{1}/_{2}$ hours of maternal efforts, she underwent an uncomplicated spontaneous vaginal delivery aided by a midline episiotomy. The placenta was delivered and was noted to be intact. Following uterine massage and intravenous oxytocin, the fundus was noted to be firm. The episiotomy was repaired without complication and the site was hemostatic. Blood loss was estimated to be 400 cc. Following delivery and repair of the episiotomy, her pulse was 70 bpm and blood pressure was 124/80 mm Hg.

Approximately 2 hours after delivery she began to complain of severe rectal pain and pressure on the right side. Her lochia remained moderate and her fundus is firm at the level of the umbilicus. Her pulse was 115 bpm and blood pressure 105/60 mm Hg. She had 200 cc of urine output in the first hour postpartum and 30 cc of urine output in the last hour.

➤ What is the most likely diagnosis?

➤ What is your next step?

➤ What are potential complications of the patient's disorder?

ANSWERS TO CASE 9:
Puerperal Vulvovaginal Hematoma

Summary: This is a 28-year-old woman, G1P1, who had a spontaneous vaginal delivery over a midline episiotomy following a prolonged second stage of labor. In the early postpartum period she developed acute onset of pain out of proportion to her episiotomy repair. She also manifested clinical signs of hypovolemia, despite a firm fundus and absence of vaginal bleeding.

➤ **Most likely diagnosis:** Puerperal vulvovaginal hematoma.

➤ **Next step:** Thorough examination (including vaginal and rectal examination and possible evaluation of the uterine cavity) to evaluate for sources of blood loss and pain.

➤ **Potential complications:**
  ➤ Short-term: severe hemorrhage (including retroperitoneal hematoma), transfusion, coagulopathy.
  ➤ Long-term: infection, scarring/disfigurement, dyspareunia.

ANALYSIS

Objectives

1. Describe the potential clinical presentations of puerperal vulvovaginal hematomas.
2. Describe the evaluation and management of puerperal vulvovaginal hematomas.
3. Discuss risk factors for, and prevention of, puerperal vulvovaginal hematomas.
4. Summarize complications associated with puerperal vulvovaginal hematomas.

Considerations

In a postpartum patient experiencing perineal or rectal pain greater than that expected following a vaginal delivery, an immediate evaluation for vulvovaginal hematomas is necessary. The tachycardia and decreasing urine output also indicate developing hypovolemia. This patient has three risk factors for puerperal hematoma—primiparous status, prolonged second stage, and episiotomy.

APPROACH TO
Puerperal Vulvovaginal Hematomas

DEFINITIONS

HEMATOMA: A localized mass of extravasated, often clotted blood that is confined to a space or potential space. In the postpartum period, such a mass may be small or large and may vary in location as described in the Clinical Approach section.

JACKSON-PRATT DRAIN: A closed-system drain consisting of a flat white perforated ribbon to be placed in the bed of a hematoma cavity following evacuation of blood and clot. The ribbon connects to a short length of plastic tubing which can be exited through a separate stab wound in the perineum and connected to a "hand grenade" suction device. Such a drain is felt by some investigators to be an important adjunct in the management of moderate-to-large vulvovaginal hematomas.

CLINICAL APPROACH

Incidence   The incidence of puerperal hematomas varies from 1/1500 to 1/309 deliveries; "large" hematomas have been reported to occur in approximately 1/4000 vaginal deliveries.[1-3] The reported incidence varies due to lack of reporting "small" hematomas, lack of agreement regarding the definition of what constitutes a hematoma, and the prevalence of risk factors in a particular population.

Classification   Puerperal hematomas are often classified according to location:

1. Vulvar (anterior triangle or posterior triangle [ischiorectal area])
2. Vaginal
3. Vulvovaginal (involving both areas)
4. Subperitoneal

An alternate classification is based on location relative to the levator musculature. Infralevator hematomas are limited by the levator ani, and the perineal body typically prevents these hematomas from spreading across the midline. Additionally, fascial planes prevent involvement of the thigh. Infralevator hematomas are the most common types following vaginal delivery. Supralevator hematomas, by definition, are located above the levator plate, and due to the potential for considerable extension into the retroperitoneal space, may be associated with significant blood loss.

Risk Factors   Episiotomy is the most common risk factor for puerperal hematomas; episiotomy was performed in 85% to 93% of the reported cases of puerperal hematomas.[4] Both midline and mediolateral episiotomy have been associated with puerperal hematomas, with higher risk associated with the latter.[5] Additionally, vaginal lacerations and instrumental vaginal delivery have also been associated with the development of hematomas.[3,5] Other risk factors that have been associated with hematomas include primiparity, multiple gestations, preeclampsia, prolonged second stage, and coagulopathy.

Presentation   The clinical presentation in patients with puerperal hematomas is primarily due to hemorrhage, most commonly involving the pudendal artery and its branches. Additionally, branches of the uterine artery may be responsible for vaginal hematomas. Subperitoneal hematomas may occur due to vascular injury to the uterine arteries or other vessels in the pelvis. Vascular injury may be immediate or delayed due to pressure necrosis and resultant vascular injury with subsequent hematoma formation.[1] The majority of patients with puerperal hematomas will present within 24 hours of delivery.

A large amount of blood may accumulate in the paravaginal and ischiorectal spaces as the anatomy of these spaces involves predominantly soft tissue. As a result, blood loss is often underestimated. Most patients with vulvovaginal hematomas will present with an ischiorectal mass, bruising, and perineal or rectal pain. Other symptoms may include fever, ileus, and extremity pain, although these are much less common in patients presenting within the first 24 hours (see Figure 9–1).

An important characteristic regarding clinical presentation is that pain associated with an infralevator hematoma is typically more severe than that expected relative to vaginal delivery or repair of a laceration or episiotomy. Supralevator hematomas, however, may present with signs and symptoms secondary to significant hypovolemia resulting from retroperitoneal hemorrhage. Supralevator hematomas are uncommonly associated with vaginal delivery, but may occur secondary to uterine scar rupture in trials of labor following previous cesarean section.

Treatment

Initial Considerations   The management approach for a woman with a puerperal hematoma is controversial, with opinions differing based on perceived size of the hematoma as well as in the use of drains. Observation only has been suggested in some reports, particularly for "small" vulvovaginal hematomas (described as < 3 cm in diameter).[3,5] Observation has also been described for a hematoma in the retropubic space following spontaneous vaginal delivery which had not initially responded to drainage.[6] Risks associated with a conservative approach in the setting of larger hematomas include infection, profuse hemorrhage, necrosis, and possibly mortality; therefore, operative intervention in this setting is often recommended. It is critical to remember

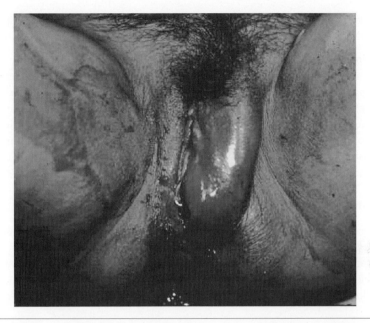

Figure 9–1. Left-sided vulvar hematoma in a patient who had a spontaneous vaginal delivery and coagulopathy due to acute fatty liver of pregnancy. *(Reproduced, with permission, from Cunningham FG, Leveno KJ, Bloom SL, et al. Williams Obstetrics. 23rd ed. New York, NY: McGraw-Hill; 2010.)*

that blood loss is often significantly underestimated in these cases, and delay in diagnosis and treatment can have catastrophic results.

Operative Approach   For vulvovaginal hematomas, an incision should be made of appropriate size (often 5-10 cm in length) to gain access to the hematoma. All clots should be removed and the area irrigated copiously. In most settings, a diffuse oozing tissue bed will be identified as opposed to discrete bleeding vessels which could be ligated or cauterized. A layered closure should then be performed to provide hemostasis and close dead space. A vaginal pack can be used if considered necessary; placement of the pack should be done with care to prevent disruption of the closure of the hematoma site and to avoid creation of additional bleeding sites as the vaginal mucosa is often friable and the patient may also be at risk for coagulopathy. Broad-spectrum antibiotics are indicated due to the risk of infection, and transfusion of blood products is often necessary.

The use of drains in the setting of a vulvovaginal hematoma is also not clearly established. The theoretical advantage of placement of drains include further elimination of dead space, reduction of pressure and possible resultant tissue necrosis, and removal of necrotic tissue and blood that may provide a source of infection.[7,8] Varied approaches to drainage have been described, including placement of a Penrose drain brought out through the introitus and a closed system Jackson-Pratt drain exiting through a separate perineal site.[7]

Angiographic Embolization   Angiographic embolization has been described for various obstetric and gynecologic conditions, including management of postpartum hemorrhage and leiomyomatous uteri. Embolization has also been described in the management of vulvovaginal hematomas, mainly in the setting of hematomas not responsive to initial therapy.[9,10] Theoretically, embolization may also be an option for management of supralevator hematomas, since embolization has been used to successfully control severe retroperitoneal bleeding in other clinical scenarios.[11-13]

Summary

Puerperal hematomas can be associated with significant morbidity, and possible mortality. Although prevention is desirable, an index of suspicion is imperative, particularly if risk factors are present. Prompt recognition and intervention, including antibiotics and transfusion, if indicated, will often lead to satisfactory results.

Comprehension Questions

9.1   A 23-year-old woman, G2P1, underwent an uncomplicated vacuum delivery. During the repair of her second-degree laceration, an expanding 4.5-cm right vaginal sidewall hematoma is noted. Her vital signs are within normal limits. What is the best treatment option?

A. Immediate incision over the hematoma, layered closure, and placement of drain
B. Packing the vagina
C. Observation for expansion
D. Vaginal ultrasound
E. Immediate blood transfusion

9.2   A 36-year-old woman, G1P0, underwent induction for severe preeclampsia. Her antepartum course was notable for obesity and gestational diabetes. She underwent a low forceps delivery for fetal distress of a 4000-g male infant. What are her risk factors for a puerperal hematoma?

A. Obesity
B. Large-for-gestational-age infant
C. Forceps delivery
D. Chronic hypertension

9.3   A 27-year-old woman, G3P2, is 4 hours postpartum from a sponta-
       neous vaginal delivery complicated by an 8-cm vulvovaginal
       hematoma, which was incised, evacuated, and repaired; no expansion
       was noted. The vagina was packed overnight and she was given broad-
       spectrum antibiotics. She is currently receiving 2 units of packed red
       blood cells due to hypovolemia associated with an estimated blood loss
       of 1200 cc. She developed a temperature to 100.8°F. Which of the fol-
       lowing is the most likely cause of her fever?
       A. Preeclampsia
       B. Deep venous thrombosis
       C. Infection of the hematoma bed
       D. Transfusion reaction
       E. Pneumonia

ANSWERS

9.1   **A.** The hematoma is greater than 3 cm and was discovered during
       episiotomy repair. Because the hematoma is expanding, the preferred
       approach would be to incise over the hematoma site, evacuate
       the clot, perform a layered closure, and place a Jackson-Pratt drain.
       A vaginal pack should then be placed to maintain pressure on the
       vaginal suture line. Transfusion should be based on the patient's
       clinical status.

9.2   **C.** Risk factors for puerperal hematomas include episiotomy, opera-
       tive delivery, vaginal lacerations, prolonged second stage, preeclamp-
       sia, multiple gestation, and clotting abnormalities. This patient was
       diagnosed with preeclampsia and underwent an operative vaginal
       delivery. A laceration was not described in this scenario; however, if
       one were to have occurred, that would also be a risk factor.

9.3   **D.** The patient is currently undergoing a transfusion and non-
       hemolytic febrile reactions are common. A fever in a patient under-
       going blood transfusion must be promptly evaluated and monitored.
       Infection of the hematoma bed is a common complication of puer-
       peral hematomas and broad-spectrum antibiotics are recommended.
       However, at only 4 hours postpartum, infection of the hematoma site
       would be unlikely.

Clinical Pearls

See US Preventive Services Task Force Study Quality levels of evidence in Case 1

➤ Observation should be reserved for nonexpanding hematomas less than 3 cm (Level III).

➤ Be prepared for volume replacement with crystalloids and blood products as hematomas can expand rapidly and blood loss is often underestimated (Level III-3).

➤ A generous incision to evacuate the hematoma and elimination of dead space through layered closure and possible drain placement are key components of operative intervention in the management of puerperal hematomas (Level II-2).

REFERENCES

1. Pieri RJ. Pelvic hematomas associated with pregnancy. *Obstet Gynecol.* 1958;12:249-258.
2. Lyons AW. Postpartum hematoma. *N Engl J Med.* 1949;240:461-463.
3. Sotto LS, Collins RJ. Perigenital hematomas; analysis of 47 consecutive cases. *Obstet Gynecol.* 1958;12:259-263.
4. McElin TW, Bowers VM Jr, Paalman RJ. Puerperal hematomas; a report of 73 cases and review of the literature. *Am J Obstet Gynecol.* 1954;67:356-366.
5. Sheikh GN. Perinatal genital hematomas. *Obstet Gynecol.* 1971;38:571-575.
6. Fieni S, Berretta R, Merisio C, Melpignano M, Gramellini D. Retzius' space haematoma after spontaneous delivery: a case report. *Acta Biomed.* 2005;76:175-177.
7. Zahn CM, Hankins GDV, Yeomans ER. Vulvovaginal hematomas complicating delivery. Rationale for drainage of the hematoma cavity. *J Reprod Med.* 1996;41:569-574.
8. You WB, Zahn CM. Postpartum hemorrhage: abnormally adherent placenta, uterine inversion, and puerperal hematomas. *Clin Obstet Gynecol.* 2006;49:184-197.
9. Villella J, Garry D, Levine G, Glanz S, Figueroa R, Maulik D. Postpartum angiographic embolization for vulvovaginal hematoma. A report of two cases. *J Reprod Med.* 2001;46:65-67.
10. Chin HG, Scott DR, Resnik R, Davis GB, Lurie AL. Angiographic embolization of intractable puerperal hematomas. *Am J Obstet Gynecol.* 1989;160:434-438.
11. Akpinar E, Peynircioglu B, Turkbey B, Cil BE, Balkanci F. Endovascular management of life-threatening retroperitonal bleeding. *ANZ J Surg.* 2008;78:683-687.
12. Tulsyan N, Kashyap VS, Greenberg RK, et al. The endovascular management of visceral aneurysms and pseudoaneurysms. *J Vasc Surg.* 2007;45:276-283.
13. Velmahos GC, Toutouzas KG, Vassiliu P, et al. A prospective study on the safety and efficacy of angiographic embolization for pelvic and visceral injuries. *J Trauma.* 2002;53:303-308.

Case 10

A 24-year-old G1P0 at 39 weeks' gestation was admitted to the hospital for induction of labor secondary to Class A2 gestational diabetes. Diabetes was diagnosed at 28 weeks when all four values on a 3-hour oral glucose tolerance test were elevated. She was initially treated with glyburide, but due to persistent fasting hyperglycemia she was placed on a traditional split-mixed insulin regimen. The estimated fetal weight on admission was 3600 g and the cervix was long and closed. After three doses of misoprostol the examination had changed to fingertip and 50% effaced. A Foley catheter was inserted into the cervix and left in place for 12 hours. When it was removed, the cervix was 2 cm dilated and still 50% effaced. Presentation was confirmed by ultrasound to be vertex and oxytocin was initiated at 8 o'clock on hospital day 2. Membranes were artificially ruptured 12 hours later and over the next 8 hours, the patient reached complete dilation. After 3 hours of pushing, the fetal head delivered spontaneously. One minute later the shoulders were delivered with a combination of McRoberts maneuver and suprapubic pressure. There was a fourth-degree extension of her midline episiotomy. The infant had Apgar scores of 5 and 7 and weighed 4050 g. The placenta was manually extracted, following which the fundus was noted to be markedly atonic. Unusually heavy bleeding necessitated immediate measures to control. Estimated blood loss prior to treatment was 1000 mL.

➤ What is the diagnosis?

➤ What are the important precipitating factors?

➤ What are the primary and secondary measures that might be used to control bleeding?

ANSWER TO CASE 10:
Postpartum Hemorrhage

Summary: This is a primigravid woman with gestational diabetes who underwent medically indicated induction of labor. The induction was long, but did culminate in vaginal delivery. The delivery was complicated by heavy bleeding and a fourth-degree extension of a midline episiotomy.

> **Diagnosis:** Postpartum hemorrhage.

> **Important precipitating factors:** Uterine atony is by far the most important cause of postpartum hemorrhage. Risk factors for atony present in this case include induction of labor, prolonged labor, and possibly uterine overdistention by a large fetus. Other risk factors for atony not present in this case include polyhydramnios, multiple gestation, rapid labor, chorioamnionitis, and a history of atony with a previous delivery. Besides atony, there is the potential for retained products of conception after manual extraction of the placenta. Also, blood loss can be increased by bleeding from the episiotomy site.

> **Primary and secondary measures to control bleeding:** These will be explained in greater detail in the clinical approach section that follows. Measures can be grouped as medical (compression, oxytocin, methylergonovine, other uterotonic agents), surgical (uterine compression sutures, vessel ligation, hysterectomy), and other (vessel embolization, packing).

ANALYSIS

Objectives

1. Anticipate the likelihood of postpartum hemorrhage in light of risk factors present before delivery.
2. Develop an organized approach to the management of postpartum hemorrhage.
3. Outline appropriate blood volume replacement.

Considerations

In this chapter, the term "postpartum hemorrhage" is restricted to bleeding caused by and/or: uterine atony, genital tract lacerations, and retained products of conception (placenta or membranes). Uterine inversion, placenta accreta, and amniotic fluid embolism are uncommon obstetrical conditions that are associated with postpartum bleeding, but these conditions are not included in the discussion of postpartum hemorrhage in this chapter. Antepartum hemorrhage includes placental abruption, placenta previa, and most cases of rupture of both scarred and unscarred uteri, as well as causes of bleeding like abortion, ectopic, and hydatidiform mole that are most often encountered in the first trimester; all of these antepartum complications are likewise excluded from consideration here. The majority of cases of postpartum hemorrhage that complicate vaginal delivery can be managed medically. Disseminated intravascular coagulation (DIC) can incite bleeding de novo, but more often it enhances bleeding due to any of the conditions mentioned above. The possibility of DIC must be kept in mind by all obstetricians managing postpartum hemorrhage due to the three causes discussed in this chapter.

APPROACH TO
Postpartum Hemorrhage

DEFINITIONS

POSTPARTUM HEMORRHAGE (PPH): Several definitions are used in the literature (need for transfusion, drop in hematocrit more than 10%), but none are completely satisfactory.[1] For ease of understanding, PPH is defined herein as estimated blood loss after vaginal delivery more than 500 cc or after cesarean delivery more than 1000 cc. Using these definitions the approximate incidence is 5%.

UTERINE ATONY: Failure of uterine smooth muscle fibers in the myometrium to contract after delivery. Normally myometrial contraction constricts the spiral arterioles supplying especially the placental bed, but with atony, this mechanism does not function properly. Because uterine blood flow at term is approximately 600 mL/min, atony can lead to rapid loss of a large volume of blood, eventually leading to hemorrhagic shock and death if not managed expeditiously.

DISSEMINATED INTRAVASCULAR COAGULATION (DIC): This diagnosis is suspected clinically when blood fails to clot, diffusely oozing from cut or raw surfaces and usually does not respond to surgical measures to control bleeding. The mechanism producing DIC may be either consumption of coagulation factors or dilution secondary to volume replacement with fluids that contain no coagulation factors, or often both. Laboratory indicators of DIC include three or more of the following: platelet count less than 100,000/mm^3, increased prothrombin time, increased partial thromboplastin time, decreased fibrinogen, increased fibrin degradation products, or increased D-dimer (bearing in mind that pregnancy itself may falsely elevate D-dimer level).

CLINICAL APPROACH

Because of the inaccuracy of visual estimates of blood loss, **the diagnosis of postpartum hemorrhage is often not identified** until the patient develops hypovolemic shock. In other words, the early recognition of significant hemorrhage requires vigilance. Multiple investigators have shown that early recognition and intervention leads to better clinical outcomes including less transfusions, less need for surgical management, and less blood loss as determined by drop in hemoglobin. The identification of hypovolemia is a clinical diagnosis. Physician and nurse skill in patient volume assessment are important to facilitate timely intervention.

The most common etiology for postpartum hemorrhage is uterine atony, and risk factors[2] have been well documented (Table 10–1). Hence, in those patients with multiple risk factors, the physician should be prepared for postpartum hemorrhage; nevertheless, serious hemorrhage often occurs in the absence of risk factors.

There are some investigators that promote active management of the third stage of labor to decrease the likelihood of PPH. Maneuvers such as massage of the uterus and judicious traction of the cord even prior to separation may enhance the onset of uterine contractions and decrease the incidence of uterine atony. These measures are certainly important in developing countries where pharmacological agents or blood products are not widely available. In the United States, active management of the third stage should be balanced against the possibility of uterine inversion.

Immediately after delivering the placenta the uterine fundus should be palpated through the abdominal wall. Assessment of vaginal bleeding and a systematic review of the clinical parameters for volume status are paramount at this stage. If the uterine fundus is soft and boggy, bimanual compression and a call for help should be initiated simultaneously. Oxytocin should be infused

---

Table 10–1 RISK FACTORS FOR UTERINE ATONY

Uterine overdistention
Multiple gestations
Polyhydramnios
Macrosomia
Grand multiparity
Abnormal labor
Rapid labor
Prolonged labor
Prolonged use of oxytocin
Chorioamnionitis
General anesthesia
Past history of postpartum hemorrhage

---

briskly intravenously and the situation should be reevaluated. If the uterus has not become firm, additional measures should be implemented. These may include placing another large-bore IV line, inserting a Foley catheter in the bladder, exploring the uterine cavity to rule out retained placenta or membranes, and inspecting for lacerations.[3]

The obstetrician should assess whether the vaginal bleeding is arising from the cervix, distal to the cervix, or above the level of the cervix. Pressure or ring forceps should be placed on lacerations if identified, but the operator continues to assess for further bleeding. In other words, sometimes patients will have significant uterine bleeding in addition to a cervical or vaginal laceration.

During the initial 2 to 3 minutes of postdelivery assessment, early postpartum atony or lacerations should be quickly identified and aggressively addressed. Rapid laboratory tests including hemoglobin, hematocrit, coagulation profile, and especially cross-matching blood are not critical at this juncture (see the section that follows on blood transfusion).

With persistent atony and ongoing bleeding, two other, interrelated considerations arise: which additional uterotonic agent(s) to try and whether to begin transfusing blood. In the absence of hypertension, Methergine (methylergonovine) 0.2 mg IM is a suitable choice and can be repeated once. 15-Methyl prostaglandin F2 alpha (Hemabate) 250 µg IM is usually tried next. There is no theoretical or practical advantage gained by intramyometrial injection. Up to eight doses can be given, but rarely is this done in practice. If one or two doses do not improve uterine tone and decrease bleeding, most obstetricians would take the next step in the algorithm. Moreover, Hemabate is expensive. Some investigators recommend the use of rectal (preferred) or oral misoprostol in doses up to 1000 µg, but the published experience is relatively small. Finally, if at the initial examination of the fundus it is found to be firm, the uterine cavity should be explored for retained products and the possibility of uterine rupture. The vagina and cervix should be carefully inspected for lacerations and, if found, appropriately repaired. Retained products and genital tract lacerations together contribute around 20% of cases of postpartum hemorrhage. The woman in the case presented had a fourth degree perineal laceration which likely added to her blood loss.

Decision to Transfuse

Adequate uterine perfusion is a requirement for delivery of all uterotonic agents to their site of action. Blood transfusion may therefore be required; transfusion may be chosen earlier in the management scheme if bleeding is very heavy or hypotension is present.

The decision to transfuse is a crucial one. Lack of recognition of hemorrhagic shock until late, delaying transfusion until the patient is hypotensive and suffering from tissue ischemia, is one of the leading reasons for maternal mortality. Yet, requesting blood products from the blood bank in unwarranted circumstances is costly, and can lead to unindicated transfusions. The issues that the obstetrician should take into account in deciding whether to transfuse include (1) patient's starting hemoglobin level, (2) rapidity of the bleeding, (3) estimated blood loss and clinical volume status based on systematic assessment, (4) response to therapy, (5) etiology of bleeding and likelihood of remedy, and (6) availability of blood products and time required to obtain blood. There is no blood test or single parameter that gives the answer to the question: "Should this patient be transfused?" There is likely no other circumstance that relies more on physician judgment and training than the patient assessment, ongoing monitoring, and timely management of hemorrhage.

If packed red blood cells are to be given, transfusion may be started with either typed and screened or O-negative blood. Waiting for blood to be cross matched is not advisable for most cases of obstetrical hemorrhage and trying to anticipate which women may require transfusion and cross matching blood in advance is both impractical and costly. If multiple units of packed cells are transfused, for example with an estimated blood loss more than 2 L, it may be indicated to transfuse fresh frozen plasma (FFP) to ensure adequate coagulation factors are present to prevent dilutional DIC. FFP contains about 700 mg of fibrinogen in 250 mL. Cryoprecipitate contains 200 mg fibrinogen in 15 mL, but the need for multiple units would expose the recipient to many donors. A recent report from Parkland Hospital (Alexander et al)[4] describes transfusion of whole blood (which obviously contains coagulation factors) for massive hemorrhage cases, but whole blood is not available at many centers.

If medical management of uterine atony fails, subsequent steps may be influenced by a woman's desire for future fertility. When sterilization is requested, the threshold to proceed with hysterectomy in the setting of severe hemorrhage requiring transfusion is often lower.

Two nonsurgical options have been championed by a few investigators in the recent literature. The first is balloon tamponade[5], with several different types of "balloons" recommended. Currently popular is the Bakri balloon which holds up to 500 cc, puts uniform pressure on the uterine cavity (possibly an improvement over the old method of packing the uterus with gauze), and allows for egress of blood through a channel in the middle of the balloon.

The second nonsurgical option is to have interventional radiology embolize the uterine arteries. This option is severely limited by the requirement for expertise and availability of radiology personnel. Until recently, the procedure was considered relatively safe. The report by Maassen et al[6] cited in the references describes two significant complications related to the procedure: development of vesicovaginal fistula in one woman and migration of gelfoam particles to the external iliac artery compromising blood flow to the woman's leg! Given that the entire series of women undergoing embolization numbered only 11, these two complications take on added significance.

Surgical Management

If medical management of uterine atony fails, subsequent steps may be influenced by a woman's desire for future fertility. When sterilization is requested, the threshold to proceed with hysterectomy in the setting of severe hemorrhage requiring transfusion is often lower. Once the abdomen is open (for example, at the time of cesarean delivery), the first step in surgical control of hemorrhage is bilateral uterine artery ligation. Next would be a compression suture like the B-Lynch stitch (see Figure 10–1) or multiple squares. An infrequent intervention could be administration of recombinant activated factor VII. This is only considered for very serious hemorrhage when other measures have failed. An appropriate dose is 90 µg/kg intravenously. The "court of last resort" is hysterectomy, which is described more fully in Case 6.

In conclusion, the approach to a woman with postpartum hemorrhage requires the implementation of a clinical algorithm that is well designed and carefully executed, analogous to the algorithm for managing shoulder dystocia.

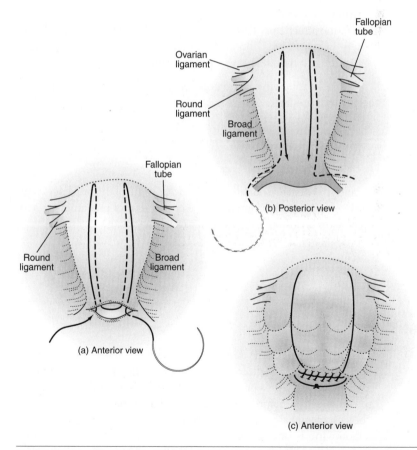

Figure 10–1. The B-lynch stitch is used to form an external compression of the uterus using suture. (Reproduced, with permission, from DeCherney AH, Nathan L, Goodwin TM, et al. Current Diagnosis & Treatment: Obstetrics & Gynecology. 10th ed. New York, NY: McGraw-Hill; 2007:483.)

Keeping in mind that uterine blood flow is 600 cc/min, the management must also be expeditious. Contemporary obstetric practice requires immediate access to a blood bank. Postpartum hemorrhage remains one of the leading causes of maternal death, both nationally and worldwide.

Comprehension Questions

10.1   With regard to the management of postpartum hemorrhage, which of the following statements is true?
       A. The most common and most effective route of administration of Hemabate (15-methyl prostaglandin F2 alpha) is intramyometrial.
       B. Methergine (methylergonovine) is no longer indicated in an algorithm for managing uterine atony.
       C. Uterine artery embolization involves negligible maternal morbidity.
       D. Use of the Bakri balloon appears to be a reasonable step before resorting to hysterectomy for uterine atony.

10.2   Which of the following blood components contains the most fibrinogen per unit volume?
       A. Packed red blood cells
       B. Fresh frozen plasma (FFP)
       C. Cryoprecipitate
       D. Platelet concentrates

10.3   When all other reasonable measures to control hemorrhage have failed, what is the appropriate intravenous dose of recombinant activated factor VII to give to a woman weighing 70 kg?
       A. 6 µg
       B. 6 mg
       C. 60 mg
       D. 6 g

ANSWERS

10.1   **D.** The Bakri balloon, despite relatively few reported experiences, appears to be a good alternative to packing the uterus with gauze. In a woman who desires preservation of fertility, use of the balloon is a reasonable step before resorting to hysterectomy. As for the other choices, Hemabate is more commonly given intramuscularly, methylergonovine is only contraindicated if the patient is hypertensive, and there are serious risks reported with uterine artery embolization.

10.2   **C.** Cryoprecipitate contains 200 mg of fibrinogen in 15 mL. The next best answer, FFP, contains 700 mg in 250 mL.

10.3   **B.** This question requires a little arithmetic. The recommended dose of recombinant factor VIIA is 90 µg/kg. Multiplying by 70 gives a dose of 6300 µg or 6.3 mg. The other choices are obviously too little or too much.

Clinical Pearls

See US Preventive Services Task Force Study Quality levels of evidence in Case 1

➤ Whether at vaginal or cesarean delivery, the value of bimanual compression (not massage) is underemphasized. For vaginal delivery, the operator's fist is placed in the anterior vaginal fornix and the abdominal hand folds the fundus forward. At cesarean delivery, a reasonably long (5-10 min) trial of bimanual compression should precede any attempt to place uterine compression sutures (B-Lynch). Such sutures will often prove unnecessary after pressure is released (Level III).

➤ If vaginal bleeding persists despite a well-contracted fundus, undiagnosed genital tract laceration (including uterine rupture) should be suspected. Thorough inspection of the birth canal, especially of the cervix, and manual exploration of the uterine cavity should be performed (Level II-3).

➤ In performing bilateral uterine artery ligation, the operator should take care not to place the stitch too low on the lower uterine segment, nor too wide into the broad ligament. Ureteral injury may result (Level II-2).

➤ When serious hemorrhage is encountered, and medical measures appear to be unsuccessful, keep in mind that drugs must be delivered to the site of action. Restoration of circulating blood volume is crucial (Level II-3).

➤ Peripartum hysterectomy for hemorrhage should not be undertaken unless the patient has been transfused first with blood. This advice is a corollary to the preceding pearl (Level III).

REFERENCES

1. Postpartum hemorrhage. ACOG *Practice Bulletin.* 2006;108:1039-1047.
2. Sosa CG, Althabe F, Belizan JM, Buekens P. Risk factors for postpartum hemorrhage in vaginal deliveries in a Latin-American population. *Obstet Gynecol.* 2009; 113:1313-1319.
3. Yeomans ER, Gilstrap LC. Postpartum hemorrhage. In: Gibbs RS, Karlan BY, Haney AF, Nygaard I (eds). *Danforth's Obstetrics and Gynecology.* 10th ed. Philadelphia, PA: Lippincott Williams & Wilkins, 2008;452-461.
4. Alexander JM, Sarode R, McIntire DD, Burner JD, Leveno KJ. Whole blood in the management of hypovolemia due to obstetric hemorrhage. *Obstet Gynecol.* 2009;113:1320-1326.
5. Georgiou C. Balloon tamponade in the management of postpartum haemorrhage: a review. *BJOG.* 2009;116:748-757.
6. Maassen M, Lambers M, Tutein Nolthenius R, van der Valk P, Elgersma O. Complications and failure of uterine artery embolization for intractable postpartum haemorrhage. *BJOG.* 2009;116:55-61.

Case 11

During an emergency cesarean section for breech presentation in labor on a patient with no prenatal care, a 25-year-old female obstetrics-gynecology resident receives a needle stick on her index finger during closure of the fascia. She was wearing a single pair of gloves, and felt the suture needle prick her skin. No obvious blood was noted on her skin after the procedure, however. The resident expresses her concern to you, the attending physician, about the risk of HIV infection since the patient had an unknown status. She confides in you that she has been immunized against hepatitis B and tetanus, and had a negative HIV test at her new OB visit within the last month. She is currently 10 weeks pregnant.

➤ How should you proceed to determine her risk of acquiring HIV through this needle stick?

➤ What should the resident be advised to do at this time, and what would be different if the patient was known to be HIV positive?

➤ What are the potential complications for this patient?

ANSWERS TO CASE 11:
HIV Exposure During Pregnancy

Summary: This 25-year-old resident at 10 weeks pregnant has sustained a needle stick and is at risk of acquiring HIV and hepatitis C.

➤ **Most likely diagnosis:** Risk of acquiring HIV, hepatitis C.

➤ **Next step:** The patient's HIV and hepatitis C status should be immediately determined. If the HIV status is positive, the resident should be offered advice regarding postexposure prophylaxis (PEP) for HIV.

➤ **Potential complications:** Seroconversion to HIV; side effects of PEP to the resident and to the fetus.

ANALYSIS

Objectives

1. Be able to advise patients about HIV risk after various exposures.
2. Understand the risks and benefits of PEP in pregnancy.
3. Be able to counsel an HIV-positive pregnant patient regarding means to reduce vertical transmission.
4. Understand recommendations for intrapartum HIV prophylaxis.

Considerations

1. Risk of HIV after various exposures

The average resident reports almost 8 needlesticks over the time of a residency and 99% have reported at least one needlestick. Risk factors for needlestick accidents include lack of sleep and long work hours. Overall the average HIV transmission risk after mucus membrane exposure is approximately 0.09% and between 0.23% and 0.33% after percutaneous exposure to HIV-infected blood. The risk of transmission differs by type of injury and likely reflects the amount of viral exposure (Table 11–1).

An exposure that may place a health care worker at risk for HIV infection is defined by the Centers for Disease Control and Prevention (CDC) as a percutaneous injury (needlestick or laceration involving a sharp object) or contact of mucus membranes or nonintact skin with blood, tissue, or body fluids (including semen and vaginal secretions) that may be infected. Fluids not considered infectious (unless in the presence of blood) include feces, saliva, sputum, nasal secretions, urine, sweat, tears, and vomitus.

A low-risk injury is one that involves a solid needle, is artificial in nature, and the source patient has a viral load less than 1500 copies/mL.

Table 11–1 RISK OF ACQUIRING HIV WITH DIFFERENT EXPOSURES

RISK FACTOR	ODDS RATIO
Needle placed in the source patient's artery or vein	4.3
Exposure to source patient who died of AIDS within 2 mo	5.6
Device visibly contaminated with source patient's blood	6.2
Deep injury	15.2

Mucocutaneous exposures are generally considered low risk unless it involves a large volume of blood or the source patient has a viral load greater than 1500 copies/mL. High-risk exposures include those involving visible blood on a hollow needle or exposure to a needle that was in the artery or vein of the source patient.

Chlorhexidine, chloroxylenol, iodophor, and alcohol-based agents are virucidal against HIV, hepatitis C virus, and hepatitis B virus. Percutaneous exposure should be washed thoroughly with one of these agents. Mucocutaneous exposures should be flushed generously with water and eyes need to be copiously irrigated with saline or water.

Each institution is required by the Occupational Safety and Health Administration (OSHA) to have their own policy regarding management of exposures to various infectious agents and this should be reviewed. In general the clinical scenario and time of exposure should be documented. Relevant clinical information about the source patient should be documented including risk factors for HIV infection. Serologic test results should be obtained from the source patient for HIV, hepatitis B, and hepatitis C. Selecting the appropriate HIV-PEP regimen may be complex so it is strongly recommended that prior to starting a regimen, consultation occurs with an infectious diseases specialist who has expertise in antiretroviral therapy and HIV transmission. Resources for consultation include: PEPline at telephone 888-448-4911 or http://www.ucsf.edu/hivcntr/Hotlines/; HIV Antiretroviral Pregnancy Registry at http://www.apregistry.com/index.htm; and HIV/AIDS Treatment Information Service at http://aidsinfo.nih.gov.

Regardless of whether PEP has been administered, the healthcare worker should be offered postexposure counseling (including psychologic counseling), testing, and medical evaluation. Antibody testing using ELISA should be used for seroconversion monitoring at baseline, 6 weeks, 12 weeks, and 6 months after exposure. Testing at 12 months should be performed in those individuals that become infected with hepatitis C after exposure to a source patient that was coinfected with HIV and hepatitis C. Extended follow-up for 12 months is also warranted if the clinical judgment of the person's health care provider deems it necessary. In addition, HIV testing should be performed on any exposed individual who has an illness compatible with an acute retroviral syndrome regardless of the interval since exposure.

In the setting of PEP the healthcare worker should be monitored for drug toxicity by testing (complete blood count and renal and hepatic function tests) at baseline and 2 weeks after starting PEP. Counseling should also be provided on the importance of completing the prescribed regimen. The exposed individual should be advised to use precautions to prevent second-ary transmission during the first 6 to 12 weeks after exposure. This includes avoiding blood or tissue donations, breast-feeding, or pregnancy. Information regarding potential drug interactions, toxicities, side effects, measures to minimize those side effects, and drugs that should not be taken with PEP should be provided. Particular attention and immediate notifica-tion should be made with the health care provider if any of the following occur: rash, fever, back or abdominal pain, hematuria, dysuria, or symptoms of hyperglycemia.

2. **Understanding the risks and benefits of postexposure prophylaxis (PEP) in pregnancy**

    Medications used in PEP to HIV include nucleoside and non-nucleoside reverse transcriptase inhibitors (NRTIs, NNRTIs), nucleotide reverse tran-scriptase inhibitors (NtRTIs), protease inhibitors, and more recently an infusion inhibitor. The CDC recommendations depend on level of expo-sure risk (Tables 11–2 and 11–3). Persons that are placed on PEP should complete four full weeks of medications. Due to side effects, 17% to 47% of individuals on PEP do not complete the entire 4-week regimen. Approximately 41% will experience one or more symptoms, most com-monly nausea (26.5%) and fatigue (22.8%).

    The most commonly used two-drug regimens include two nucleosides. Zidovudine (ZDV) and lamivudine (3TC), also known in combination as Combivir, are taken twice daily. Tenofovir (TDF) and emtricitabine (FTC) are available in a once-daily combined formulation named Truvada. Common side effects of Combivir include GI upset, headaches, and malaise. Truvada is better tolerated, but there is less experience with this drug combination for PEP. Uncommon side effects of Truvada include rash, diarrhea, and weakness. Three-drug regimens usually involve adding a pro-tease inhibitor such as Kaletra (lopinavir/ritonavir). Most protease inhibitors can cause GI upset and are cytochrome P450 inducers, so care should be taken if on other medications (Table 11–4).

    While the effects of antiretroviral drugs in pregnancy and on the devel-oping fetus are limited, there is growing data regarding the safety of many of these medications. There are, however, anti-HIV medications which should be avoided in pregnancy including the following:

    Efavirenz is Class D and significant malformations (anencephaly, anoph-thalmia, and cleft palate) have been associated with its use in monkeys

Table 11-2 RECOMMENDED HIV PEP FOR PERCUTANEOUS INJURIES

EXPOSURE TYPE	HIV-1	HIV-2	UNKNOWN SOURCE	HIV NEGATIVE
Low-risk	2-drug PEP.	Expanded ≥ 3-drug PEP.	Generally no PEP; however consider 2-drug PEP if source with risk factors or exposure to infected person is likely.[a]	No PEP.
High-risk	Expanded ≥ 3-drug PEP.	Expanded ≥ 3-drug PEP	Generally no PEP; however consider 2-drug PEP if source with risk factors or exposure to infected person is likely.[a]	No PEP.

[a]"Consider" indicates PEP is optional and decision to initiate PEP is based on discussion of risks and benefits with treating clinician.

receiving efavirenz during the first trimester at a dose comparable to human therapeutic exposure. There have also been three case reports of neural tube defects in humans after first-trimester exposure. Its use should be avoided in the first trimester and women of childbearing potential must be counseled on the risks and avoidance of pregnancy.

Table 11-3 RECOMMENDED HIV PEP FOR MUCOCUTANEOUS MEMBRANE EXPOSURE

EXPOSURE TYPE	HIV-1	HIV-2	UNKNOWN SOURCE	HIV NEGATIVE
Small volume (few drops)	2-drug PEP.	2-drug PEP.	No PEP.	No PEP.
Large volume (major splash)	2-drug PEP.	Expanded ≥ 3-drug PEP.	Generally no PEP; however consider 2-drug PEP if source with risk factors or exposure to infected person is likely.[a]	No PEP.

[a]"Consider" indicates PEP is optional and decision to initiate PEP is based on discussion of risks and benefits with treating clinician.

Table 11–4 PRIMARY SIDE EFFECTS AND TOXICITIES ASSOCIATED WITH ANTIRETROVIRAL AGENTS

CLASS AND AGENT	SIDE EFFECT AND TOXICITY
NRTIs (nucleoside reverse transcriptase inhibitors)	
Zidovudine (Retrovir, ZDV, AZT)	Anemia, neutropenia, nausea, headache, insomnia, muscle pain/weakness
Lamivudine (Epivir, 3TC)	Abdominal pain, nausea, diarrhea, rash, and pancreatitis
Stavudine (Zerit, d4T)	Peripheral neuropathy, headache, diarrhea, nausea, pancreatitis, insomnia, elevated liver function tests (LFTs), anemia, neutropenia
Didanosine (Videx, ddI)	Pancreatitis, lactic acidosis, neuropathy, diarrhea, abdominal pain, nausea
Emtricitabine (Emtriva, FTC)	Headache, nausea, vomiting, diarrhea, rash, skin discoloration
NtRTIs (nucleoside analogue reverse transcriptase inhibitors)	
Tenofovir (Viread, TDF)	Nausea, diarrhea, vomiting, flatulence, and headache
NNRTIs (non-nucleoside reverse transcriptase inhibitors)	
Efavirenz (Sustiva, EFV)	Rash (including Steven-Johnson), insomnia, somnolence, dizziness, nightmares, and teratogenicity
Protease inhibitors	
Indinavir (Crixivan, IDV)	Abdominal pain, nephrolithiasis, and indirect hyperbilirubinemia
Nelfinavir (Viracept, NFV)	Diarrhea, nausea, abdominal pain, weakness, and rash
Ritonavir (Norvir, RTV)	Weakness, diarrhea, nausea, elevated cholesterol/triglycerides, oral paresthesia, taste alteration
Saquinavir (Invirase, SQV)	Diarrhea, abdominal pain, nausea, hyperglycemia, elevated LFTs
Atazanavir (Reyataz, ATV)	Nausea, headache, rash, abdominal pain, diarrhea, vomiting, indirect hyperbilirubinemia
Lopinavir/Ritonavir (Kaletra) LPV/RTV	Diarrhea, fatigue, headache, nausea, increased cholesterol/triglycerides
Fusion inhibitor	
Enfuvirtide (Fuzeon, T-20)	Local site reaction, bacterial pneumonia, insomnia, depression, peripheral neuropathy, cough

Delavirdine and zalcitabine (which is no longer available in the United States) are not recommended secondary to rodent studies showing potential for teratogenicity and developmental toxicity.

Nevirapine is a Class B drug and while there is no evidence of human teratogenicity, there is increased risk of rash-associated, and potential fatal liver toxicity among those with CD4 counts more than $250/mm^3$ when first initiating therapy.

The use of didanosine (Class B) and stavudine (Class B) individually have a good safety record in pregnancy. However, fatal cases of lactic acidosis have been reported when used together.

Tenofovir is a Class B drug but there is insufficient data to recommend its use. Studies in monkeys have shown decreased fetal growth and reduction in fetal bone density. Clinical studies in humans have shown bone demineralization with chronic use, especially in children. There is also significant placental passage in humans so the clinical significance is unknown.

Reyataz (atazanavir) is a Class B drug with theoretical concerns regarding increased indirect bilirubin levels which may exacerbate physiologic hyperbilirubinemia in the neonate even though transplacental passage is very low. Insufficient data currently exists to recommend its use.

Other drugs that are not recommended as of yet due to insufficient data include: darunavir, fosamprenavir, tipranavir, enfuvirtide, maraviroc, and raltegravir.

3. **Counseling an HIV-positive pregnant patient regarding means to reduce vertical transmission**

Standard criteria for initiation of antiretroviral therapy in the treatment-naïve patient according to the Department of Health and Human Services (DHHS) in 2008 are as follows: presence of an AIDS-defining illness or a CD4 count of less than 350 cells/mm, patients with HIV-associated nephropathy, or patients coinfected with hepatitis B. Clinical scenarios delineated and published by the *Public Health Service Task Force (2008)* help to describe optimal management strategies for women that are of childbearing age and are HIV positive. All scenarios reaffirm the importance of providing antiretroviral drugs during pregnancy, labor and to the infant to decrease vertical transmission. In all scenarios neonatal administration of zidovudine should be administered for 6 weeks started within 6 to 12 hours after birth.

Women receiving antiretroviral drugs that reduce HIV viral loads to less than 1000 copies/mL have a very low risk of transmission. However, viral load is not the determining factor when deciding the use of antiretroviral drugs in pregnancy because transmission can occur even at low or undetectable levels. Combination antiretroviral regimens are more effective than single-drug regimens in reducing transmission during pregnancy, so prophylactic antiretroviral drugs should be offered to all HIV-infected pregnant women, regardless of CD4 count or viral load.

Unadjusted for mode of delivery, women receiving antiretroviral therapy have an approximate 1.2% risk of vertical transmission. Among women with a viral load of less than 1000 copies/mL the transmission rate was 0.5% to 0.8% regardless of mode of delivery. ACOG has recommended that a scheduled cesarean delivery (prior to labor or ROM) at 38 weeks should be considered for all HIV-infected women with viral loads of more than 1000 copies/mL around the time of delivery. For women with a viral load less than 1000 copies/mL, data regarding the benefit of scheduled cesarean delivery has not been sufficient to prove this as the recommended mode of delivery. Prior to cesarean section zidovudine should be administered intravenously for at least 3 hours.

Factors that increase risk of transmission include elevated viral load, decreased CD4 count, and prolonged rupture of membranes. The risk of transmission increases 2% over the baseline risk for each hourly increment following membrane rupture. Therefore, assuming a baseline risk for transmission of 1%, the risk at 1 hour would be theoretically 1.02% and would increase to 1.16% at 8 hours post rupture of membranes.

4. **Recommendations for intrapartum prophylaxis**

Intrapartum management of the HIV-infected mother includes avoiding instrumentation and assisted second-stage delivery, and avoidance of placement of fetal scalp electrode and rupturing of membranes when possible. In addition an episiotomy should not be used if possible. Zidovudine is the antiretroviral drug of choice in maternal intrapartum and neonatal postpartum regimens (Tables 11–5 and 11–6).

HIV-infected women of childbearing age, but who are not currently pregnant and have indications for antiretroviral therapy should initiate therapy as per adult treatment guidelines. Drugs that have teratogenic potential or insufficient data to use in pregnancy should be avoided.

The HIV-infected woman who is antiretroviral naïve and does not require treatment for her own health should still be offered antiretroviral therapy during pregnancy and in the intrapartum period to decrease the risk of vertical transmission. Drug resistance testing is recommended prior to initiating drug therapy. One can consider delaying therapy initiation until after completion of the first trimester to decrease the risk of teratogenicity. The previously listed contraindicated drugs should be avoided, and the antiretroviral regimen used prenatally should be continued during the intrapartum period with ZDV given as a continuous infusion while

Table 11–5 MATERNAL INTRAPARTUM/POSTPARTUM

DRUG	DOSING	DURATION
Zidovudine (ZDV, AZT)	2 mg/kg IV over 1 h, followed by continuous infusion of 1 mg/kg per hour.	Onset of labor until delivery of infant.

Table 11–6 NEONATAL		
DRUG	**DOSING**	**DURATION**
> 35 wk infant zidovudine (ZDV, AZT)	2 mg/kg orally (or 1.5 mg/kg intravenously) started as close to birth as possible, then every 6 h.	Birth to 6 wk.
30-35 wk infant zidovudine (ZDV, AZT)	2 mg/kg orally (or 1.5 mg/kg intravenously) started as close to birth as possible, then every 12 h, advanced to every 8 h at 2 wk of age.	Birth to 6 wk.
< 30 wk zidovudine (ZDV, AZT)	2 mg/kg orally (or 1.5 mg/kg intravenously) started as close to birth as possible every 12 h, advanced to every 8 h at 4 wk of age.	Birth to 6 wk.

other agents are continued orally. Drug therapy should be discontinued postpartum unless there is an indication for continued therapy.

The patient that is HIV-infected and antiretroviral naïve who has indications for antiretroviral therapy for maternal health reasons should also have drug resistance testing prior to initiation of therapy. Therapy should be started in this group of patients immediately even if medications must begin during the first trimester.

The infected mother who is receiving antiretroviral therapy and becomes pregnant should continue her regimen if it is suppressing the virus unless she is taking efavirenz or other potentially teratogenic drugs in the first trimester. Also to be avoided is the combination of didanosine and stavudine which have the potential for adverse effects to the mother. If viremia is not being successfully suppressed, drug resistance testing should be done. As a general rule drug therapy should not be halted in the first trimester. As with other HIV-positive patients, zidovudine should be given as a continuous infusion during labor while other antiretroviral agents are continued orally and in the postpartum period.

The pregnant woman who is HIV-infected and has had prior exposure to antiretroviral therapy but is not receiving therapy at the time of conception should have a complete history. Assessment should be made as to whether antiretroviral therapy is necessary for the health of the mother. Antiretroviral therapy should be started after resistance testing and continued as described in the preceding discussion during the intrapartum and postpartum period if indicated.

The HIV-infected woman who has received no antiretroviral therapy prior to presenting in labor should have one of the following regimens instituted: (1) zidovudine given to the mother intravenously and the infant for 6 weeks started within 6 to 12 hours after birth; or (2) zidovudine given as a continuous infusion during labor plus single-dose nevirapine at labor onset with single dose nevirapine plus zidovudine for the infant for 6 weeks. This regimen increases the risk of nevirapine resistance. Evaluation of the mother in the postpartum period should be undertaken to assess need for continued antiretroviral therapy.

An HIV-infected mother who presents after 36 weeks, is not on antiretroviral therapy, and in whom the viral load and CD4 count is unknown and will likely not be available prior to delivery should be started on antiretroviral therapy. She should be counseled that a scheduled cesarean section will likely reduce vertical transmission risk. The cesarean section should be scheduled at 38 weeks' gestation on the best available dating information. Prior to surgery zidovudine should be started 3 hours prior to surgery and the infant should be treated as discussed in the preceding discussion. Prophylactic antibiotics at the time of cesarean section are recommended and continued antiretroviral therapy in the postpartum period is dictated by the CD4 count and viral load when they become available.

The HIV-infected woman who has elected a scheduled cesarean delivery but who presents in early labor or soon after rupture of membranes should have intravenous zidovudine started immediately. The decision to allow vaginal delivery or proceed to cesarean section should be made in the context of available clinical information such as how rapidly labor is progressing and how long membrane rupture has occurred.

Rapid testing for women in labor who presents with unknown HIV status is available and accurate. This allows the pregnant women to learn her HIV status and receive antiretroviral prophylaxis during labor and be referred for further workup postpartum. Antiretroviral therapy should be started immediately after a positive rapid HIV test result.

HIV transmission via breast milk has been well-documented and there is no safe way to treat breast milk to eliminate the virus and allow safe breastfeeding. The Public Health Service does not recommend breastfeeding for HIV-infected women in the United States, where safe and affordable alternatives are available.

Comprehension Questions

11.1   A 30-year-old surgical resident who is 10 weeks' pregnant is stuck by a needle from a patient who is known to be HIV positive. Which of the following serological testing for the source patient is appropriate?
   A. Hepatitis A
   B. Hepatitis C
   C. Cytomegalovirus
   D. Herpes simplex virus

11.2   Which of the following antiretroviral drugs or drug combinations has the best safety profile in pregnancy?
   A. Efavirenz
   B. Delavirdine
   C. Didanosine with stavudine
   D. Nelfinavir

11.3   Which of the following should be a part of intrapartum management of an HIV-infected mother?
   A. Intravenous administration of zidovudine as part of medication in labor
   B. Early rupture of membranes
   C. Placement of a scalp electrode
   D. Instrumentation to assist second-stage of labor

ANSWERS

11.1   **B.** Regardless of whether PEP has been administered, the health care worker should be offered postexposure counseling (including psychological counseling), testing, and medical evaluation. Antibody testing using ELISA should be used for seroconversion monitoring at baseline, 6 weeks, 12 weeks, and 6 months after exposure. It is not required that the source patient be offered counseling. Hepatitis B and C and HIV viral load should be performed on the source patient.

11.2   **D.** While not the preferred protease inhibitor to be used in pregnancy, nelfinavir is the only above mentioned drug that has demonstrated a good safety profile for the mother and infant and has not demonstrated human teratogenicity. Efavirenz has been associated with anencephaly, neural tube defects, anophthalmia, and cleft palate. Rodent studies have shown potential for carcinogenicity and teratogenicity with the use of delavirdine. There have been cases of fatal lactic acidosis with the use of didanosine and stavudine in combination.

11.3   **A.** Intravenous administration of zidovudine is the cornerstone of therapy to decrease HIV vertical transmission. The Pediatric AIDS Clinical Trials Group protocol (PACTG) 076 demonstrated that the use of zidovudine in the antepartum and intrapartum periods and then administration to the newborn decreased transmission by approximately 70%. Intrapartum management of the HIV-infected mother includes avoiding instrumentation and assisted second-stage delivery as well as avoidance of placement of a fetal scalp electrode and artificial rupture of membranes if possible. In addition an episiotomy should not be used if possible.

Clinical Pearls

See US Preventive Services Task Force Study Quality levels of evidence in Case 1

➤ Any pt who experiences a needle stick should be offered post exposure counseling (Level III).

➤ Nelfinavir is the protease inhibitor that has been shown to have a good safety profile for the mother and infant (Level II-2).

➤ Route of delivery for HIV infected pregnant women depends on the viral load and prenatal medication use (Level II-3).

REFERENCES

1. Scheduled cesarean delivery and the prevention of vertical transmission of HIV infection. ACOG Committee Opinion Number 234, May 2000. *Obstet Gynecol.* 2001;73:279-281.
2. Baggaley RF, Boily MC, White RG, Alary M. Risk of HIV-1 transmission for parenteral exposure and blood transfusion: a systematic review and meta-analysis. *AIDS.* 2006;20:805-812.
3. Boyce JM, Pittet D. Guideline for hand hygiene in health-care settings. Recommendations of the healthcare infection control practices advisory committee and HICPAC/SHEA/APIC/IDSA hand hygiene task force. *MMWR Recomm Rep.* 2005;51(RR-16):1-45.
4. Bulterys M, Jamieson DJ, O'Sullivan MJ, et al. Rapid HIV-1 testing during labor: a multicenter study. *JAMA.* 2004;292:219-223.
5. Cardo DM, Culver DH, Ciesielski CA, et al. A case-control study of HIV seroconversion in health care workers after percutaneous exposure. *NEJM.* 1997;337:1485-1490.
6. CDC. Updated US Public Health service guidelines for the management of occupational exposures to HIV and recommendations for postexposure prophylaxis. *MMWR.* 2005;54: 1-17.
7. CDC. Antiretroviral postexposure prophylaxis after sexual, injection-drug use, or other nonoccupational exposure to HIV in the United States. *MMWR.* 2005;54:1-19.

8. Conner EM, Sperling RS, Gelber R, et al. Reduction of maternal-infant transmission of human immunodeficiency virus type 1 with zidovudine treatment. Pediatric AIDS Clinical Trials Group Protocol 076 Study Group. *NEJM*. 1994;331:1173-1180.

9. Cooper ER, Chaurat M, Mofenson LM, et al. Combination antiretroviral strategies for the treatment of pregnant HIV-1 infected women and prevention of perinatal HIV-1 transmission. *J Acquir Immune Defic Syndr Hum Retrovirol*. 2002:55:592-597.

10. DHHS Panel on Retroviral Guidelines for Adults and Adolescents-A working group of the Office of AIDS Research Advisory Council. Guidelines for the use of antiretroviral agents in HIV-1 infected adults and adolescents. AIDSinfo.nih.gov January, 2008. 1-127.

11. European Collaborative Study. Mother-to-child transmission of HIV infection in the era of highly active antiretroviral therapy. *Clin Infect Dis*. 2005;40:458-465.

12. Makary MA, Al-Attar A, Holzmueller CG, et al. Needlestick injuries among surgeons in training. *NEJM*. 2007;356:2693-2699.

13. Parkin JM, Murphy M, Anderson J, El-Gadi S, Forster G, Pinching AJ. Tolerability and side-effects of post-exposure prophylaxis for HIV infection. *Lancet*. 2000;355:722-723.

14. Public Health Service Task Force. Recommendations for use of antiretroviral drugs in pregnant HIV-infected women for maternal health and interventions to reduce perinatal HIV transmissions in the United States. AIDSinfo.nih.gov July, 2008. 1-98.

15. Shapiro D, Tuomala R, Pollack H, et al. Mother-to child HIV transmission risk according to antiretroviral therapy, mode of delivery, and viral load in 2895 US women (PACTG 367). 11th Conference on retroviruses and Opportunistic Infections; February 8-11, 2004; San Fancisco, CA. Abstract 99.

Case 12

A 17-year-old primigravida presents in labor with no prenatal care. By her LMP, she is 39 weeks' gestation, but bedside ultrasound reveals a symmetrically grown fetus with normal amniotic fluid volume, estimated fetal weight of 2300 g, and estimated gestational age of 34 weeks. She denies medical problems or drug usage prior to or during pregnancy. Her vital signs are normal and she rapidly progresses from 6 cm dilation to spontaneous vaginal delivery of a 2390 g male infant with Apgar score of 7/8. On examination of the neonate, the pediatrician estimates the gestational age to be 39 to 40 weeks and notes hepatosplenomegaly and a petechial rash over the infant's trunk and extremities.

➤ What is the most likely diagnosis?

➤ What is your next step?

➤ What are potential complications of the patient's disorder?

ANSWERS TO CASE 12:

Congenital Infection of the Neonate

Summary: This 17-year-old primigravida with a negative medical history delivered a symmetrically growth-restricted infant at term with evidence of thrombocytopenia and hepatosplenomegaly after a pregnancy with no prenatal care.

➤ **Most likely diagnosis:** Congenital cytomegalovirus infection.

➤ **Next step:** Evaluate patient for acute, chronic infection.

➤ **Potential complications:** Potential infectivity to other patients, staff; risk of recurrence in subsequent pregnancy; long-term effects to neonate.

ANALYSIS

Objectives

1. Recognize the prenatal patient at risk for delivering an infant with a congenital infection.
2. Understand noninvasive and invasive testing appropriate to evaluate the potentially infected prenatal patient.
3. Describe the labor management of the patient at risk for a congenitally infected neonate.
4. Discuss the risk of recurrence of congenital infection in subsequent pregnancies.

Considerations

While most pregnant patients who deliver congenitally infected infants have had no identifiable risk factors before delivery, specific situations occur that do pose additional risk. In addition to routine testing at the initial prenatal visit for hepatitis B, syphilis, gonorrhea, *Chlamydia*, HIV, and rubella, careful history at that time may reveal risk factors for, or prior infection with, other potential pathogens including group B β-hemolytic *Streptococcus* (GBS), herpes simplex virus (HSV), hepatitis C, and toxoplasmosis. During pregnancy, a nondescript viral type illness may indicate the presence of toxoplasmosis, parvovirus, hepatitis B or C, or CMV that, depending on the trimester, could pose devastating effects on the fetus.

The congenitally infected fetus may demonstrate impaired growth in a symmetrical fashion, as opposed to the asymmetrically growth-restricted infant whose impaired growth is due to placental inadequacy. The congenitally infected fetus may also demonstrate anomalies including hydrops, intracranial calcifications, ventriculomegaly or hydrocephalus, cardiac anomalies, and bony abnormalities.

At delivery, the neonate that is small for gestational age without obvious prenatal etiology, has consistently low Apgar scores at 5 and 10 minutes with no evidence of intrapartum cause, and/or has a rash or petechiae should be brought to the attention of the pediatrician for further evaluation for potential congenital infection. An ongoing discussion between the obstetrician and pediatrician should ensue to determine if isolation of neonate or mother is warranted, and if further maternal testing would assist the pediatrician in determining the underlying cause of the neonate's appearance at birth.

APPROACH TO
Congenital Infection of the Neonate

If not previously performed at her first prenatal visit, the patient whose previous child has been affected with a congenital infection should be evaluated for the potential for recurrence. The development of maternal antibodies to rubella and parvovirus protect future fetuses and make the recurrence of toxoplasmosis and hepatitis B unlikely. Hepatitis C and HSV become much less likely to recur with the presence of maternal antibodies, and the potential for antibiotic-induced eradication of syphilis, gonorrhea, *Chlamydia*, and *Listeria* makes recurrence of these infections potentially preventable. Antibiotic prophylaxis to reduce vaginal colonization with GBS reduces the risk of neonatal infection with this bacteria, and antenatal and intrapartum prophylaxis with appropriate antivirals reduces the risk of vertical transmission with HIV.

Table 12–1 lists various agents responsible for congenital infection, the baseline population risk of congenital infection, the method to confirm diagnosis, and risk of congenital infection with an acute infection during pregnancy if no treatment is offered (or available). While routine screening is obtained for many of these infectious agents, others will be detected only with a high index of suspicion. Table 12–2 lists reasons why a potential agent that causes congenital infection may come to the attention of the obstetrician and necessitate further testing.

CMV Infection

Cytomegalovirus (CMV) is the most common congenital infection worldwide. It is found in many secretions, and daycare centers are common locations of acquisition of the infection. Primary infection with CMV is associated with a higher viral load and a risk factor for congenital infection. After the primary infection, the virus can be dormant and have periodic reactivation. Viral shedding occurs despite the presence of IgG antibody. Pregnant women are often asymptomatic; however, 10% to 15% of infected women

Table 12–1 INCIDENCE OF CONGENITAL INFECTION AND DETECTION METHODS

AGENT	INCIDENCE OF CONGENITAL INFECTION	METHOD TO DETECT RISK OF FETAL/ NEONATAL INFECTION	RISK OF CONGENITAL INFECTION
Rubella	Rare	Amniocentesis/PCR	80-100 (first trimester); 10-20 (second trimester); 60 (third trimester)
Hepatitis B virus	~1/100,000	HBsAg+ with/without HBeAg+ mother at time of delivery	70%-90% if mother HBsAg and HBeAg +; 10%-20% if mother HBsAg +, HBeAg −
Hepatitis C virus	Rare	Maternal HCV antibodies and/or HCV-RNA.	4.6%-10%; 2-7× higher if co-infected with HIV
Gonorrhea	Up to 2% of pregnant women infected	Nucleic acid amplification tests; nucleic acid hybridization	30% risk of ophthalmia neonatorum without prophylaxis
Chlamydia	Up to 12% of pregnant women infected	Nucleic acid amplification tests; nucleic acid hybridization	50% if chlamydial cervicitis
Syphilis	8.5/100,000	Maternal serology	60%-90% in untreated maternal primary, secondary syphilis
GBS	0.5-1/1000	Vaginal/rectal culture	If mother vaginal/ rectal + : 50% rate of neonatal colonization and 1% rate of early onset sepsis
Toxoplasmosis	3/1000	Maternal serology; amniotic fluid PCR	17% in first trimester; 25% in second trimester; 65% in third trimester
CMV	1.5-20/1000	Maternal serology with IgG avidity; amniotic fluid PCR	50% with primary infection in any trimester

(Continued)

Table 12–1 INCIDENCE OF CONGENITAL INFECTION AND DETECTION METHODS (CONT.)

AGENT	INCIDENCE OF CONGENITAL INFECTION	METHOD TO DETECT RISK OF FETAL/ NEONATAL INFECTION	RISK OF CONGENITAL INFECTION
Parvovirus B19	1-2/100	Maternal serology; amniotic fluid PCR	With maternal seroconversion, 3.9% will have hydrops
HIV	< 400 annually in United States	Maternal serology	26%
Herpes simplex virus	1:3200	Viral culture or PCR assay of lesion	30%-50% if subclinically shedding virus from infection acquired during third trimester compared to 3% of symptomatic reactivation of HSV during labor
Listeria	Rare	Bacterial culture	50%-100%
Enterovirus	Rare	Viral culture or PCR assay	Up to 3% during seasonal outbreaks

develop a mono-like illness with fatigue, lymphadenopathy, elevated liver function tests, fever, and pharyngitis.

Primary infection, associated with higher viral load, is associated with a 40% to 50% fetal transmission, and can lead to significant morbidity and mortality. Reactivation is associated with only a 1% risk of vertical transmission. With such a high prevalence of CMV infection, thankfully, most neonates are asymptomatic. Only 5% manifest the severe congenital syndrome of IUGR, microcephaly, intracranial calcifications, mental retardation, sensorneural deficits, hepatosplenomegaly, and jaundice. Nevertheless, some of the asymptomatic neonates will develop learning disabilities or neurological deficits later in childhood.

The diagnosis of maternal infection with CMV is established with paired acute and convalescent titers. CMV-specific IgM antibody is diagnostic of acute infection; also a fourfold rise in IgG titer is likewise diagnostic. Viral culture is not generally helpful. Suspicion of fetal infection is raised by IUGR, microcephaly, cerebral calcifications, ascites, hyperechoic bowel, and oligohydramnios. Amniotic fluid assay for PCR of the CMV DNA is considered the test of choice.

Table 12–2 FINDINGS THAT SUGGEST NEED FOR FURTHER EVALUATION FOR INFECTION

AGENT	ROUTINE PRENATAL SCREENING? (Y/N)	FINDINGS THAT INDICATE NEED FOR FURTHER EVALUATION
Rubella	Yes	Rash, suboccipital adenopathy, seroconversion; US evidence of IUGR, congenital heart disease
Hepatitis B virus	Yes	Maternal jaundice, elevated LFTs
Hepatitis C virus	No	Acute non-A, non-B hepatitis
Gonorrhea	Yes	Positive screen; vaginitis
Chlamydia	Yes	Positive screen; cervicitis
Syphilis	Yes	Positive serology; hydrops, polyhydramnios, stillbirth
GBS	Yes	Intrapartum fever; UTI
Toxoplasmosis	No	Ventriculomegaly; IUGR, ascites, lymphadenopathy
CMV	No	Ventriculomegaly; microcephaly, IUGR, intracranial calcification; echogenic bowel
Parvovirus B19	No	Maternal seroconversion followed by fetal hydrops
HIV	Yes	Maternal serology
Herpes simplex virus	No	Lesions or symptoms during pregnancy
Listeria	No	Fever, premature birth, stillbirth
Enterovirus	No	Hydrops; decreased fetal movement; fetal tachycardia

The treatment of a pregnant woman infected by CMV is supportive. In situations where a primary infection that is discovered, the patient should be offered amniocentesis testing. Counseling should be careful since although the transmission with primary infection is high, the likelihood of a normal neonate is also very high. There is currently no vaccine. Antiviral therapy has not been shown to decrease vertical transmission. Some limited data suggest that CMV-specific IgG may decrease vertical transmission, although more studies are needed. The focus on congenital CMV is currently prevention. Antiviral therapy to the infected neonate may decrease the risk of later sequelae.

Other Infections

When an agent that may cause congenital infection has been identified during a pregnancy, it is important to determine if therapy is indicated and if specific prenatal evaluations should be avoided to minimize infectious risk to the fetus. Table 12–3 lists infectious agents, whether therapy is available, and the risk of congenital infection if optimal therapy is administered. Table 12–4 lists those infectious agents and activities that may affect the risk of vertical transmission. The patient will often inquire about the safety of lactation and the possibility of congenital infection. Aside from maternal HIV infection or cracked/bleeding nipples where blood-borne pathogens may be an issue, breast-feeding is safe.

When a fetus is suspected of having acquired a congenital infection, the potential effects of that infection should be discussed with the parents. While there are many determinants of the severity of fetal infection including the nature of the infectious agent, general rules are that primary maternal infections and earlier trimester of acquisition seem to be most important.

Once the neonate is delivered and the pediatricians have determined the presence of a congenital infection, the parents should be informed about the risk of recurrence and activities they may undertake to reduce or prevent recurrence. Table 12–5 lists various agents and the effects of congenital infection and risk of recurrence in subsequent pregnancies.

Table 12–3 RISK OF CONGENITAL INFECTION WITH OPTIMAL THERAPY

AGENT	POTENTIAL THERAPY? (Y/N)	RISK OF CONGENITAL INFECTION WITH OPTIMAL PERINATAL THERAPY
Rubella	No	> 80% in first trimester; rare > 16 wk
Hepatitis B virus	Hepatitis B immune globulin (HBIG), HB vaccine after birth	1%-2% if mother HBsAg +, HBeAg −; 5%-10% if HBsAg and HBeAg +
Hepatitis C virus	No	4.6%-10%; 2-7× higher if coinfected with HIV
Gonorrhea	Yes	< 5%
Chlamydia	Yes	5%-20% risk of pneumonia
Syphilis	Yes	< 5% risk of congenital infection
GBS	Yes	Rare
Toxoplasmosis	Yes	Spiramycin reduces by 60%
CMV	Yes	16%
Parvovirus B19	Yes	PUBS may treat fetal anemia
HIV	Yes	< 1%-2%
Herpes simplex virus	Yes	1%-2%
Listeria	Yes	Unknown
Enterovirus	No	Up to 3% during seasonal outbreaks

Table 12–4 ACTIVITIES THAT MAY AFFECT VERTICAL TRANSMISSION

AGENT	DOES AMNIOCENTESIS INCREASE, DECREASE, OR NOT EFFECT RISK OF VERTICAL TRANSMISSION?	DOES AROM INCREASE RISK OF VERTICAL TRANSMISSION?	SHOULD FSE BE AVOIDED?	IS CESAREAN SECTION INDICATED IN PRESENCE OF INFECTION?	MAY MOTHER BREAST-FEED?
Rubella	No effect	No	No effect	No	Yes
Hepatitis B virus	No/low effect	Possibly	May increase	No	Yes
Hepatitis C virus	No/low effect	Possibly	May increase	No	Yes, unless nipples are cracked or bleeding
Gonorrhea	No effect	May increase with prolonged rupture of membrane (ROM)	Scalp abscess if active infection	No	Yes
Chlamydia	No effect	May increase with prolonged ROM	No effect	No	Yes
Syphilis	No effect	No effect	No effect	No	Yes
GBS	No effect	May increase with prolonged ROM	May increase	No	Yes

(Continued)

Table 12–4 ACTIVITIES THAT MAY AFFECT VERTICAL TRANSMISSION (CONT.)

AGENT	DOES AMNIOCENTESIS INCREASE, DECREASE, OR NOT EFFECT RISK OF VERTICAL TRANSMISSION?	DOES AROM INCREASE RISK OF VERTICAL TRANSMISSION?	SHOULD FSE BE AVOIDED?	IS CESAREAN SECTION INDICATED IN PRESENCE OF INFECTION?	MAY MOTHER BREAST-FEED?
Toxoplasmosis	No effect	No effect	No effect	No	Yes
CMV	No effect	Possibly	No effect	No	Yes
Parvovirus B19	No effect	No effect	No effect	No	Yes
HIV	No definite effect	May increase with prolonged ROM	Yes	Yes, when viral load is > 1000 copies/mL	No
Herpes simplex virus	No effect	May increase with prolonged ROM	Yes	Yes	Yes
Listeria	No effect	No effect	No	No	Yes
Enterovirus	No effect	No effect	No	No	Yes

Table 12–5 EFFECTS OF CONGENITAL INFECTION AND RISK OF RECURRENCE

AGENT	EFFECTS OF CONGENITAL INFECTION	RISK OF RECURRENCE
Rubella	IUGR, deafness, cataracts, CHD, mental retardation	Extremely rare
Hepatitis B virus	Cirrhosis, hepatocellular carcinoma	Extremely rare
Hepatitis C virus	Chronic liver disease	4.6%-10%; 2-7× higher if coinfected with HIV
Gonorrhea	Ophthalmia neonatorum	Depends on TOC
Chlamydia	Ophthalmia neonatorum; pneumonia	Depends on TOC
Syphilis	IUGR; stillbirth; bony abnormalities	Depends on TOC
GBS	Pneumonia/sepsis/meningitis	Based on colonization and prophylaxis in subsequent pregnancy
Toxoplasmosis	Chorioretinitis; hydrocephalus	Extremely rare
CMV	Seizures, chorioretinitis, sensorineural hearing loss	2-20/1000
Parvovirus B19	Stillbirth if anemia severe; no long-term effects expected	Extremely rare
HIV	HIV; AIDS	< 1%-2%
Herpes simplex virus	Skin/eye/mucus membrane involvement; CNS involvement; disseminated infection	3%
Listeria	Preterm birth; stillbirth	Extremely rare
Enterovirus	Myocarditis; encephalitis	Extremely rare

Comprehension Questions

12.1   A 27-year-old G2P1 woman at 8 weeks' gestation is seen for her first
       prenatal visit. Her first pregnancy was complicated by a neonate with
       congenital toxoplasmosis. Which of the following statements dealing
       with recurrence is the most appropriate?
       A. "You should have your housecats tested for toxoplasmosis."
       B. "The risk of recurrence is extremely low."
       C. "We will need to retest you for toxoplasmosis antibodies."
       D. "You will need prophylactic antibiotics near term."

12.2   The most common fetal presentation of parvovirus B19 infection is
       which of the following?
       A. Hypoplastic left heart
       B. Skeletal dysplasia
       C. Ventriculomegaly
       D. Hydrops fetalis

12.3   A 24-year-old G1P1 woman is inquiring about whether it is acceptable
       for her to breast-feed. Breast-feeding is contraindicated in which of
       the following maternal infections?
       A. HIV
       B. Hepatitis B virus
       C. Hepatitis C virus
       D. Group B *Streptococcus*
       E. Syphilis

12.4   Which of the following organisms cannot be completely eradicated
       from the pregnant woman with antibiotics?
       A. *Neisseria gonorrhea*
       B. *Chlamydia trachomatis*
       C. *Treponema pallidum*
       D. Group B *Streptococcus*

ANSWERS

12.1   **B.** Patients with a history of delivering a neonate with congenital
       toxoplasmosis develop antibodies to the parasite. These antibodies
       enable them to convey immunity to future pregnancies and can be
       reassured that recurrence of congenital infection is extremely rare.
       Testing cats for toxoplasmosis provides no useful information to aid
       with pregnancy management, and maternal antibody status will be
       positive (because of her history) and thus not necessary to evaluate.

12.2   **D.** Fetal parvovirus infection causes severe anemia and myocarditis, both of which may be responsible for congestive heart failure and hydrops. Structural anomalies are not associated with congenital parvovirus infection.

12.3   **A.** Because of the availability of clean water and infant formula, breast-feeding in developed countries is contraindicated in women who are HIV positive. In developing nations with poor or contaminated water supplies and erratic availability of appropriate formula, breastfeeding is sometimes recommended.

12.4   **D.** Group B *Streptococcus* resides in the vagina and rectum, and is rarely eradicated with antibiotics. Thus, during each pregnancy, even with a history of antibiotic therapy, reevaluation of the vaginal and rectal flora is indicated.

Clinical Pearls

See US Preventive Services Task Force Study Quality levels of evidence in Case 1

➤ The fetus with no structural anatomic abnormalities found to have nonimmune hydrops fetalis should be evaluated for congenital infection (Level II-3).

➤ The neonate with low Apgar score, growth restriction, and petechiae should be carefully evaluated by pediatrics for congenital infection (Level II-2).

➤ Maternal HIV rarely results in an infected neonate when antenatal and intrapartum evaluations and antiviral medications are appropriately administered (Level I).

➤ Invasive diagnostic procedures, such as amniocentesis, may be offered in all situations of maternal infection, after careful counseling with the parents regarding actual and theoretical risks (Level III).

➤ Cesarean section solely because of the presence of maternal infection is indicated only in selected cases of HIV and HSV (Level I).

➤ The most common congenital infection is cytomegalovirus (Level II-2).

REFERENCES

1. Adler SP, Nigro G, Pereira L. Recent advances in the prevention and treatment of congenital cytomegalovirus infections. *Semin Perinatol.* 2007 Feb;31(1):10-18.
2. Alexander JM, Sheffield JS, Sanchez PJ, et al: Efficacy of treatment for syphilis in pregnancy. *Obstet Gynecol.* 1999;93:5.
3. Bialek SR, Armstrong GL, Williams IT. Hepatitis C virus. In: Long S, ed. *Principles and Practice of Pediatric Infectious Diseases*. 3rd ed. Philadelphia, PA: Churchill Livingstone; 2008.

4. Brown ZA, Gardella C, Wald A, Morrow RA, Corey L. Genital herpes complicating pregnancy. *Obstet Gynecol.* 2005;106:845-856.

5. Centers for Disease Control and Prevention: Achievements in public health: elimination of rubella and congenital rubella syndrome—United States, 1969-2004. *MWR.* 2005;54:279-282.

6. Centers for Disease Control and Prevention. *Sexually Transmitted Disease Surveillance, 2006.* Atlanta, GA: US Department of Health and Human Services, November 2007.

7. Darville T. Chlamydia trachomatis. In: Long S, ed. *Principles and Practice of Pediatric Infectious Diseases.* 3rd ed. Philadelphia, PA: Churchill Livingstone; 2008.

8. de Jong E, de Haan TR, Kroes ACM, Beersma MFC, Oepkes D, Walther FJ. Parvovirus B19 infection in pregnancy. *J Clin Virol.* 2006;36:1-7.

9. Gambarin-Gelwan M. Hepatitis B in pregnancy. *Clin Liver Dis.* 2007;11:945-963.

10. Geisler WM, James AB. Chlamydial and gonococcal infections in women seeking pregnancy testing at family-planning clinics. *Am J Obstet Gynecol.* 2008;198:502.e1-502.e4.

11. MacDonald PDM, Whitwam RE, Boggs JD, et al. Outbreak of listeriosis among Mexican immigrants as a result of consumption of illicitly produced Mexican-style cheese. *Clin Infect Dis.* 2005 Mar 1;40(5):677-682.

12. Mendelson E, Aboudyb Y, Smetana Z, Tepperberg M, Grossman Z. Laboratory assessment and diagnosis of congenital viral infections: rubella, cytomegalovirus (CMV), varicella-zoster virus (VZV), herpes simplex virus (HSV), parvovirus B19 and human immunodeficiency virus (HIV). *Reprod Toxicol.* 2006;21:350-382.

13. Modlin JF, Polk BF, Horton P, et al: Perinatal echovirus 11 infection: risk of transmission during a community outbreak. *N Engl J Med.* 1981;305:368-371.

14. Montoya J, Rosso F. Diagnosis and management of toxoplasmosis. *Clin Perinatol.* 2005;32:705-726.

15. Munro SC, Hall B, Whybin LR, et al. Diagnosis of and screening for cytomegalovirus infection in pregnant women. *J Clin Microbiol.* 2005 Sept;4713-4718.

16. Nigro G, Adler SP, La Torre R, et al. Passive immunization during pregnancy for congenital cytomegalovirus. *N Engl J Med.* 2005;353:1350-1362.

17. Ouellet A, Sherlock R, Toye B, Fung KF. Antenatal diagnosis of intrauterine infection with coxsackievirus B3 associated with live birth. *Infect Dis Obstet Gynecol.* 2004;12(1):23-26.

18. Pembrey Lucy, Newell Marie-Louise, Tovo Pier-Angelo, and the EPHN Collaborators. The management of HCV infected pregnant women and their children. *J Hepatol.* 2005;43:515-525.

19. Tang JW, Aarons E, Hesketh LM, et al. Prenatal diagnosis of congenital rubella infection in the second trimester of pregnancy. *Prenat Diagn.* 2003;23:509-512.

20. Viral hepatitis in pregnancy. ACOG Practice Bulletin No. 86. American College of Obstetricians and Gynecologists. *Obstet Gynecol.* 2007;110:941-955.

21. Watts DH. Management of human immunodeficiency virus infection in pregnancy. *N Engl J Med.* 2002;346:1879-1891.

Case 13

A 22-year-old G2P1 woman is seen in the office at 18 weeks' gestation after noting a week of anorexia, nausea, vomiting, and dark-colored urine. She also feels her skin and sclera have become jaundiced. She has noted mild pruritus, but no right upper quadrant (RUQ) pain or pharyngitis. She has been your patient for a number of years and has no history of prescription medications, drug or alcohol abuse, blood transfusions, or sexually transmitted infections (STIs). She knows no one with a similar illness and is monogamous with her husband. She works as a scrub tech in your hospital and has received the full hepatitis B immunization series. She cannot remember the last time she was stuck by a needle in the operating room (OR), but was recently exposed to blood of a liver transplant patient when it soaked through the cuff of her surgical gown.

She denies travel other than a week's trip to the beach 1 month ago where she ate both fried shrimp and raw oysters. Her 2-year-old daughter attends day care and neither her daughter nor her husband has been noted to be sick recently.

➤ What is the most likely diagnosis?

➤ What is your next step?

➤ What are the potential complications of the patient's disorder?

ANSWERS TO CASE 13:
Hepatitis A During Pregnancy

Summary: This 22-year-old patient became jaundiced with nausea, vomiting, and pruritus after ingesting raw shellfish within the previous month and may have contracted hepatitis A by the fecal-oral route. Alternatively, this patient may have contracted hepatitis A from contact with her asymptomatic daughter who possibly became infected at the day care center (epidemics possible in day cares where a portion of the children require diaper changes; the majority of infected children are either asymptomatic or have subclinical infection).

➤ **Most likely diagnosis:** Hepatitis A.

➤ **Next step:** Obtain hepatitis serologies and liver function tests in order to make an exact diagnosis and other laboratory studies in order to determine severity of illness and whether hospitalization is required.

➤ **Potential complications:** Care for acute viral hepatitis in pregnancy is entirely supportive. Fulminant hepatitic failure in pregnancy is rare, but patients with a prolonged prothrombin time (PT) and other evidence of acute hepatitic failure should be hospitalized. Patients should be educated on preventive measures and behaviors that will prevent transmission of hepatitis infection to others.

ANALYSIS

Objectives

1. Be able to advise patients about hepatitis risk after various exposures.
2. Understand the evaluation of the pregnant patient with evidence of liver disease.
3. Be able to counsel a hepatitis-positive patient about means to reduce vertical or postpartum transmission.
4. Understand recommendations for prophylaxis against various forms of hepatitis.

Considerations

This 22-year-old, G2P1 presented at 18 weeks' gestation with signs and symptoms of acute hepatitis including anorexia, nausea, vomiting, dark urine, jaundice, and mild pruritus. She had received the full hepatitis B vaccination series, which generates immunity to hepatitis B in over 90% of recipients. Immunity to hepatitis B infection (HBV) also prevents acquisition of hepatitis D (HDV) infection. She had no history of recent needlesticks or blood transfusions, intravenous drug abuse, sexually transmitted diseases, and is in a monogamous relationship, thus making her at low risk for contracting hepatitis C (HCV). Her only stated possible risk factor for HCV was her recent exposure to blood via exposure to a liver transplant patient's blood which soaked through her cuff (in the United States, liver failure due to chronic HCV is the most common indication for liver transplantation). However, she would have to have had a break in her skin for this blood-soaked cuff to place her at risk for contracting HCV. This patient denied travel to foreign countries where hepatitis E (HEV) is endemic, thus making HEV highly unlikely. She does have a risk factor for HAV by virtue of her history of having eaten raw oysters (or other raw or undercooked shellfish); the fried shrimp should have posed no risk since they were well-cooked unless they happened to be handled by a restaurant worker actively infected with HAV who had used substandard hygienic measures (inadequate hand-washing after using the bathroom) after the shrimp were prepared. In this circumstance, any food (not just shellfish) may be a vector for infection if handled by an infectious food service worker after it has been prepared. HAV is transmitted via fecal-oral route. Alternatively, a less obvious risk factor for HAV infection may have been the fact that her 2-year-old daughter is in day care; outbreaks of HAV in day care centers have been well documented, though they are decreasing as adoption of the Advisory Committee on Immunization Practices (ACIP) recommendation for routine infant vaccination for HAV is becoming more common. The majority of HAV infections in children are asymptomatic or are subclinical. This patient may have contracted HAV after fecal-oral contamination from her daughter after changing a diaper. In a study of adults who did not have an identifiable source, 52% lived in a household with a child younger than 6 years of age. Since this patient is not taking any prescription medications, a drug-induced hepatitis is excluded. Because this patient is in the mid-second trimester of pregnancy, pregnancy complications such as acute fatty liver of pregnancy and HELLP syndrome which may cause gastrointestinal signs and symptoms are not part of the differential diagnosis.

Since this patient's history is most consistent with an acute viral hepatitis, serologies should be done to make a specific diagnosis, including hepatitis B surface antigen (HBsAg), IgM antibody to hepatitis B core antigen (IgM anti-HBc), IgM antibody to hepatitis A (IgM anti-HAV), and antibody to hepatitis C (anti-HCV). Anti-HCV should be repeated if serologies fail to establish a diagnosis and no other cause can be found, since anti-HCV may not be present until 6 to 10 weeks after the onset of symptoms. In this patient, only the IgM anti-HAV would return positive, establishing a diagnosis of acute hepatitis A infection.

Other laboratories that should be drawn in this patient include serum aminotransferases (AST and ALT), fractionated bilirubin levels, complete blood cell count and differential, and a prothrombin time. An elevated PT signifies more extensive liver damage and confers a worse prognosis, and the degree of liver damage does not always correlate with the size of elevations in serum aminotransferase levels.

In this patient who presented with signs and symptoms of acute HAV infection, immunoprophylaxis with immunoglobulin (Ig) or hepatitis A vaccine would not be helpful or necessary; she will develop a natural lifelong immunity as her infection resolves. However, close family contacts such as her husband and child are at risk for acute infection and should receive immunoprophylaxis (if they are not already vaccinated or do not already have natural immunity).

Because this patient is experiencing an acute HAV infection at 18 weeks' gestation, she is likely to resolve her infection within 2 months and should not be infectious at the time of her expected delivery. However, even if a patient acquired acute HAV later in gestation and was still infectious at the time of delivery, cesarean delivery should be reserved for the usual obstetric indications. Mothers with acute infection may breast-feed safely by observing strict hygienic measures that would prevent fecal-oral transmission to her child.

APPROACH TO
Hepatitis A During Pregnancy

There are five major viral causes of hepatitis: hepatitis A, B, C, D, and E. All produce clinically indistinguishable illness which can vary from asymptomatic to symptomatic but resolving, to fulminate hepatic failure and death. Acute infection with hepatitis B, C, and D sometimes may lead to chronic infection and chronic liver disease with resultant risks of progression to cirrhosis, progressive hepatic failure, and hepatocellular carcinoma. Infection with hepatitis A and E viruses never produces a chronic infectious carrier state. Thus, infection with these viruses does not convey a risk for progression to cirrhosis and hepatocellular cancer. **Hepatitis E is the only one of these viral infections whose course seems to be unfavorably altered by pregnancy; the case fatality ratio in the gravid population is approximately 10% to 20% compared to 1% to 2% in a nonpregnant adult population.**

Since there are no acceptable specific therapies for any of the acute viral hepatitides in pregnancy and because there are no acceptable treatment regimens for chronic hepatitis during pregnancy, the obstetrician/gynecologist's most effective means of impacting maternal and fetal/neonatal outcome is through primary prevention of maternal disease acquisition. Prevention can be via education of patients in avoidance of high-risk behaviors that increase the risk for acquisition of viral hepatitis and via appropriate vaccinations. Additionally, prevention by timely administration of immunoprophylaxis when an exposure has occurred or may occur in the future (travel to an endemic area) may prevent occurrence of a viral hepatitis episode.

Hepatitis Risk Factors and Prophylaxis

The risk factors for various hepatitis viruses vary and are not identical. There are no immunoprophylactic treatments available for hepatitis C and E; immunoprophylaxis is available for HAV, HBV, and HDV infection (by virtue of HBV immunoprophylaxis).

Infection with HAV is almost always via the fecal-oral route. Both sporadic and epidemic infections are described; epidemics are facilitated by conditions of overcrowding and poor personal hygiene. Outbreaks may occur at restaurants anytime an infected cook or waitstaff mishandles food and transmits virus onto that food after substandard hand-washing techniques (fecal-oral contamination). Specific food sources that are at higher risk of harboring HAV virus include raw or undercooked shellfish and uncooked produce such as green onions and strawberries. Persons at increased risk for HAV infection include those traveling to or moving from countries with intermediate or high endemicity of HAV infection and users of illicit drugs (whether injectable or not). HAV may also be contracted by ingestion of contaminated well water or other infected water supplies.

Primary prevention of HAV infection is by vaccination and/or administration of Ig. The vaccine is inactivated, carries no risk of causing disease, and is safe for administration during pregnancy. There are two different hepatitis A vaccine preparations available in the United States with a third vaccine being a combination of hepatitis A and hepatitis B vaccine. Travelers to endemic areas are considered protected if they have received the initial HAV vaccine dose four or more weeks prior to travel. If travel to endemic areas is necessary before 4 weeks has elapsed, Ig (0.02 mL/kg) should be given at a different injection site (usually contralateral anatomic site).

HBV is most efficiently transferred as a blood-borne illness. Other important modes of transmission include perinatal (most common source of HBV infection worldwide) and via intimate sexual contact. Thus, any exposure to infected blood products via intravenous drug use (needle-sharing), needle-sticks, etc. places an individual at risk for acquisition of acute HBV infection. Exposure to infected blood through mucous membranes or broken skin also may result in infection. Other risk factors for HBV infection include individuals with multiple sexual partners, individuals who use intravenous drugs, and individuals who have sexual partners that engage in high-risk behaviors. Epidemiologic studies suggest that the majority of perinatal infections occur either intrapartum or postpartum, although up to 10% of these infections may be hematogenously spread in utero. These in utero infections may thus only be prevented by primary prevention of maternal infection. There is some limited literature to suggest that maternal administration of lamivudine or maternal administration of HBIG may decrease the risk for in utero (transplacental) hepatitis B infection. However, such treatment is not currently generally recommended in the United States. Perinatal transmission is relatively uncommon in America and western Europe, but is a very frequent mode of transmission in Asia and many developing nations where the seroprevalence of HBsAg positivity and incidence of the chronic carrier state are high. Prevention of perinatal HBV infection is important since 90% of infected neonates will develop chronic HBV infection and 25% will ultimately die from either cirrhosis or hepatocellular carcinoma. Semen and saliva, while not as efficient as blood, are other possible sources of infection. Individuals who are sexually intimate with infected people are at substantial risk of acquiring hepatitis B if they have not been actively or passively immunized. In developed nations where neonates will be given HBIG and hepatitis B vaccine, breastfeeding by HBsAg-positive mothers is not contraindicated.

Adult prophylaxis for HBV infection consists of three IM injections (deltoid, not gluteal) at 0, 1, and 6 months. Five years after vaccination, 80% to 90% of healthy vaccines have protective anti-HBs levels. Even after anti-HBs levels become undetectable, some protection appears to persist (those individuals should have Ig administered for new situations in which postexposure prophylaxis would be indicated). Because the incidence of new HBV infection in the United States continued to rise after the introduction of the vaccine and targeting of "high-risk" groups, universal childhood HBV vaccination has now been recommended. If an unvaccinated individual has an exposure to HBV, postexposure prophylaxis consists of a combination of HBIG (0.06 mL/kg) and a full HBV vaccination series. When HBIG and HBV vaccine are administered at the same time they should be given at different anatomic sites. Immunoprophylaxis should be given as soon as possible after the exposure and is not recommended if more than 14 days have elapsed since the occurrence of an at-risk sexual encounter. For newborns born to HBsAg-negative mothers, routine vaccination with the three shot hepatitis B vaccine is recommended. The first dose should be given prior to hospital discharge followed by doses at 1 to 2 months and 6 to 18 months, respectively. For newborns born to HBsAg-positive mothers or to mothers whose HBsAg status is unknown, the recommendation is to give HBIG and the first dose of hepatitis vaccine within 12 hours of delivery at different anatomic sites followed by the 1 to 2 month and 6 to 18 month doses.

HCV is primarily contracted by intravenous exposure to infected blood. High-risk groups are similar to those of HBV, intravenous drug users, hemophiliacs, and patients who attend sexually transmitted disease clinics. Persons who are recommended for HCV screening include ever users of injectable illicit drugs, persons who received a blood product transfusion before 1987 or from a known HCV positive donor, persons who received an organ transplant before 1992, hemodialysis patients, and persons requiring care for an STI including HIV. The incidence of transfusion-associated hepatitis C (then called non-A non-B hepatitis) began falling in the late 1980s with the introduction of anti-HBc and ALT screening and has now fallen to trivial levels (1/1,000,000) with the use of the newer anti-HCV assays. As a result, sharing of infected needles has become a much more important source of hepatitis C infection. Although many individuals with hepatitis C infection have no identifiable risk factor, sexual and perinatal transmission are not thought to be important contributors, unless there is coinfection with HIV. Factors associated with increased risk for perinatal transmission include high maternal HCV viral loads, coinfection with HIV (HAART therapy appears to decrease this risk by reducing HCV viral load) intravenous drug use, and placement of a fetal scalp electrode. Duration of rupture of membranes for greater than 6 hours has been less convincingly shown to be a risk factor. Gestational age at delivery, mode of delivery, and the presence of chorioamnionitis have not been shown to be risk factors for vertical transmission. High-risk groups should be considered for HCV screening but universal screening is currently not recommended in either the gravid or nonpregnant population. There are no vaccines or well-established prophylactic treatments for postexposure prophylaxis for adults or newborns at risk for HCV infection.

HDV infection only occurs as coinfection or superinfection with HBV. In the United States, HDV infection most often occurs in intravenous drug users, hemophiliacs, and other individuals frequently exposed to infected blood. Individuals who have moved from endemic areas and are HBsAg positive should also be considered for HDV testing, especially if they have symptoms of hepatitis. Hepatitis D may be effectively prevented by prevention of hepatitis B infection.

Hepatitis E infection occurs primarily in the developing areas of Asia, India, Central America, and Africa and is acquired via fecal-oral infection. Infection occurs most commonly after fecal contamination of water supplies caused by natural disasters such as floods, monsoons, and typhoons. HEV differs from HAV in that person-to-person transmission of infection is very rare, even to close contacts. HEV is not often encountered in the United States outside of recent immigrants or recent travelers from endemic areas. No vaccines or postexposure prophylactic treatments are available to prevent HEV infection.

Clinical Considerations

Therapies for chronic HBV and HCV infection are not offered to pregnant patients due to concerns for possible teratogenicity of ribavirin. These patients, however, should receive counseling and inform sexual, household, and needle-sharing contacts of their infectious status and refrain from behaviors such as sharing of toothbrushes, razors, and needles which could have blood on them and serve as vectors for infection. Additionally, infected patients should be educated that hepatitis viruses can remain stable and infectious even after long periods in the outside environment such as on countertops, even when blood is not visible on the infected surface. Thus, blood and infected secretions should be meticulously cleaned with a 1:100 dilution of household bleach in tap water. Patients with chronic HBV, HCV, or HDV should be followed by a physician experienced in the evaluation and management of liver disease and should be referred for postpartum evaluation if they do not have such a physician involved in their care. There is inadequate data available to quantify the risk for vertical transmission with various intrapartum management maneuvers such as artificial rupture of membranes, fetal scalp electrode placement, or operative vaginal delivery. However, a 2002 NIH Consensus Statement recommended against the use of fetal scalp electrodes and many academic institutions avoid procedures that may potentially expose the neonate's bloodstream to infection from maternal blood or body secretions, especially for chronic HCV patients whose neonates do not have any known effective prophylactic treatments available to them.

Amniocentesis in viremic patients may theoretically cause fetal infection by either maternal-fetal blood exchange via damaged fetal vessels in the placenta or by fetal swallowing of infected amniotic fluid after transplacental trauma from the amniocentesis needle. Though available information in the literature demonstrates that the risk for vertical transmission of HBV and HCV with amniocentesis appears to be low, the data are not conclusive. Currently, the available data appear to show a low risk for fetal infection in HBsAg-positive patients but perhaps a higher risk in the HBeAg-positive population. There is insufficient data to evaluate level of risk in patients undergoing chorionic villus sampling where the likelihood of maternal-fetal blood exchange is much higher than with non-transplacental amniocentesis. Given this limited data set and the potentially dire consequences of in utero HBV or HCV infection, it seems prudent to discuss and exhaust noninvasive screening options with these patients and avoid invasive diagnostic procedures unless there is a well-established risk that outweighs the risk of vertical transmission. In the rare cases where an invasive diagnostic procedure is deemed necessary in an HBsAg-positive patient, consider HBIG immunoprophylaxis (especially in the more infectious HBeAg patient), although data that would support or refute this recommendation is currently unavailable.

Breast-Feeding

Unless there are fissures or abrasions on the breast that would increase neonatal exposure to maternal blood, breast-feeding with hepatitis is not contraindicated. Patients with HAV infections should use appropriate hygienic precautions that prevent fecal-oral spread of infection. As long as the neonate receives appropriate HBIG and HBV vaccination, breast-feeding has not been observed to increase the risk for vertical transmission of HBV. Current recommendations support no increase in vertical transmission in asymptomatic chronic HCV. However, there does appear to be an increased risk for vertical transmission of HCV in patients with high HCV viral loads (exact level considered high has not been established). Thus, in patients with typically high viral loads such as new acute HCV infections and symptomatic recurrent infections, breast-feeding should probably be proscribed. Even though there is no immunoprophylaxis for HCV and HEV, breast-feeding has not been shown to increase the risk for childhood HCV and HEV infection.

In fact, in reported cases of HEV where infected local water supplies were the likely source of infection, breast-feeding would likely decrease the risk for the infant acquiring disease decreasing exposure to the infected water source.

Laboratory Evaluation

Serum aminotransferases (AST and ALT) typically rise to 400 to 4000 IU or more and precede increases in serum bilirubin levels. Increased serum bilirubin usually consists of both direct and indirect fractions; scleral icterus and jaundice are typically visible with bilirubin levels greater than or equal to 2.5 mg/dL. An initial lymphopenia and neutropenia is followed by an atypical lymphocytosis. A prothrombin time (PT) should always be checked since clotting factor administration may be necessary and severity of liver damage does not always correlate with elevations in serum transaminases. An elevated PT level signifies more extensive liver damage and a worse prognosis. A variety of nondiagnostic and nonspecific elevations in laboratory values also may occur with acute viral hepatitis including elevations in serum IgG and IgM, anti-smooth muscle antibodies, antinuclear antibody, heterophil antibodies, and elevations in rheumatoid factor. The presence of rheumatoid factor-positive arthritis can give rise to a false-positive serologic diagnosis of both acute hepatitis A and B, based on the laboratory findings of a false-positive IgM anti-HAV or IgM anti-HBc.

The serologic diagnosis of acute viral hepatitis can be made with four serologic tests which include HBsAg, IgM anti-HAV, IgM anti-HBc, and anti-HCV. Currently there are no good diagnostic serologies available outside the research setting for acute hepatitis D and E. A diagnostic algorithm can then be applied (Table 13–1). It should be noted that anti-HCV may never become detectable in 20% to 30% of acute hepatitis C infections and may disappear after recovery from acute infections. Because a false-positive anti-HCV ELISA serology can occur, a confirmatory recombinant immunoblot assay (RIBA) should be considered, especially in patients without an identifiable risk factor for hepatitis C. Viremias (acute or chronic) may be tested by measuring HAV RNA, HBV DNA, HCV RNA, and HDV RNA.

Testing of patients suspected of having chronic viral hepatitis should include HBsAg and anti-HCV. Though almost all textbooks recommend testing HBsAg-positive patients for HBeAg and anti-HBe to evaluate the degree of infectivity, this testing serves no practical value for the pregnant patient whose neonate should be given HBIG and HBV vaccination series regardless of these results and who themselves are not eligible for pegylated interferon or ribavirin therapy (FDA category X) for chronic HBV or HCV infection while they are pregnant. Testing for hepatitis D (anti-HDV) can be helpful in the clinical settings of acute fulminant hepatitis, severe chronic cases, acute exacerbations in patients with chronic HBV infection, and in areas of the world where HDV is endemic. Additionally, patient with frequent percutaneous exposures (intravenous drug users) should be tested for hepatitis D.

Table 13–1 SIMPLIFIED DIAGNOSTIC APPROACH IN PATIENTS PRESENTING WITH ACUTE HEPATITIS

		SEROLOGIC TESTS OF PATIENT'S SERUM		
HBsAg	IgM anti-HAV	IgM anti-HBC	Anti-HCV	DIAGNOSTIC INTERPRETATION
–	+	–	–	Acute hepatitis A
+	–	+	–	Acute hepatitis B
–	–	+	–	Acute hepatitis B (HBsAg below detection threshold)
–	–	–	+	Acute hepatitis C
+	+	+	–	Acute hepatitis A and B
–	+	+	–	Acute hepatitis A and B (HBsAg below detection threshold)
+	+	–	–	Acute hepatitis A superimposed on chronic hepatitis B
+	–	–	–	Chronic hepatitis B

Data from Fauci AS, Braunwald E, Kaspar DL, Hauser SL. *Harrison's Principles of Internal Medicine. 17th ed.* New York: McGraw-Hill, 2008.

Comprehension Questions

13.1 A 25-year-old woman G1P0 at 15 weeks' gestation is noted to have an active hepatitis infection. She asks whether she can breast-feed. Which of the following statements is most accurate?

  A. She may breast-feed if it is hepatitis A but she should not breast-feed if it is hepatitis B.

  B. She may breast-feed if it is hepatitis C.

  C. She may breast-feed in the case of hepatitis A and B, but should not breast-feed with hepatitis C.

  D. She should not breast-feed with any of the viruses.

  E. There is insufficient information to render an opinion.

13.2.   A 36-year-old G2P1 woman at 15 weeks' gestation is noted to have an increased risk of fetal aneuploidy. She is infected with hepatitis C. Which of the following statements regarding invasive diagnostic techniques such as CVS or amniocentesis in HBV and HCV infected patients on vertical transmission to the fetus is true?

   A. There is no evidence of increased vertical transmission in these procedures.

   B. This is some evidence of increased vertical transmission with both procedures.

   C. The evidence indicates an increased risk of vertical transmission with HBV but not with HCV.

   D. The evidence indicates that CVS carries a greater vertical transmission than amniocentesis.

13.3.   The most effective method of improving neonatal outcomes with regards to hepatitis infections in pregnancy is which of the following?

   A. Treatment of acute viral infection with antiviral agents such as lamivudine.

   B. Separation of the baby from a mother with an acute hepatitis infection.

   C. Patient education or avoidance of risk behaviors and appropriate vaccinations and postexposure prophylaxis to the neonate.

   D. The use of passive immunization for the pregnant patient has been shown to improve neonatal outcome.

ANSWERS

13.1   **B.** There is no contraindication with breast-feeding with any of the hepatitis virus infections.

13.2   **B.** The literature indicates that there may be an increased risk of vertical transmission with HBV and HCV with invasive prenatal testing.

13.3   **C.** Patient education, avoidance of risk behaviors, and appropriate vaccination to the neonate is the best strategy to improve neonatal outcome. Antiviral medication is not indicated solely for pregnancy, but may generally be used if indicated. The baby does not need to be separated from the infected mother. Immunization is not helpful once the patient has developed an infection.

Clinical Pearls

See US Preventive Services Task Force Study Quality levels of evidence in Case 1

➤ Clinical course of hepatitis is unaltered by pregnancy except in cases of hepatitis E, where there is a 10- to 20-fold increased risk for fulminant hepatitis leading to death (Level II-2).

➤ Breast-feeding is acceptable with all types of acute viral hepatitis with precautions that normally minimize risk of transmission (Level II-2).

➤ Only supportive care is available for acute viral hepatitis and there are no specific treatments currently available for acute hepatitis in pregnancy (Level III).

➤ Vaccines for hepatitis A and B are safe in pregnancy, hepatitis B vaccine reduces the risk of hepatitis D, and there are currently no vaccines available for hepatitis C and hepatitis E (Level III).

➤ HBV infection acquired perinatally results in an 85% to 95% chance of chronic infection in the neonate with a 25% to 30% lifetime risk of serious or fatal liver disease (Level II-2).

➤ HBIG and hepatitis B vaccinations series reduces the neonatal transmission rate by 85% to 95% (Level I).

➤ High HCV viral titers, preterm premature rupture of the membranes, and internal fetal monitoring are risk factors for neonatal acquisition for HCV infection, although there are no well-established preventive measures for neonatal HCV infection, and routine HCV screen is not recommended (Level III).

➤ Patients at high risk for HCV infections such as HIV-positive patients, intravenous drug users, and patients with multiple sexual partners should be considered for HCV testing (Level III).

➤ For hepatitis C, there is no proven decreased risk of neonatal infection conferred by cesarean delivery as opposed to vaginal delivery (Level II-2).

REFERENCES

1. Airoldi J, Berghella V. Hepatitis C in pregnancy. *Obstet and Gynecol Surv.* 2006;61(10):666-672.
2. Alexander JM, Ramus R, Jackson G, Sercely B, Wendel GD Jr. Risk of hepatitis B transmission after amniocentesis in chronic hepatitis B carriers. *Infect Dis Obstet Gynecol.* 1999;7:283-286.
3. Centers of Disease Control and Prevention. A comprehensive immunization strategy to eliminate transmission of hepatitis B virus infection in the United States: Recommendations of the Advisory Committee on Immunization Practices (ACIP); Part I. Immunization of infants, children, and adolescents. *MMWR.* 2005;54(No. RR-16):1-34.

4. Centers for Disease Control and Prevention. A comprehensive immunization strategy to eliminate transmission of hepatitis B virus infection in the United States: Recommendations of the Advisory Committee on Immunization Practices (ACIP); Part II: Immunization of Adults. MMWR. 2006;55(No. RR-16):1-33.

5. Centers for Disease Control and Prevention. Recommendations for prevention and control of hepatitis C virus (HCV) infection and HCV-related chronic disease. MMWR. 1998;47(no. RR-19):1-39.

6. Delamare C, Carbonne B, Heim N, et al. Detection of hepatitis C virus RNA (HCV RNA) in amniotic fluid: a prospective study. J Hepatol. 1993;31:416-420. (Level II-2)

7. Ferrero S, Lungaro P, Bruzzone BM, Gotta C, Bentivoglio G, Ragni N. Prospective study of mother-to-infant transmission of hepatitis C virus: a 10-year study. Acta Obstet Gynecol Scand. 2003;82:229-234. (Level II-2)

8. Hussaini SH, Skidmore SJ, Richardson P, Sherratt LM, Cooper BT, O'Grady JG. Severe hepatitis E infection during pregnancy. J Viral Hepat. 1997;4:51-54. (Level III)

9. Ko TM, Tseng LH, Chang MH, et al. Amniocentesis in mothers who are hepatitis B virus carriers does not expose the infant to an increased risk of hepatitis B virus infection. Arch Gynecol Obstet. 1994;225:25-30.

10. Kumar R, Shahul F. Role of breast-feeding in transmission of hepatitis C virus to infants of HCV-infected mothers. J Hepatol. 1998;29:191-197.

11. Li SM, Shi MF, Yang YB, et al. Effects of hepatitis B immunoglobulin on interruption of HBV intrauterine infection. World J Gastroenterol. 2004;10:3215-3217. (Level I)

12. Prevention of Hepatitis A through active or passive immunization. Recommendations of the Advisory Committee of Immunization Practices (ACIP). MMWR. 2006;55 (No.RR-7):1-23.

13. Updated US Public Health Service Guidelines for the management of occupation exposures to HBV, HCV, HIV and recommendations for post-exposure prophylaxis. MMWR. 2001;50(RR-11):1-42.

14. van Zonneveld M, van Nuren AB, Niesters HG, et al. Lamivudine treatment during pregnancy to prevent perinatal transmission of hepatitis B virus infection. J Viral Hepat. 2003;10:294-297.

15. Viral Hepatitis in Pregnancy. ACOG Practice Bulletin No. 86. American College of Obstetricians and Gynecologists. Obstet Gynecol. 2007;110:941-955.

Case 14

A 23-year-old G1P0 at 34 weeks' gestation by first-trimester sonography presents with a 3-day history of malaise, anorexia, nausea, and vomiting. Her prenatal course has been uncomplicated to date. She denies a history of medical problems and surgeries.

On physical examination, the patient appears ill, with jaundice. Vitals: temperature, 98.9°F; BP, 120/78 mm Hg; pulse, 105 bpm; respiratory rate, 18 breaths per minute, lungs clear, cardiac regular rhythm. HR, 99 beats per minute with grade 2/4 systolic ejection murmur. Fundal height is 33 cm; epigastric tenderness is noted without guarding or rebound. Extremities are without edema or tenderness. The fetal heart rate tracing shows a baseline of 150 seconds, moderate variability, positive accelerations, no decelerations. Irregular contractions every 10 to 25 minutes are noted on tocodynamometer, although the patient does not perceive them. Her cervix is closed and long on digital examination. Bedside ultrasound shows fetal biometry consistent with 34 weeks, anterior placenta, and normal amniotic fluid.

During the evaluation, the patient has three episodes of emesis. Intravenous fluids with potassium repletion are started and antiemetics are administered. Laboratory results are as follows: Hgb 12 mg/dL, Hct 33%, WBC 19 × 10³/µL, platelet count 127,000/mm³, AST 482 IU/L, ALT 402 IU/L, conjugated bilirubin 5.2 mg/dL, total bilirubin 6.0, LDH 302, serum creatinine 1.1 mg/dL, serum glucose 51 mg/dL, K⁺ 3.0 mEq/L. Amylase, lipase, ammonia, uric acid, and coagulation studies are within normal range. Urine analysis is only remarkable for specific gravity 1.03 and large ketones but otherwise negative.

➤ What is the differential diagnosis?

➤ What is the most likely diagnosis?

➤ What are the maternal risks associated with this diagnosis?

➤ What are the fetal risks associated with this diagnosis?

ANSWERS TO CASE 14:
Acute Fatty Liver of Pregnancy

Summary: This is a 23-year-old G1 at $34^0/_7$ weeks' gestation with malaise, nausea, vomiting, abdominal tenderness as well as clinical and laboratory evidence of liver dysfunction.

> **Differential diagnosis:** In the second and third trimester, acute fatty liver of pregnancy (AFLP), intrahepatic cholestasis of pregnancy (IHCP), and severe preeclampsia with HELLP (hemolysis, elevated liver enzymes, low platelets) should be considered in a patient with evidence of liver dysfunction. Other conditions that may occur at any gestational age include viral hepatitis, pancreatitis, drug toxicity, cholelithiasis or rarely, malignancy. Conditions associated with nausea, vomiting, and abdominal pain that should also be considered in the differential include pyelonephritis, appendicitis, and hyperemesis gravidarum (HEG), however, these are less likely in this case.

> **Most likely diagnosis:** The most likely diagnosis is AFLP given this patient's symptoms, evidence of liver dysfunction, and hypoglycemia.

> **Maternal risks associated with this diagnosis:** Maternal complications include pulmonary edema, coagulopathy, acute renal failure, infection, pancreatitis, diabetes insipidus (DI), hepatic encephalopathy, coma, liver transplantation, and maternal death.

> **Fetal risks associated with this diagnosis:** Fetal demise is a potential complication with AFLP if the diagnosis is delayed and delivery is not expedited. Prematurity complications are increased due to risk of both spontaneous and iatrogenic preterm birth. The fetus may also be affected with a fatty acid oxidation disorder.

ANALYSIS

Objectives

1. Recognize the clinical presentation of AFLP.
2. Become familiar with the evaluation and management.
3. Understand genetic implications associated with AFLP.

Considerations

It is not uncommon for pregnant women to present with nonspecific symptoms of nausea, vomiting, and malaise. In most instances, these symptoms may be attributed to normal pregnancy or hyperemesis gravidarum (HEG), especially during first trimester. Other times symptoms are secondary to a benign, self-resolving process such as a viral syndrome. On rare occasions such as this, nonspecific symptoms may represent a serious and potentially life-threatening condition.

Acute fatty liver of pregnancy (AFLP) should always be in the differential for any patient who presents in the third trimester with nausea, vomiting, and abdominal pain. Although the incidence of AFLP is reportedly 1 in 7000 to 1 in 16,000 pregnancies[1-10] (Level III), this may very well be an overestimation from published case series derived from tertiary referral centers.

Often times, there is a delay in diagnosis as there are overlapping clinical and laboratory findings of AFLP with other conditions. The major diagnosis that must be excluded is preeclampsia (HELLP syndrome). Although the frequency of hypoglycemia is variable with AFLP, its presence may help to distinguish it from HELLP syndrome. Another laboratory abnormality seen with **AFLP** that is not seen with HELLP syndrome is a **markedly reduced antithrombin III levels.** However, routine testing for antithrombin III is not practical since it may take several days to obtain results. In the absence of hypertension and proteinuria, the diagnosis of HELLP syndrome is also less likely; however, it is important to note that approximately 15% and 10% of HELLP syndrome occurs in the absence of hypertension and proteinuria, respectively. Hemolysis occurs in both conditions but is more common with HELLP syndrome than with AFLP. On the other hand, jaundice, coagulopathy, and impaired renal function are more common with AFLP than with HELLP syndrome. Liver biopsies from cases of HELLP syndrome reveal periportal hemorrhage and fibrin deposition which is in contrast to the microvesicular fatty infiltration seen with AFLP[11] (Level III). Fortunately, the management of both conditions is similar in that delivery is indicated when either is suspected.

Another pregnancy-specific condition associated with liver dysfunction that needs to be considered in the third trimester is intrahepatic cholestasis of pregnancy (IHCP). The predominant symptom with IHCP is pruritus (without a rash) which helps to distinguish it from AFLP. Other conditions that need to be considered that are coincidental to pregnancy and can occur at any gestational age include viral hepatitis, cholelithiasis, pancreatitis, drug-induced toxicity, and, rarely, thrombotic thrombocytopenic purpura (TTP) and hemolytic uremic syndrome (HUS). It is also important to note that pyelonephritis and acute appendicitis must be considered with any patient that presents with nausea, vomiting, and abdominal pain. Because management strategies and outcomes differ among these conditions, obtaining the correct diagnosis is of the utmost importance.

The diagnosis of AFLP is most commonly made by clinical symptoms and laboratory findings. In this ill-appearing patient with emesis, abdominal tenderness, jaundice, liver impairment, and hypoglycemia, the most likely diagnosis is AFLP. Renal insufficiency, hemolysis, hemoconcentration, and leukocytosis are also evident in this patient and are not uncommon with AFLP. Hospitalization is indicated as this condition is progressive and sudden deterioration of both mother and fetus may occur at any time. The ultimate treatment is delivery after maternal stabilization. As long as maternal and fetal status is stable and reassuring, this patient is a good candidate to undergo induction of labor. Cesarean delivery should be reserved for the usual obstetrical indications or if delivery is not affected within a reasonable time and maternal and/or fetal status deteriorates.

APPROACH TO
Acute Fatty Liver of Pregnancy

AFLP affects women of all ages, race, and geographic areas. It is more common in nulliparas with a male fetus and in multiple gestations[1,11] (Level III). It usually manifests in the third trimester with onset between 28 to 38 weeks' gestation[2-6,13] (Level III). Although rare, earlier cases have been reported in the second trimester[12-14] (Level III). Less often, symptoms may not develop until the first few days of the postpartum period[2,10] (Level III).

The typical patient appears ill with nonspecific symptoms for 1 to 2 weeks. The most common symptoms are **nausea and vomiting (75%), abdominal pain (50%), jaundice (37%), and malaise (31%)**[2,6,7,10] (Level III). **Half of women with AFLP may also have preeclampsia** at presentation or at some point during their disease course[7,10] (Level III). Patients occasionally present with altered mental status due to hepatic encephalopathy. On physical examination, the patient may have hypertension, tachycardia (secondary to dehydration), low-grade fever, mild jaundice, and/or epigastric tenderness. In cases of severe coagulopathy, bleeding may be evident from multiple sites. Although less common (15%-20% cases), patients may actually be asymptomatic at the time of presentation or they may present for other reasons[11] (Level III). Some patients may present with preterm contractions/labor or with decreased fetal movement (secondary to maternal acidosis).

As the disease progresses, additional complications may arise. Marked **hypoglycemia** may occur with variable frequency, developing in 17% to 100% of women due to impaired gluconeogenesis from liver dysfunction[2,6,7] (Level III). A recent review of 16 cases of AFLP from three tertiary centers showed a 50% incidence of hypoglycemia[10] (Level III). Hypoglycemia has also been found to be more common in the postpartum period. Additional maternal complications are **hepatic encephalopathy (60%), acute renal failure (50%), disseminated intravascular coagulopathy (DIC) (55%), pulmonary edema/acute respiratory distress syndrome (ARDS) (25%), and infection**[2,6,7,10] (Level III). **Acute pancreatitis may complicate 15%** of cases and confers a poor prognosis. This complication may occur later in the disease process and is associated with hyperglycemia[9] (Level III). Transient central **diabetes insipidus** in first week after delivery has also been reported. The mechanism for this is unknown but it is presumably from elevated vasopressinase levels which results in prodigious urine output[15] (Level III).

Laboratory evaluation usually reveals parameters consistent with liver dysfunction. Prolonged clotting times, reduced fibrinogen as well as antithrombin III levels are associated with coagulopathy. Hyperbilirubinemia is usually of the conjugated type and has been reported to be in the range of 5 to 10 mg/dL. Liver enzymes (aspartate transaminase, alanine transaminase) are mildly elevated, rarely exceeding 1000 U/L. Endothelial exudation activation may cause hemoconcentration, leukocytosis, and thrombocytopenia. Hemolysis is likely from impaired cholesterol synthesis which contributes to erythrocyte membrane damage. LDH levels may vary from 250 to 4000 IU/L. As renal failure progresses, metabolic acidosis with elevated creatinine and uric acid levels is common. Either hypoglycemia or hyperglycemia may be present with the latter occurring in association with pancreatitis. In 12 cases of AFLP complicated by pancreatitis, the average peak for amylase was 552 U/L (range 26-113 U/L) and lipase 1866 U/L (range 100-5869 U/L)[9] (Level III). Elevated ammonia levels are more common with progressive liver failure. Table 14–1 shows a summary of laboratory findings of 169 women with AFLP taken from six published studies.

Computed tomography (CT), magnetic resonance imaging (MRI), and ultrasound imaging of the liver have limited usefulness and therefore the diagnosis of AFLP is made by clinical and laboratory evaluation. Hepatic imaging is helpful in excluding other disorders that may be confused with AFLP when the diagnosis is unclear. It is useful in detecting suspected complications of AFLP such as a pancreatic pseudocyst or hemorrhagic pancreatitis. The finding of fat on CT or ultrasound has been reported in cases of AFLP. This finding is nonspecific[16] (Level III). The gold standard for diagnosis is the presence of microvesicular fatty infiltration of hepatocytes on liver biopsy. In patients without this diagnostic feature, special staining with oil red O on frozen section or electron microscopy can help to confirm the diagnosis of AFLP[11] (Level III). Liver biopsy may be considered *after* coagulopathy has been corrected in those in whom the diagnosis remains in question; however, it is rarely used in clinical practice.

Once the diagnosis of AFLP is made, delivery is recommended regardless of gestational age. Antenatal corticosteroids to induce lung maturity can be administered as soon as preterm birth is anticipated if gestational age < 34 weeks. Delivery should not be delayed to complete a full course of antenatal steroids once the diagnosis is made as maternal and fetal status may deteriorate trying to accomplish this. Consultation with maternal-fetal medicine and neonatology is advised. Although there is no definitive treatment, maternal stabilization with supportive care is a mainstay of management.

Table 14–1 LABORATORY FINDINGS IN 169 WOMEN WITH AFLP

STUDY	N	WBC (×10³/μL)	FIBRINOGEN (mg/dL)	PLATELET (×10³/μL)	AST (IU/L)	ALT (IU/L)	T.BILIRUBIN (mg/dL)	D. BILIRUBIN (mg/dL)	GLUCOSE (mg/dL)	CR (mg/dL)	AMMONIA (μmol/L)	LDH (IU/L)
Reyes[a]	12	18.5 (8.5-34.2)	NA	NA	NA	315 (28-1200)	9.1 (1.8-17.3)	6.4 (0.64-12)	NA	NA	NA	NA
Usta[a]	14	NA	139 (37-110)	126	1067 (200-3670)	NA	NA	NA	NA	2.4 (1.1-3.6)	NA	NA
Castro[a]	28	NA	125 (32-446)	113 (11-186)	210 (45-1200)	NA	NA	NA	NA	2.5 (1.1-5.2)	NA	NA
Pereira[b]	32	NA	NA	123 (25-262)	99 (25-911)	NA	8.3 (3.7-37.5)	NA	NA	2.7 (1.1-8.6)	NA	NA
Vigil-De Gracia[a]	10	27.4 (8.5-34.2)	136 (15-345)	76 (21-179)	444 (85-1025)	392 (107-900)	11 (1.5-27)	NA	37 (6-59)	NA	NA	993 (379-1503)
Fesenmeier[a]	16	NA	NA	151 (33-303)	523 (120-2371)	423 (43-1504)	NA	5.8 (0.9-11.9)	81 (11-159)	2.4 (0.5-4.4)	69.7 (15-150)	1438 (244-3922)
Knight[b]	57	20.7 (8.5-46.5)	NA	122 (14-436)	310 (37-3198)	300 (21-1156)	NA	5.9 (1.0-39.6)	56 (18-148)	1.9 (0.7-4.5)	73 (22-121)	NA

[a]Mean values
[b]Median values

It is important to monitor vital signs and repeat laboratory tests every 6 to 8 hours or more frequent as needed. Transfusion of blood products may be necessary for correction of clinical coagulopathy and anemia. Serial glucose monitoring is also recommended with intravenous glucose infusion in order to maintain blood glucose levels > 60 mg/dL. It also is important to correct any electrolyte abnormalities and reduce high ammonia levels with lactulose when necessary. Continuous fetal monitoring to asses fetal well-being is also recommended. It is important to note that the fetal status may deteriorate rapidly, likely secondary to maternal acidosis or uteroplacental insufficiency or both[11] (Level III).

Induction of labor is very reasonable in the absence of other indications that may preclude vaginal delivery. Vaginal delivery is optimal in a patient with AFLP who is at very high risk of hemorrhage and postoperative complications from AFLP. Cesarean delivery should be considered for the usual obstetrical indications or if maternal/fetal status deteriorates necessitating expeditious delivery. Anesthesia should be based on coexisting coagulopathy. If preeclampsia develops, magnesium sulfate should be administered for seizure prophylaxis.

Intensive care unit admission may be necessary intrapartum or postpartum for several reasons including maternal stabilization as well as close monitoring of laboratory abnormalities and complications that may develop in the postpartum period. Although clinical improvement is expected 2 to 3 days after delivery, laboratory abnormalities may continue for 7 to 10 days[7] (Level III). Fulminant liver failure and need for liver transplant is very rare but has been reported.

The maternal mortality rate in older studies was reportedly in the order of 60% to 70%. In more recent case series, the maternal mortality rate has been found to be lower, in the range of 1.8% to 20%[3,4,9,10,17] (Level III, Level II-2). Prompt diagnosis and aggressive treatment of associated complications may contribute to improved maternal outcome. Perinatal mortality is approximately 13% based on the most recent literature[10] (Level III); however, neonatal morbidity remains high due to prematurity complications.

Molecular advances have improved our understanding of the pathogenesis of AFLP. Several reports have provided evidence to support an association between AFLP and an inherited fatty acid oxidation disorder of **long-chain 3-hydroxyacyl-CoA dehydrogenase (LCHAD)** deficiency in the fetus. This enzyme catalyzes the third step in the β-oxidation of fatty acids in mitochondria by facilitating the formation of 3-ketoacyl-CoA from 3-hydroxyacyl-CoA. With deficiency of the enzyme, the latter metabolite accumulates in the fetus and enters the maternal circulation causing hepatic fat deposition and impaired liver function.

The most common mutation of LCHAD deficiency associated with AFLP that has been studied is **E474Q** (or GC1528C). In a study of 24 families, Ibdah and colleagues examined the association between LCHAD deficiency in children and severe liver disease in their mothers. Of the 19 children that were found to be homozygous for E474Q or compound heterozygous (E474Q plus a different mutation on the other allele), the majority of these mothers developed AFLP, HELLP syndrome, or both during their pregnancy involving these children. Thus based on this study, carrying a fetus with LCHAD deficiency is associated with a 79% risk of developing AFLP or HELLP syndrome with the former having a stronger association than the latter[18] (Level II-2). A subsequent prospective study confirmed this association and it is suggested that 1 in 5 women who develop AFLP may carry an LCHAD deficient fetus[19] (Level II-2). Whether the pathogenesis of AFLP and HELLP syndrome is related remains unclear. At present, 17 mutations of β-oxidation have been identified raising the possibility that other defects may be associated with ALFP but are less well studied to date.

Molecular testing for the most common mutation, E474Q, and known genetic variants are available for women who develop AFLP, their partner, or their infants. This information is important for counseling a couple regarding their risk of having an affected fetus with LCHAD deficiency. With an autosomal recessive pattern of inheritance, a heterozygous couple has a 25% chance of having an affected fetus. Prenatal diagnosis by enzyme assay of amniocytes or chorionic villus samples may be available for an at-risk couple. Infants or children with LCHAD deficiency are at risk of developing fatal nonketotic hypoglycemia, defects in urea cycle formation, cardiomyopathy, or progressive neuromyopathy[18] (Level II-2). The recurrence risk of AFLP in subsequent pregnancies (whether or not there is an associated inherited fatty acid oxidation defect) is likely to be increased but difficult to quantify based on the available literature.

Comprehension Questions

14.1   A 35-year-old woman G1P0 at 35 weeks' gestation is noted to have BP in the 160/100 range and 3+ proteinuria. Her blood pressures during pregnancy were 120/70. The SGOT is 80 IU/L and SGPT 100 IU/L. The serum bilirubin is 0.2 mg/dL and serum glucose level is 90 mg/dL. The hemoglobin level is 12 g/dL and platelet count 120,000/mm^3. Which of the following is the most likely diagnosis?

A. Acute fatty liver of pregnancy
B. Acute cholestasis of pregnancy
C. HELLP syndrome
D. Hepatitis
E. Preeclampsia

14.2. A 29-year-old G2P1 woman at 34 weeks' gestation presents with fatigue, nausea and vomiting, and abdominal pain. The patient has an evaluation and is diagnosed with acute fatty liver of pregnancy. Which of the following is thought to be the etiology of this condition?

A. Estrogen effect on the liver decreasing transport of bile salts
B. Sludge in the gall bladder leading to delayed transit
C. Long chain fatty acid metabolism defect
D. Variant of preeclampsia

ANSWERS

14.1. **D.** This scenario is most consistent with preeclampsia. In acute fatty liver of pregnancy, the liver function tests usually show an elevated bilirubin and the glucose is low. Acute cholestasis is not usually associated with hypertension. HELLP syndrome would have thrombocytopenia (platelets < 100,000), and hepatitis is associated with transaminase enzymes in the 1000s.

14.2. **C.** AFLP is thought to be due to an inherited fatty acid oxidation disorder of **long-chain 3-hydroxyacyl-CoA dehydrogenase (LCHAD)** deficiency in the fetus. This enzyme catalyzes the third step in the β-oxidation of fatty acids in mitochondria by facilitating the formation of 3-ketoacyl-CoA from 3-hydroxyacyl-CoA. With deficiency of the enzyme, the latter metabolite accumulates in the fetus and enters the maternal circulation causing hepatic fat deposition and impaired liver function. Although many patients with AFLP have preeclampsia, it is not thought to be a variant of preeclampsia.

Clinical Pearls

See US Preventive Services Task Force Study Quality levels of evidence in Case 1

➤ AFLP is a rare condition in the third trimester associated with significant maternal and perinatal morbidity (Level III).

➤ The major diagnosis that must be excluded is preeclampsia (HELLP syndrome) (Level III).

➤ Although there is no definitive treatment, maternal stabilization with supportive care is a mainstay of management (Level III).

➤ One in five women who develop AFLP may carry an LCHAD deficient fetus (Level II-3).

➤ Molecular testing for the most common mutation, E474Q, and known genetic variants should be offered for women who develop AFLP, their partner, or their infants (Level III).

REFERENCES

1. Davidson KM, Simpson LL, Knox TA, D'Alton ME. Acute fatty liver of pregnancy in triplet gestation. *Obstet Gynecol.* 1998;91:806-808. (Level III)
2. Usta IM, Barton JR, Amon EA, Gonzalez A, Sibai BM. Acute fatty liver of pregnancy: An experience in the diagnosis and management of fourteen cases. *Am J Obstet Gynecol.* 1999;181:389-395. (Level III)
3. Vigil-De Garcia P, Lavergne JA. Acute fatty liver of pregnancy. *Int J Gynaecol Obstet.* 2001;72:193-195. (Level III)
4. Pereira SP, O'Donohue J, Wendon J, Williams R. Maternal and perinatal outcome in severe pregnancy related liver disease. *Hepatology.* 1997;26:1258-1262. (Level III)
5. Reyes H. Acute fatty liver of pregnancy. A cryptic disease threatening mother and child. *Clin Liver Dis.* 1999;3:69-81. (Level III)
6. Castro MA, Fasset MJ, Reynolds TB, Shaw KJ, Goodwin TM. Reversible peripartum liver failure: A new perspective on the diagnosis, treatment, and cause of acute fatty liver of pregnancy, based on 28 consecutive cases. *Am J Obstet Gynecol.* 1999;181:389-395. (Level III)
7. Reyes H, Sandoval L, Wainstein A, et al. Acute fatty liver of pregnancy: A clinical study of 12 episodes in 11 patients. *Gut.* 1994;35:101. (Level III)
8. Mabie WC. Acute fatty liver of pregnancy. *Gastroenterol Clin North Am.* 1992;21: 951-959. (Level III)
9. Moldenhauer JS, O'Brien JM, Barton JR, Sibai B. Acute fatty liver of pregnancy associated with pancreatitis: a life-threatening complication. *Am J Obstet Gynecol.* 2004;190:502-505. (Level III)
10. Fesenmeir MF, Coppage KH, Lambers DS, Barton JR, Sibai BM. Acute fatty liver in 3 tertiary care centers. *Am J Obstet Gynecol.* 2005;192:1416-1419. (Level III)
11. Sibai BM. Imitators of severe preeclampsia. *Obstet Gynecol.* 2007;109(4):956-966. *This is an excellent review of the different conditions that share many of the clinical and laboratory findings of patients with severe preeclampsia-eclampsia (Level III).*
12. Buytaert IM, Elewaut GP, Van Kets HE. Early occurrence of acute fatty liver in pregnancy. *Am J Gastroenterol.* 1996;91:603-604. (Level III)
13. Monga M, Katz AR. Acute fatty liver in the second trimester. *Obstet Gynecol.* 1999;93:811-813. (Level III)
14. Suzuki S, Watanabe S, Araki T. Acute fatty liver of pregnancy at 23 weeks of gestation. *BJOG.* 2001;108:223-224. (Level III)
15. Kennedy S, Hall PM, Seymour AE, Haque W. Transient diabetes insipidus and acute fatty liver of pregnancy. *Br J Obset Gynecol.* 1994;101:387. (Level III)
16. Castro M, Ouzounian J, Colletti P, et al. Radiologic studies in acute fatty liver of pregnancy. A review of the literature and 19 new cases. *J Reprod Med.* 1996;41:839. (Level III)
17. Knight M, Nelson-Percy C, Kurinczuk JJ, and on behalf of UK obstetric surveillance system (UKOSS). A prospective national study of acute fatty liver of pregnancy in the UK. *Gut.* 2008;57:951-956. *This is the largest population-based study of a cohort of women with AFLP which showed improved maternal and fetal outcomes than previously reported (Level II-2).*
18. Ibdah JA, Bennett MJ, Rinaldo P, et al. A fetal fatty-acid oxidation disorder as a cause of liver disease in pregnant women. *N Engl J Med.* 1999;340:1723-1731. *A cohort of 24 children with 3-hydroxyacyl-CoA dehydrogenase deficiency underwent DNA amplification and nucleotide-sequence analyses to identify the alpha subunit of the*

trifunctional protein. Seventy-nine of heterozygous mothers developed AFLP or HELLP syndrome while carrying fetuses with Glu474Gln mutation (Level II-2).

19. Yang Z, Yamada J, Zhao Y, Strauss AW, Ibdah JA. Prospective screening for pediatric mitochondrial trifunctional protein defects in pregnancies complicated by liver disease. JAMA. 2002;288:2163-2166.

A cohort study of 108 samples of maternal blood from women who developed AFLP or HELLP syndrome was tested. Mutations causing LCHAD deficiency were detected in 19% of women with a history of AFLP but only one with HELLP syndrome. The authors concluded that in approximately one out of five pregnancies complicated by AFLP the fetus had LCHAD deficiency (Level II-2).

Case 15

A 29-year-old G1P0 African American female at 34 weeks' gestation arrives at the hospital via ambulance with a history of a seizure at home witnessed by her husband. She has a history of chronic hypertension. The husband reports that over the preceding 2 days, she has been complaining about a worsening frontal headache, unrelieved by acetaminophen. On arrival to labor and delivery, she is postictal. Her blood pressure at admission is 180/116 mm Hg, with 4+ proteinuria. Her fundal height is 31 cm. After arrival, she has another tonic-clonic seizure involving both the upper and lower extremities. An ultrasound shows a fetus with an estimated fetal weight of 2000 g at the fifth percentile for gestational age.

➤ What is the most likely diagnosis?

➤ What are the next management steps?

➤ What are the potential complications of the patient's condition?

ANSWERS TO CASE 15:
Eclampsia

Summary: A 29-year-old G1P0 at 34 weeks' gestation with history of chronic hypertension with new onset seizure, elevated blood pressure, and proteinuria. The fetus measures in the fifth percentile for estimated fetal weight.

➤ **Most likely diagnosis:** Eclampsia.

➤ **Next management step:** Obtain IV access and administer intravenous magnesium sulfate, control blood pressure with intravenous agents.

➤ **Potential complications:** Include intrauterine growth restriction, abruption, DIC, renal dysfunction, liver dysfunction, intracranial hemorrhage, and stillbirth.

ANALYSIS

Objectives

1. Recognize the risk factors for preeclampsia/eclampsia.
2. Know how to administer magnesium sulfate to prevent seizures and to treat recurrent seizures.
3. Know the agents available for the treatment of recurrent seizures.
4. Understand the varied clinical presentations of the eclamptic patient.
5. Describe other clinical conditions that are part of the differential diagnosis of a seizure in pregnancy.

Considerations

This is a 29-year-old primigravida with chronic hypertension presenting at 34 weeks with new onset seizure, hypertension, and proteinuria.

The first priority is to stabilize the patient with respect to controlling the seizure and hypertension.

Eclampsia is the occurrence of a seizure in a patient with preeclampsia. The exact cause of eclampsia is unknown. Eclampsia occurs in approximately 0.5% of patients with mild preeclampsia and in 2% of patients with severe preeclampsia. The combination of seizures, hypertension, edema, and proteinuria make the diagnosis of eclampsia relatively certain. However, patients with eclampsia may present with a wide range of signs and symptoms. Although hypertension is typically associated with eclampsia, up to 16% may not present with hypertension. 10% of patients developing eclampsia prior to 32 weeks' gestation will not have hypertension.

Table 15–1 RISK FACTORS FOR THE DEVELOPMENT OF PREECLAMPSIA
History of fetal growth restriction, abruptio placentae
Multifetal gestation
Hydrops fetalis
Unexplained fetal growth restriction
Antiphospholipid antibody syndrome or inherited thrombophilia
Nulliparity
Age > 40 y or < 18 y
Chronic hypertension
Family history of preeclampsia
Preeclampsia in a previous pregnancy
Chronic renal disease
Vascular or connective tissue disorder
Diabetes mellitus
High body mass index

Although eclampsia is usually associated with proteinuria, it may be absent in up to 14% of cases. Edema, also typically associated with eclampsia, may be absent in 25% of women.

The clinician should be aware of certain symptoms that may be helpful in the diagnosis of eclampsia. These include persistent headaches (frontal and occipital), photophobia, altered mentation, visual changes, and epigastric, or right upper quadrant pain.

Risk factors for developing eclampsia are the same as for preeclampsia (Table 15–1). Eclamptic seizures may occur antepartum, intrapartum, or postpartum. Antepartum eclamptic convulsions occur in 38% to 53% of those patients with eclampsia and 11% to 44% occur postpartum.[1] Almost all cases of postpartum eclampsia occur within the first 2 days postpartum. If there is a seizure more than 48 hours postpartum, a thorough neurological workup should be undertaken.[2] This should include imaging of the brain and cerebrovascular anatomy, lumbar puncture, and lab tests to evaluate possible metabolic abnormalities. Approximately 90% of eclamptic seizures occur after 28 weeks' gestation and approximately 8% occur between 21 and 28 weeks' gestation. Only 1% to 2% of cases of eclampsia occur at 20 weeks' gestation or less; these may be associated with placental abnormalities such as molar pregnancies or hydropic changes. The occurrence of a seizure at ≤ 20 weeks' gestation also mandates a thorough neurologic workup.

APPROACH TO
Eclampsia

DEFINITIONS

ECLAMPSIA: Refers to the onset of convulsions in a woman with preeclampsia. Such convulsions are not attributable to an underlying seizure disorder or to other causes. It is prudent to remember that eclampsia can sometimes occur with minimal blood pressure elevation and little or no proteinuria, that is before preeclampsia has been clinically diagnosed.

CORTICAL BLINDNESS: Loss of vision due to vasogenic edema occurring most commonly in the occipital cortex. The diagnosis is made on imaging studies of the brain.

MAGNESIUM SULFATE: The consensus drug of choice for the treatment and prevention of eclampsia. The actual drug administered is magnesium sulfate septahydrate, of which elemental magnesium is 10% by weight.

Etiology

The exact cause of eclampsia is not known. Autopsies of individuals who have died from eclampsia usually show some cerebral pathology in the form of infarction, edema, and/or hemorrhage. Eclamptic patients may exhibit numerous neurologic abnormalities including focal deficits, cortical blindness and even coma; fortunately, these will rarely be permanent.

Differential Diagnosis of Eclampsia

When evaluating a pregnant patient with a seizure, other etiologies should be considered (see Table 15–2).[1]

Management of Eclampsia

The goals of management are:
1. Prevention of maternal injury and hypoxia
2. Prevention of recurrent seizures
3. Control of hypertension
4. Delivery of fetus and placenta

During the convulsions or immediately afterward, care should be taken to prevent maternal injury, maintain airway patency, and maternal oxygenation. The patient should be in the lateral decubitus position to minimize aspiration, and the side rails of the bed should be in the upright position. Maternal oxygenation should be maintained with supplemental oxygen.

Table 15–2 DIFFERENTIAL DIAGNOSIS OF ECLAMPSIA

Cerebrovascular accident
Hypertensive crisis
Space occupying lesions of the brain
Epilepsy
Metabolic disorders
Infection of the CNS
Illicit drug use
Thrombotic thrombocytopenic purpura
Gestational trophoblastic disease
Thrombophilia
Vasculitis
Reversible posterior leukoencephalopathy syndrome (RPLS)
Post-dural puncture syndrome

Magnesium sulfate is the drug of choice for the treatment and prevention of seizures and is given at an initial loading dose of 6 g intravenously over 15 minutes followed by a maintenance infusion of 2 g/h.[1] An alternate dosing regimen seldom used in contemporary practice employs a 4 g IV loading dose of magnesium sulfate along with 5 g IM in each buttock followed by 5 g IM every 4 hours.[2] Magnesium levels are not necessary if there are normal reflexes and normal renal function. If hypermagnesemia develops with significant cardiorespiratory depression, 10 cc of 10% solution of calcium gluconate can be used to reverse magnesium toxicity. This should be given slowly intravenously with maternal cardiac monitoring.

After receiving magnesium sulfate, up to 10% of eclamptic patients will have a recurrent seizure. For this, an additional 2 to 4 g bolus of magnesium sulfate can be given intravenously over a 3 to 5 minute period. If after the second bolus of magnesium sulfate another seizure occurs, sodium amobarbital 250 mg can be given intravenously over 3 to 5 minutes. If seizures persist, despite these interventions, then there should be consideration of the use of paralytic agents with intubation and mechanical ventilation. Magnesium sulfate infusion should be continued for 24 hours after delivery or after the last seizure. The goal of treating hypertension should be to maintain the systolic blood pressure between 140 and 160 mm Hg and the diastolic between 90 and 110 mm Hg. Hydralazine is used to treat hypertension using boluses of 5 to 10 mg every 15 to 20 minutes intravenously (total cumulative dose usually 30 mg). Labetalol may also be used in doses of 20 to 40 mg intravenously every 15 to 20 minutes (total cumulative dose 220 mg). Less often, oral nifedipine may be used, 10 to 20 mg every 30 minutes (total cumulative dose 50 mg in 1 h). Sodium nitroprusside is an effective agent for hypertensive crisis, but seldom used in obstetrics secondary to concern for cyanide toxicity. An arterial line should be in place for any patient receiving nitroprusside. It has an immediate onset of action and a duration of action between 1 and 10 minutes. In pregnancy, the initial rate of infusion should be 0.2 μg/kg/min (lower than 0.5 μg/kg/min in the nonpregnant patient) because most preeclamptic/eclamptic patients have depleted intravascular volume.

Maternal convulsions will result in maternal hypoxemia and hypercarbia which may cause fetal heart rate abnormalities. These fetal heart rate abnormalities will usually resolve spontaneously within 10 minutes. After the cessation of the convulsions, if the fetal heart rate abnormalities persist after 15 minutes, other complications such as abruption should be considered. Eclampsia is not an indication for cesarean delivery. The mode of delivery should be based on gestational age, fetal status, presence of labor, and cervical Bishop score. With a gestational age of less than 30 weeks, absence of labor, and a Bishop score of less than 5, most would proceed to cesarean delivery.

Either epidural analgesia or systemic opioids can be used for pain relief. Delivery is the definitive treatment for eclampsia.

Maternal Complications

Maternal death has increased in patients with eclampsia, the most common cause of intracranial hemorrhage (see Figure 15–1). Other complications that are increased include placental abruption, pulmonary edema, acute renal failure, disseminated intravascular coagulopathy, aspiration pneumonia, and cardiopulmonary collapse.[3] Additional complications are listed in Table 15–3.

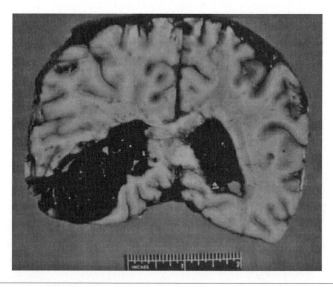

Figure 15–1. A fatal hypertensive intracerebral hemorrhage in a primigravid woman with eclampsia. *(Reproduced, with permission, from Cunningham FG, Leveno KJ, Bloom SL, et al. Williams Obstetrics. 23rd ed. New York, NY: McGraw-Hill; 2010.)*

Table 15–3 MATERNAL AND NEONATAL OUTCOMES ASSOCIATED WITH ECLAMPSIA
Cardiopulmonary arrest
Abruption
Pulmonary edema
Aspiration pneumonia
Disseminated intravascular coagulation
Acute renal failure
Liver hematoma
Perinatal death
HELLP syndrome
Preterm birth

Perinatal Complications

Perinatal mortality is also increased and varies from 5% to 12%. Preterm delivery occurs in up to 50%.

Recurrence Risk

The recurrence risk for eclampsia in a subsequent pregnancy is 2%. However, the risk of preeclampsia in a subsequent pregnancy is 25%.

Comprehension Questions

15.1   Which of the following is most accurate regarding eclampsia?
   A. Hypertension is nearly always present prior to an eclamptic seizure.
   B. Proteinuria may be absent in approximately 14% of eclamptics.
   C. Fetal bradycardia during an eclamptic seizure is generally an indication for cesarean section.
   D. The majority of eclamptic seizures occur in the postpartum period.

15.2   A patient weighing 70 kg has an eclamptic seizure and has been given a 6-g loading dose of magnesium sulfate and then placed on a 2 g/h infusion. She has another seizure 30 minutes later. Which of the following should be the next step in management?
   A. Immediately prepare for cesarean section.
   B. Administer additional magnesium sulfate 2 g IV over 2 to 3 minutes.
   C. Obtain a stat CT of the head.
   D. Perform an ultrasound to evaluate the placenta for abruption.

15.3   A 26-year-old woman at 34 weeks' gestation is admitted with a BP of
         180/120 mm Hg and is noted to have a 3-minute tonic-clonic seizure.
         Which of the following management approaches is most appropriate?
         A. Prevent maternal hypoxia and injury, administer magnesium sul-
            fate, control blood pressure, decide on mode of delivery.
         B. Prepare for immediate cesarean section, control blood pressure,
            administer magnesium sulfate after cesarean section.
         C. Administer magnesium sulfate and wait for its effect on BP; if no
            change after 30 minutes, then administer antihypertensive agents.
         D. Administer magnesium sulfate, use an intravenous antihyperten-
            sive agent to control BP to achieve a target of systolic blood pres-
            sure (SBP) of 120 and diastolic blood pressure (DBP) of 80 range,
            decide on mode of delivery.

15.4   During an eclamptic seizure, the fetal heart rate shows a heart rate of
         150 beats per minute and persistent late decelerations. Which of the
         following should be the appropriate response?
         A. Immediate delivery via cesarean section.
         B. Allow in utero resuscitation and observe for 10 to 15 minutes, if
            the fetal heart rate pattern continues to be nonreassuring, then
            proceed with cesarean section if the mother is stable.
         C. Allow for in utero resuscitation and after 10 minutes delivery by
            cesarean section even though the mother's BP is 190/130 mm Hg.
         D. Allow for in utero resuscitation, observe fetal heart rate pattern
            every 10 to 15 minutes, and if it continues to be nonreassuring,
            proceed with induction.

ANSWERS

15.1   **B.** Proteinuria may be absent in a significant number of patients.
         Hypertension is usually present with eclampsia although it may be
         absent in up to 16% of patients. Fetal bradycardia is usually present
         during an eclamptic seizure due to maternal respiratory difficulty and
         usually will resolve with cessation of the seizure. Immediate cesarean
         should not be performed, particularly in an unstable patient. The
         majority of seizures occur in the antepartum period.

15.2   **B.** Approximately 10% of patients will have a recurrent seizure. This
         may cause a change in the fetal status. It is best to allow for in utero
         resuscitation. Administration of an additional bolus of magnesium
         sulfate will usually be successful in treating the recurrent seizure.

15.3   **A.** Initially, the goal of managing eclampsia is to maintain maternal
         oxygenation and prevent injury. After this, magnesium sulfate for
         seizure prophylaxis should be given along with controlling the SBP
         to 140 to 160 and DBP 90 to 110 mm Hg. Only after the mother is
         stable should there be an assessment regarding mode of delivery.

15.4   **C.** The fetal heart rate pattern may be nonreassuring during and shortly after a convulsion. This will usually correct after 10 to 15 minutes. If the fetal heart rate continues to be nonreassuring, then one must consider abruption and if the mother is stable, delivery by cesarean section.

Clinical Pearls

See US Preventive Services Task Force Study Quality levels of evidence in Case 1

➤ Magnesium sulfate is the best agent for the prevention of seizures or recurrent seizures related to eclampsia (Level I).

➤ In up to 25% of cases of eclampsia, the blood pressure will be less than 140/90 mm Hg or there will be no proteinuria (Level II-2).

➤ The management of eclampsia includes stabilization of the mother, treatment and prevention of seizures, lowering of severe high blood pressure, and delivery of the baby, preferably vaginally (Level II-2).

➤ Seizures occurring greater than 48 hours postpartum should initiate a complete neurologic evaluation (Level II-3).

➤ The rate of eclampsia recurring in a subsequent pregnancy is 2% (Level II-2).

REFERENCES

1. Sibai BM. Diagnosis, prevention, and management of eclampsia. *Obstet Gynecol.* 2005 Feb;105(2):402-410.
2. Pritchard JA, Cunningham FG, Pritchard SA. The Parkland Memorial Hospital protocol for treatment of eclampsia: evaluation of 245 cases. *Am J Obstet Gynecol.* 1984 Apr 1;148(7):951-963.
3. Sibai BM, Eclampsia VI. Maternal-perinatal outcome in 254 consecutive cases. *Am J Obstet Gynecol.* 1990 Sep;163(3):1049-1055.
4. Miles JF Jr, Martin JN Jr, Blake PG, Perry KG Jr, Martin RW, Meeks GR. Postpartum eclampsia: a recurring perinatal dilemma. *Obstet Gynecol.* 1990 Sep;76(3 Pt 1):328-331.

Case 16

A 36-year-old G3P2002 Hispanic female at 36 weeks' gestation is sent from her physician's office to the obstetrical triage unit for mildly elevated blood pressures. The patient denies headache, visual abnormalities, or right upper quadrant pain. She has no uterine contractions or vaginal bleeding. Her blood pressure in the first trimester was in the 100/60 mm Hg range. On examination today, her BP is 156/98 mm Hg, HR 98 beats per minute, temperature 98.4°F, and RR 12. Her heart and lung examinations were normal. The fetal heart tones are in the 135 beats per minute range with accelerations. There are no uterine contractions. The vaginal examination reveals that the cervix is closed, long, and presenting part is cephalic. The CBC shows a hemoglobin level of 11 g/dL, platelet (plt) 80,000/mm^3, and glucose 98 mg/dL, serum glutamic oxaloacetic transaminase (SGOT) 400 IU/L and serum glutamic pyruvic transaminase (SGPT) 440 IU/L, and lactate dehydrogenase (LDH) 1000 mg/dL. Serum creatinine level is 0.8 mg/dL.

➤ What is the most likely diagnosis?

➤ What are your next steps?

➤ What additional lab tests are indicated at this stage?

ANSWERS TO CASE 16:
HELLP Syndrome

Summary: A 36-year-old G3P2002 Hispanic female at 36 weeks' gestation has a BP of 156/98 mm Hg. Her cervix is unfavorable and presenting part is cephalic. The patient has thrombocytopenia (plt 80,000), glucose 98 mg/dL, SGOT 400 IU/L and SGPT 440 IU/L, and LDH 1000 mg/dL. Serum creatinine level is 0.8 mg/dL.

> **Most likely diagnosis:** Hemolysis, elevated liver enzymes, low platelets (HELLP) syndrome.

> **Next steps:** Admission to labor and delivery unit, begin magnesium sulfate as prophylaxis against convulsions, assess and stabilize maternal condition, particularly blood pressure and coagulation abnormalities (DIC screen), and consider the best option for delivery.

> **Lab tests: A DIC screen should be obtained.** The blood bank should be contacted for possible need for blood products. Currently, there is no overt sign of bleeding or coagulopathy, and no transfusion is needed. The hemoglobin level and platelet count should be monitored, and the platelet count should be above 20,000/mm^3 to guard against spontaneous hemorrhage, and above 50,000/mm^3 for surgical hemostasis.

ANALYSIS

Objectives

1. Be able to describe the clinical presentation of HELLP syndrome.
2. Be able to describe the differential diagnosis of HELLP syndrome including causes of abnormal liver function tests.
3. Be able to describe the complications of HELLP syndrome.
4. Describe the treatment of HELLP syndrome including management of the blood products.

Considerations

The clinical presentation of patients with HELLP syndrome is highly variable and is considered a variant of preeclampsia. Patients may present with nonspecific symptoms or subtle signs of preeclampsia. Not all women (12%-18% cases) with HELLP syndrome have hypertension.[1] Generally, patients who present with HELLP syndrome are older, multiparous, white females who present at less than 35 weeks gestation.[2]

Patients usually present remote from term, complaining of epigastric or right upper quadrant pain, some have nausea or vomiting, and others have nonspecific viral syndrome-like symptoms. Most patients (90%) give a history of malaise for the past few days before presentation and some will have nonspecific viral syndrome-like symptoms.[3] A subset of patients with severe thrombocytopenia may present with bleeding from mucosal surfaces, hematuria, petechial hemorrhages, or ecchymosis.

There is no strict definition of HELLP syndrome. Criteria for HELLP syndrome is hemolysis (abnormal peripheral blood smear, LDH > 00 U/L, total bilirubin > 1.2 mg/dL); elevated liver enzymes (AST > 70 U/L); and low platelets (< 100,000/mm^3), low serum haptoglobin levels.[4] Peripheral blood smear may show schistocytes, burr cell, and echinocytes. There is no consensus in the literature regarding the liver function test to be used or the degree of elevation in these tests to diagnose elevated liver enzymes.[3]

The differential diagnoses of HELLP syndrome is extensive and may be found in Table 16–1. Because some patients with HELLP syndrome may present with gastrointestinal, respiratory, or hematologic symptoms in association with elevated liver enzymes or low platelets in the absence of hypertension or proteinuria, many cases of HELLP syndrome will initially be misdiagnosed.[3] HELLP is most commonly confused with two other medical conditions, acute fatty liver of pregnancy (AFLP), and thrombotic thrombocytopenic purpura/ hemolytic uremic syndrome (TTP/HUS).[5] The differentiation among HELLP, AFLP, and TTP/HUS is based on specific laboratory findings and slight differences in clinical presentation. An effort should be made to attempt to identify an accurate diagnosis given that management strategies may differ among these conditions. Patients with acute fatty liver of pregnancy typically present with nausea, vomiting, abdominal pain, and jaundice. Most patients will have

Table 16–1 DIFFERENTIAL DIAGNOSIS OF HELLP SYNDROME

Acute fatty liver of pregnancy
Hemolytic uremic syndrome
Thrombotic thrombocytopenic purpura
Systemic lupus erythematosis
Appendicitis
Hyperemesis gravidarum
Idiopathic thrombocytopenia
Gastroenteritis
Viral hepatitis
Pancreatitis
Gallbladder disease
Glomerulonephritis
Hemorrhagic or septic shock

prolonged PT and PTT with low fibrinogen and low serum glucose.[5] TTP is an extremely rare condition during pregnancy characterized by neurologic dysfunction, fever, severe thrombocytopenia, and severe hemolysis with a very low hematocrit. The liver enzymes may be normal or slightly elevated. Patients with HUS usually present with renal failure and most cases develop in the postpartum period.[3]

The presence of HELLP syndrome is associated with an increased risk of maternal death (1%).[6] Maternal morbidities of HELLP syndrome include eclampsia, placental abruption, acute renal failure, pulmonary edema, adult respiratory distress syndrome, subcapsular liver hematoma, disseminated intravascular coagulopathy, intracerebral hemorrhage, and sepsis. There is also an increased rate of wound hematomas and the need for transfusion of blood and blood products. The development of HELLP syndrome in the postpartum period also increases the risk of renal failure and pulmonary edema.[7] Perinatal mortality and morbidities also are increased in HELLP syndrome with the reported perinatal death rate ranging from 7.4% to 20.4%.[4]

APPROACH TO
HELLP Syndrome

Management and Treatment of HELLP Syndrome

Laboratory evaluation should include a complete blood count with platelet count, a peripheral smear, coagulation studies, serum AST, creatinine, glucose, bilirubin, and LDH levels. HELLP syndrome requires the presence of all the following: platelet count less than 100,000/mm³, AST more than 70 IU/L (> 2 times upper limit for normal values), abnormal peripheral smear, LDH more than 600 IU/L, and/or bilirubin more than 1.2 mg/dL.

The clinical course of women with HELLP syndrome is characterized by usually progressive and sometimes sudden deterioration in maternal and fetal conditions. The first priority is to assess and stabilize maternal condition, particularly coagulation abnormalities.[3] Transfer to a tertiary care center with appropriate neonatal care facilities is recommended. If present, severe hypertension should be controlled as well as correction of coagulopathy (Table 16–2). A magnesium sulfate infusion should be started for the prevention of an eclamptic seizure. Computed tomography or ultrasound of the abdomen should be considered if subcapsular hematoma of the liver is suspected.

Evaluation of the fetal well-being includes nonstress testing, biophysical profile, and ultrasound to evaluate the fetal growth and rule out intrauterine growth restriction.

Table 16–2 ANTIHYPERTENSIVE MEDICATION (TO KEEP BLOOD PRESSURE < 160/100 MM HG)

Hydralazine
5 mg IV bolus, repeat as needed every 15 to 20 min for a maximum dose of 20 mg/h

Labetalol
20-40 mg IV every 10-15 min for a maximum of 220 mg over 1 h

Nifedipine
10-20 mg orally every 30 min for a maximum dose of 40 mg/h

Immediate delivery is indicated in patients more than 34 weeks' gestation age. For patients less than 34 weeks, antenatal corticosteroids should be given and delivery planned in 48 hours, provided the maternal or fetal status does not decompensate (Table 16–3).[3] Because of the significant morbidity and mortality associated with HELLP syndrome, expectant management past 48 hours is generally not advised.

Other authors recommend a more conservative approach to prolong pregnancy in cases of fetal immaturity. The aim of expectant management is to improve neonatal morbidity and mortality. There is no high-quality evidence demonstrating that overall perinatal outcome in patients with HELLP syndrome is improved with expectant management compared with pregnancies delivered after a course of glucocorticoids.[8] Expectant management of HELLP syndrome remains an investigational approach and is contraindicated in women with DIC.

The presence of HELLP syndrome is not an indication for immediate delivery by cesarean section. Patients with a favorable cervix should undergo a trial of labor. Labor may be initiated with oxytocin infusion as for routine induction in all patients with gestational age over 30 weeks' gestation. The option of prostaglandin induction or elective cesarean section should be considered in patients at less than 30 weeks' gestational age with an unfavorable cervix.[3]

Table 16–3 INDICATIONS FOR DELIVERY IN HELLP SYNDROME

- < 23 wk or limits of viability
- ≥ 34 wk
- After corticosteroid administration if < 34 wk
- Fetal distress
- Maternal distress
  - Eclampsia
  - DIC
  - Respiratory distress
  - Suspect liver hematoma

Consultation with the anesthesiology team is warranted. Epidural anesthesia should be used with caution as many anesthesiologists are reluctant to place an epidural catheter with a platelet count less than 75,000/mm³. General anesthesia is the method of choice for cesarean sections in severe thrombocytopenia. The use of pudendal block is contraindicated in the setting of HELLP syndrome.

In the presence of significant bleeding (ecchymosis, bleeding from the gums, oozing from puncture sites, wound, intraperitoneal) with HELLP syndrome and in all patients with a platelet count less than 20,000/mm³, platelet transfusion is indicated either before or after delivery. If cesarean delivery is required, platelet transfusion of approximately 5 to 10 units should be initiated on call to the operating room in patients with severe thrombocytopenia (< 50,000) before intubation. There is rapid consumption of platelets in these patients (see Table 16-4 for blood product transfusion).

The surgeon should consider placement of a drain (subfacial, subcutaneous, or both) due to generalized oozing. The risk of hematoma formation without preventive therapy is approximately 20%.[3]

Postpartum management of HELLP patients should include close hemodynamic monitoring and serial laboratory evaluations approximately every 6 hours for 48 hours. Generally, most patients show resolving disease process within 48 hours postdelivery.

Table 16–4 BLOOD COMPONENT THERAPY FOR DIC IN PREGNANCY

Fresh frozen plasma (FFP) volume = 250 mL
• Corrects PT, PTT, and fibrinogen. Use 4 units initially and then as needed.
• Each unit increases fibrinogen 5-10 mg/dL.

Cryoprecipitate (volume 35-40 mL)
• Rich in fibrinogen.
• Utilizes less volume than FFP.
• Give when fibrinogen < 100 mg/dL or if clinical hemorrhage and fibrinogen < 150 mg/dL.
• Each unit increases fibrinogen 5-10 mg/dL.

Platelets
• Transfuse if maternal platelets < 20,000/mm³ whether or not clinically bleeding.
• Transfuse if maternal platelets < 50,000/mm³ if maternal hemorrhage or cesarean delivery.
• Each pack of platelets increases platelet count by 7,000-10,000/mm³.
• Rapid consumption of platelets in the setting of DIC.

Packed RBCs
• Increases oxygen carrying capacity.
• Transfuse to keep hematocrit > 25%.
• Follow electrolytes as hemolysis and RBC transfusion may lead to hyperkalemia.

Management of DIC

DIC may complicate HELLP syndrome and is a perilous situation in which there is the simultaneous processes of accelerated formation and lysis of clots. As a result, the body consumes clotting factors more rapidly than can be produced and replaced. Definitive therapy for DIC is removal of the inciting factor. In HELLP syndrome, the inciting factor is pregnancy related, and the definitive therapy is delivery.

Comprehension Questions

16.1   When counseling patients with a history of HELLP syndrome, what do you tell them is the approximate risk of recurrence of HELLP syndrome in subsequent pregnancies?

A. < 5%
B. 15%
C. 20%
D. 50%

16.2   A patient with HELLP syndrome is noted to have repetitive late decelerations and significant vaginal bleeding. Placental abruption is suspected. During an emergency cesarean delivery, the patient starts bleeding from venipuncture and IV site, mucous membranes, and incision sites. Stat labs are sent from the operating room, resulting in decreased fibrinogen, prolonged prothrombin time, and aPTT. What is the best management?

A. Transfusion of whole blood
B. Recombinant factor VII
C. Embolization of the hypogastric arteries
D. Fresh frozen plasma

16.3   A 34-year-old G2P1 woman is at 30 weeks' gestational age. She is noted to have severe preeclampsia and is delivered by cesarean due to nonreassuring fetal heart rate patterns. Two days postoperatively, the patient is noted to have severe right upper quadrant pain, and elevated liver function tests. On CT scan, she is noted to have a 4 cm hepatic hematoma without evidence of rupture. Her BP is 140/80 mm Hg, HR 90 beats per minute. Her hemoglobin level is 11.2 g/dL and plt count of 140,000/mm^3. Which of the following is the most appropriate management of this patient?

A. Blood transfusion of 3 units of packed erythrocytes
B. Percutaneous embolization of the hepatic arteries
C. Surgical repair
D. Serial ultrasound or CT

ANSWERS

16.1 **A.** Women with a history of HELLP syndrome are at increased risk of all forms of preeclampsia in subsequent pregnancies. The rate of recurrence of HELLP syndrome is less than 5%. However, the rate of preeclampsia is approximately 20% with significantly higher rates if the onset of HELLP syndrome occurred in the second trimester. Patients who have underlying chronic hypertension have higher risks of recurrence.[9] Therefore, these patients require close monitoring during subsequent pregnancies and should be counseled on their increased risk for adverse pregnancy outcome. At this time, there is no preventive therapy for recurrent HELLP syndrome.[4]

16.2 **D.** The diagnosis of DIC is usually made clinically with confirmation made through laboratory studies. A falling fibrinogen is usually the hallmark of DIC. Prolonged PT usually occurs prior to prolongation of the aPTT. Two intravenous lines should be established and a Foley catheter should be placed. Aggressive fluid resuscitation can be accomplished while blood component therapy is given. See Table 16–4 for blood component therapy. The fluid status must be monitored closely, as hypovolemia can lead to the development of acute renal failure. Fluid overload, on the other hand, can lead to pulmonary edema.

16.3 **C.** Management of a contained hepatic hematoma should include close hemodynamic monitoring and checking coagulation status. The patient should be supported with volume replacement and blood transfusion as needed. If the size of the hematoma remains stable and the laboratory abnormalities are resolving, the patient may be discharged with outpatient follow-up. Avoidance of abdominal palpation, convulsions, or emesis should be undertaken to prevent increased intra-abdominal pressure.[10]

A ruptured subcapsular liver hematoma is a surgical emergency, and should involve liver trauma and vascular surgeons. It usually involves the right lobe. Correction of coagulopathy and massive transfusions of blood products is essential. The maternal and fetal mortality rate is over 50%.[11] The current recommendation for treating rupture of subcapsular liver hematoma in pregnancy is packing and drainage.

Clinical Pearls

See US Preventive Services Task Force Study Quality levels of evidence in Case 1

➤ The diagnostic criteria used for HELLP syndrome are variable and inconsistent (Level III).

➤ HELLP syndrome may be confused with other medical, surgical conditions or obstetric complications (Level II-3).

➤ The potential benefits of expectant management in patients remote from term remain experimental (Level II-2).

➤ The use of pudendal block is contraindicated in patients with HELLP syndrome (Level III).

➤ Epidural anesthesia should be used with caution and is contraindicated with a platelet count less than 75,000/mm³ (Level III).

➤ The use of corticosteroids to improve maternal outcome remains experimental (Level I).

REFERENCES

1. Martin JN, Rinehart B, May WL, Magann EF, Terrone DA, Blake PG. The spectrum of severe preeclampsia: comparative analysis by HELLP syndrome classification. *Am J Obstet Gynecol.* 1999;180:1373-1384.

2. Roberts JM, Funai EF. Pregnancy related Hypertension. In: Creasy RK, Resknik R, Iams JD, Lockwood CJ, Moore TR, eds. *Creasy and Resnik's maternal fetal medicine: principles and practice,* 6th ed. Philadelphia: Saunders, 2009, 651-690.

3. Sibai BM. Diagnosis, controversies, and management of the syndrome of hemolysis, elevated liver enzymes, and low platelet count. *Obstet Gynecol.* 2004;103:981-991.

4. Queenan JT (ed). *Chronic Hypertension in Pregnancy in High Risk Pregnancy.* Washington DC: American College of Obstetricians and Gynecologists, 2007.

5. Sibai BM. Imitators of severe preeclampsia. *Obstet Gynecol.* 2007;109:956-966.

6. Sibai BM, Ramadan MK, Usta I, Salama M, Mercer BM, Friedman SA. Maternal morbidity and mortality in 442 pregnancies with hemolysis, elevated liver enzymes, and low platelets (HELLP syndrome). *Am J Obstet Gynecol.* 1993;169:1000-1006.

7. Drakeley AJ, LeRoux PA, Anthony J, Penny J. Acute renal failure complicating severe preeclampsia requiring admission to an obstetric intensive care unit. *Am J Obstet Gynecol.* 2002;186:253-256.

8. Abramovici D, Friedman SA, Mercer BM, Audibert F, Kao L, Sibai BM. Neonatal outcome in severe preeclampsia at 24 to 36 weeks' gestation: does HELLP syndrome matter? *Am J Obstet Gynecol.* 1999;180:221-225.

9. Van Pampus MG, Wolf H, Mayruhu G. Long-term follow up in patients with a history of HELLP syndrome. *Hypertens Pregnancy.* 2001;20:15-23.

10. Fonseca JE, Mendez F, Catalono P, Arias F. Dexamethasone treatment does not improve the outcome of women with HELLP syndrome. A double-blind, placebo-controlled, randomized clinical trial. *Am J Obstet Gynecol.* 2005;193:1591-1598.

11. Barton, JR, Sibai BM. Gastrointestinal complications of preeclampsia. *Semin Perinatol.* 2009;33:179-188.

Case 17

An 18-year-old G1P0 Hispanic female at 28 weeks' gestation comes into the obstetrical triage unit complaining of decreased fetal movement and headache. Her prenatal history is unremarkable. Her blood pressures in the first trimester was in the 100/60 mm/Hg range. On examination, her BP is 170/110 mm Hg, HR 98 beats per minute, temperature 98.4°F, and RR 12 breaths/min. Her heart and lung examinations are normal. The abdomen is nontender and the fundal height is 27 cm. The fetal heart tones are in the 135 beats per minute range with occasional variable decelerations on external fetal monitoring. There are no uterine contractions. The vaginal examination reveals that the cervix is closed, long, and posterior. The CBC shows a hemoglobin level of 12 g/dL, plt = 110,000, glucose = 98 mg/dL, SGOT = 32 IU/L and SGPT = 28 IU/L, and LDH = 102 mg/dL. Serum creatinine level is 0.6 mg/dL. The urinalysis shows 3+ protein on dipstick.

➤ What is the most likely diagnosis?

➤ What are your next steps?

➤ What are the important considerations in managing her pregnancy?

ANSWERS TO CASE 17:

Severe Preeclampsia

Summary: An 18-year-old G1P0 Hispanic female at 28 weeks' gestation has decreased fetal movement and headache. Her BP is 170/110 mm Hg, and fundal height is 27 cm. The fetal heart tones are in the 135 beats per minute range with occasional variable decelerations without contractions. The cervix is unfavorable. The CBC shows a hemoglobin level of 12 g/dL, plt 110,000/mm³, glucose 98 mg/dL, SGOT 32 IU/L, SGPT 28 IU/L, LDH 102 mg/dL, and creatinine 0.6 mg/dL. The urinalysis shows 3+ protein on dipstick.

➤ **Most likely diagnosis:** Severe preeclampsia.

➤ **Next steps:** (1) Initiate bed rest and serial blood pressure measurements, (2) fetal ultrasound and biophysical profile, and (3) characterization of the headache to assess for severe neurologic threat.

➤ **Important management considerations:** If the patient is felt to have severe preeclampsia of sufficient threat to either maternal or fetal well-being, then magnesium sulfate should be initiated, and plans made to proceed with delivery. However, often with bed rest, the blood pressure and headache will subside. If the patient can be stabilized and fetal well-being is assured, expectant management may be considered. If expectant management is chosen, then it would be appropriate to begin magnesium sulfate, administer corticosteroids, start a 24-hour urine protein collection, and begin serial laboratory studies to evaluate the patient for HELLP syndrome.

ANALYSIS

Objectives

1. Be able to describe the diagnostic criteria of preeclampsia and severe preeclampsia.
2. Be able to describe the diagnostic and management approach to preeclampsia.
3. Be able to discuss the considerations of managing severe preeclampsia in a preterm gestation.
4. Be able to describe the complications of severe preeclampsia.

Considerations

The first responsibility of the obstetrician to any patient with preeclampsia is to stabilize the mother and assess the well-being of her fetus. This patient's severe hypertension will need to be treated aggressively if it is not responsive to bed rest alone. The goal of antihypertensive therapy is to keep the systolic blood pressure less than 160 mm Hg and the diastolic pressure less than 100 mm Hg. Apresoline (hydralazine), labetalol, or nifedipine are antihypertensive medications that are commonly used for control of blood pressure. Her platelet count of 110,000/mm^3 is concerning for HELLP (hemolysis, elevated liver enzymes, low platelets) syndrome and these labs will need to be followed closely for significant changes. Her headache is concerning for the possibility of an impending seizure. If it does not resolve with bed rest or if she has other signs of CNS irritability, such as visual disturbances, clonus, or change in mental status, then magnesium sulfate for seizure prophylaxis should be started immediately. Urinary output should be measured on an hourly basis and collected for measurement of urinary protein. Fetal assessment is also critical. Continuous electronic fetal monitoring, a biophysical profile, or Doppler assessment of the fetal vessels are common ways to assess the fetus for evidence of uteroplacental insufficiency and significant compromise. Evaluation of the fetus for intrauterine growth restriction should be done as well. Delivery is the only "cure" for her preeclampsia.

In cases of fetal immaturity (< 34 wk gestation), expectant management may be considered if the fetal status is reassuring, the maternal condition can be stabilized, and the patient is in a carefully monitored care unit with experienced nurses and physicians. The primary consideration in this case would be gaining time to administer antenatal corticosteroids for the benefit of the premature fetus. There are no maternal benefits to expectant management. Assuming that the diagnosis of severe preeclampsia is confirmed, magnesium sulfate should be started, and the patient's blood pressure should be kept less than 160/100 mm/Hg. Betamethasone or dexamethasone should be started as soon as possible. Diminished urine output is common and while excessive proteinuria (> 5 g/24 h) is indicative of severe disease, it alone is not an indication for delivery. Further decrease in her platelet count, increase in her liver enzymes, or elevation of her LDH are all signs of worsening HELLP syndrome. At this point, expectant management should be reassessed and delivery considered. Poorly controlled hypertension, seizures, evidence of pulmonary edema, placental abruption, or signs of fetal compromise would be indications for delivery irrespective of gestational age. Once a course of corticosteroids for the fetus has been completed, the situation should be reevaluated. Further delay may be considered if the maternal and fetal status are stable and the benefits of delay outweigh the risks of continuing the pregnancy. Vaginal delivery is not contraindicated, but rapid deterioration of the fetal status and/or maternal condition may dictate an expedited delivery by cesarean section. The anesthesiologist should be made aware of the mother's status and neonatology should be present for the delivery of this premature infant.

APPROACH TO

Severe Preeclampsia

Nomenclature

Preeclampsia is a complication of human pregnancies occurring in 5% to 8% of all pregnant patients, and is a leading cause of maternal and fetal morbidity and mortality. Preeclampsia is, by definition, the development of new-onset hypertension (BP ≥140/90 mm Hg) and proteinuria (greater than 300 mg/24 h) in the mother after the 20th week of gestation. Currently, preeclampsia is designated as "mild" or "severe" based on several clinical and laboratory parameters. Mild preeclampsia is defined as a systolic blood pressure ≥ 140 mm Hg and a diastolic blood pressure ≥ 90 mm Hg in a previously normotensive pregnant patient, and the presence of ≥ 300 mg of protein in a 24-hour urine collection in a patient without previous renal disease.[1] In addition to these clinical parameters, the patient should have no other complaints or laboratory abnormalities and her fetus should exhibit normal growth. Severe preeclampsia is defined as a systolic BP ≥ 160 mm Hg and/or diastolic BP ≥ 110 mm Hg, ≥ 5 g of urinary protein excretion per 24 hours, plus evidence of other organ system involvement such as impaired liver function, thrombocytopenia, oliguria (≤ 500 mL in 24 h), pulmonary edema, epigastric or right upper quadrant pain, cerebral or visual disturbances, and/or fetal growth restriction.[1] In some cases, patients with chronic hypertension may have superimposed preeclampsia. Gestational hypertension is new-onset hypertension after the 20th week of gestation without the development of proteinuria. Lastly, the development of grand mal seizures in a patient with preeclampsia is defined as eclampsia. Our discussion will focus on severe preeclampsia.

Risk Factors and Etiology

Preeclampsia is unique to human pregnancies and generally thought of as a disease of nulligravid women. Seventy-five percent of cases are seen in pregnancies near term or intrapartum.[2] These cases are generally mild and not usually associated with significant complications or adverse outcomes. Cases of severe preeclampsia are often seen in patients with underlying maternal diseases and usually occur earlier in the third trimester of pregnancy. Commonly accepted risk factors for the development of preeclampsia include maternal obesity, advanced maternal age, chronic hypertension, diabetes, multifetal gestation, and African American ethnicity.[8] A maternal history of connective tissue disease, thrombophilia, or a family history of preeclampsia also increases a person's risk of preeclampsia. Pregnancy-related risk factors include molar pregnancies, fetal triploidy, a previous pregnancy complicated by preeclampsia or gestational hypertension, and unexplained fetal growth restriction.[8] There are no tests which are reliable in predicting the onset or severity of the disease.[5]

The etiology of preeclampsia is unknown. In the early 20th century, it was thought to be caused by fetal "toxins" which crossed the placenta and entered the maternal circulation.[3] Today, it is thought of as a multifactorial process involving abnormal trophoblast invasion of the uterine vessels, immunologic intolerance, maternal maladaptation to cardiovascular or inflammatory changes of pregnancy, and genetic influences.[4] These abnormalities lead to reduced uteroplacental blood flow, endothelial cell dysfunction, an imbalance of pro- and antiangiogenic factors, and alterations in prostaglandin production.[8] The result is intense vasospasm, systemic hypertension, capillary leakage, and other changes which result in multiorgan dysfunction. While the etiology is still uncertain, several studies have looked at various treatment modalities to prevent preeclampsia. Unfortunately no reliable treatment or supplementation regimen has shown consistently favorable results.[5]

Diagnosis and Differential Diagnosis

The diagnosis of preeclampsia requires regular assessment of the pregnant patient and a high degree of suspicion. Properly performed blood pressure measurements are essential for the proper diagnosis. Measurements must be performed with the appropriate size blood pressure cuff to be accurate. The patient should be sitting and allowed to rest for a few minutes before checking her blood pressure. Judgment should not be made with just one abnormal reading, and serial measurements will often clarify the clinical picture. The patient may have several complaints or be completely asymptomatic. The hypertensive patient should be questioned for the presence of a severe, long-lasting, frontal or occipital headache, blurry vision, or scotomata. It is also important to know if she has abdominal or epigastric pain, nausea, vomiting, or decreased fetal movement. On physical examination, significant weight gain over a short period of time may be an important clinical sign, as is pronounced edema in nondependent areas. On abdominal examination one should look for right upper quadrant abdominal pain or uterine tenderness and an appropriate fundal height. While fetal growth abnormalities are not diagnostic of preeclampsia, the presence for intrauterine growth restriction in patients with preeclampsia is indicative of severe disease. Signs of hyperreflexia are worrisome for an impending seizure. Proteinuria may be variable and, if more than 1+ on a urine dipstick, a 24-hour urine collection for total urinary protein and creatinine clearance should be started. Once the patient is thoroughly evaluated and laboratory assessments are complete, a determination can then be made as to whether or not the patient has preeclampsia and if so, if it is mild or severe disease.

The differential diagnosis of preeclampsia may include pyelonephritis, cholelithiasis, appendicitis, gastroenteritis, and/or renal stones. Most of these conditions can be distinguished by a complete medical history, thorough physical examination, and appropriate laboratory studies. Although rare, other conditions may mimic severe preeclampsia. These conditions include acute fatty liver of pregnancy, thrombotic thrombocytopenic purpura, hemolytic uremic syndrome, systemic lupus erythematosus with lupus nephritis, systemic viral sepsis, and systemic inflammatory response syndrome.[6] These microangiopathic disorders have many of the same clinical and laboratory findings as severe preeclampsia with HELLP syndrome. Each disorder has some distinguishing features which can be identified if the diagnosis is suspected. Treatment strategies are based on the specific disease process and delivery may or may not be indicated.

Management

If the patient is found to have blood pressures ≥ 160 mm Hg systolic or ≥ 110 mm Hg diastolic, proteinuria ≥ 5 g in a 24-hour urine collection, oliguria (≤ 500 cc/24 h), cerebral or visual disturbances, epigastric or right upper quadrant abdominal pain, pulmonary edema, thrombocytopenia (< 100,000/mm^3), or fetal growth restriction, she/he meets the criteria for severe preeclampsia.[1] Management of severe preeclampsia calls for careful monitoring of both the maternal and fetal condition, and may be influenced by the gestational age of the fetus at the time of diagnosis. Delivery is the only cure, and the health of the mother should be the primary concern. Blood pressures should be kept below 160/100 mm Hg to avoid cerebral vascular accidents in the mother. Labetalol has replaced hydralazine as the drug of choice for treating severe hypertension in many centers. It may be given as 20 to 40 mg IV every 10 to 15 minutes for a maximum of 220 mg. Invasive cardiovascular hemodynamic monitoring is rarely necessary. Urinary output must be closely monitored for the development of severe oliguria. Urinary excretion of protein should be measured on a regular basis. Seizure prophylaxis with magnesium sulfate is recommended, especially if there are signs of CNS irritation.

Most protocols for magnesium sulfate recommend an IV bolus of 4 to 6 g over 20 minutes, followed by an infusion of 1 to 2 g per hour. This is usually continued throughout labor and for the first 24 hours of the postpartum period. The patient should be monitored closely for respiratory depression, a primary concern with magnesium sulfate therapy. Laboratory studies to screen for HELLP syndrome are important as changes in these parameters may be unrecognized clinically. The presence of right upper quadrant or epigastric abdominal pain is concerning for liver swelling and potential rupture. Severe thrombocytopenia may predispose the patient to bleeding problems and may be an indication for delivery. Platelet transfusion may be necessary if signs of coagulation problems are evident clinically, if the platelet count is < 20,000 mm^3, or if a surgical procedure is planned. If the pregnancy is more than 34 weeks of gestation in a well-dated pregnancy, there is no benefit to delaying delivery once the mother's condition is stabilized.[7] Delivery should take place in a facility that can provide neonatal support if necessary.

Severe preeclampsia is not a contraindication to a vaginal delivery. Vaginal delivery, however, is not recommended in pregnancies less than 30 weeks gestation with HELLP syndrome and a Bishop score of less than 5.[8] Pitocin (Oxytocin) or prostaglandins may be used to induce labor. Epidural anesthesia for labor is not contraindicated unless severe thrombocytopenia is present. After delivery, the disease process usually begins to improve quickly. Within the first 48 hours, many laboratory values will have begun to return to normal, urinary output should have increased dramatically, and the proteinuria usually will have diminished significantly. In spite of these improvements, seizures can still occur up to 48 hours after delivery. Magnesium sulfate should be continued for the first 24 hours postpartum or until the patient has demonstrated a significant and sustained diuresis. It may be continued longer if neurologic symptoms persist and there is ongoing concern for seizure. If HELLP syndrome was a complicating factor, those laboratory abnormalities should be followed until they begin to show improvement. Hypertension may persist after delivery for several weeks to months and may require ongoing treatment.

Management Remote from Term

Pregnancies complicated by severe preeclampsia remote from term pose more difficult clinical decisions. In these pregnancies, the desire to delay the delivery in hopes of improving the fetal outcome is understandable. Expectant management has been advocated by some authors in those pregnancies with severe preeclampsia and less than 34 weeks of gestation where the mother can be safely stabilized and there is no evidence of fetal compromise. The immediate goal of expectant management is to delay delivery for 24 to 48 hours in order to give antenatal steroids to improve fetal lung function. Longer delays may have other benefits to the fetus, especially in the case of the extremely premature infant. In a retrospective study by Sibai and others, expectant management resulted in prolonging pregnancies between 27 and 33^6/$_7$ weeks' gestation by a median of 5 days. While the neonatal outcomes were favorable, maternal morbidity was seen in 25% of mothers.[9] Conditions such as pulmonary edema, renal failure, eclampsia, DIC, or nonreassuring fetal status necessitate delivery at any gestational age once the patient is stabilized. Previable pregnancies or pregnancies at the edge of viability which are complicated by severe preeclampsia pose even more difficult moral and ethical decisions. Again, maternal well-being must be the first consideration in these difficult cases and early termination of the pregnancy may be indicated.

Complications

Much like the disease itself, the complications of severe preeclampsia are protean in nature. Complications commonly listed include pulmonary edema, renal failure, DIC, abruptio placentae, adult respiratory distress syndrome, subcapsular liver hematoma, and retinal detachment (see Table 17-1). All of these complications are more common in pregnancies complicated by HELLP syndrome. Maternal deaths are still encountered as a result of eclamptic seizures, liver rupture, or cerebral vascular accidents. Fetal and neonatal morbidity and mortality result from intrauterine growth restriction, preterm delivery, and complications associated with placental abruptions. Patients in whom preeclampsia is diagnosed early in gestation have a higher complication rate. Future pregnancies may also be complicated by preeclampsia.[10]

The syndrome of hemolysis, elevated liver enzymes, and low platelets (HELLP) deserves special consideration as this syndrome adds to the complexity of severe preeclampsia. The acronym of HELLP was coined by Weinstein in 1985, but Pritchard and others had described many features of the syndrome much earlier.[11,12] While this syndrome is usually associated with the typical features of preeclampsia, 10% to 15% of patients with HELLP syndrome will lack proteinuria or hypertension.[13] The hemolysis is due to a microangiopathic hemolytic process. The elevated liver enzymes are the result of liver ischemia and periportal necrosis. The thrombocytopenia is variable and related to platelet activation, aggregation, and consumption. Diagnostic tests for these problems include evaluation of liver enzymes (AST and ATL), a CBC and platelet count, and an LDH level. Some or all of these changes may be diagnosed in the individual patient. The clinical course is usually progressive and is associated with increased rates of maternal and fetal morbidity and mortality. Thrombocytopenia is a particularly worrisome development that predisposes the patient to significant risks. The development of a subcapsular liver hematoma and subsequent rupture often has devastating consequences. Special care and expertise are often needed to manage these very difficult cases. The abnormalities resolve fairly quickly after delivery and usually without permanent organ damage. Women with a history of HELLP syndrome have an increased risk of preeclampsia in their subsequent pregnancies, especially if the onset of the disease was in the second trimester.[14]

Table 17–1 PREGNANCY OUTCOME IN WOMEN WITH MILD AND SEVERE PREECLAMPSIA

	Hauth et al[15]		Buchbinder et al[16]		Hnat et al[17]	
	MILD (N = 217)	SEVERE (N = 109)	MILD[a] (N = 62)	SEVERE[a] (N = 45)	MILD (N = 86)	SEVERE (N = 70)
Delivery (wk)[a]						
< 37 (%)	NR	NR	25.8	66.7	14.0	33.0
< 35 (%)	1.9[b]	18.5[b]	9.7	35.6	2.3	18.6
SGA infant (%)[a]	10.2	18.5	4.8	11.4	NR	NR
Abruptio placentae (%)	0.5	3.7	3.2	6.7	0	1.4
Perinatal death (%)	1.0	1.8	0	8.9	0	1.4

[a]This study included women with previous **preeclampsia**. The other studies included only nulliparous women.
[b]These rates are for delivery at less than 34 weeks.

Comprehension Questions

17.1 Which of the following is a criteria for the diagnosis of severe preeclampsia?

A. Presence of 3+ edema

B. Maternal blood pressure > 160/110 mm Hg on two separate occasions 6 hours apart

C. The excretion of 700 mg of protein in a 24-hour urine collection

D. Decreased fetal movement

17.2 A 22-year-old G1P0 woman at 29 weeks' gestation is noted to have a diagnosis of HELLP syndrome. Which of the following finding is most likely to be present in this patient?

A. Seizures/convulsions

B. Oliguria

C. Low platelets

D. Subcapsular liver hematoma

17.3   Magnesium sulfate is given to the preeclamptic patient for which of
        the following?
        A. Control blood pressure
        B. Improve urinary output
        C. Reduce peripheral edema
        D. Prevent seizures

17.4   A 28-year-old nullipara at 29 weeks' gestation is diagnosed with severe
        preeclampsia based on persistent blood pressures of 220/140 mm Hg
        range and 3+ proteinuria. Her first-trimester blood pressures were in
        the 100/60 mm Hg range. She is counseled regarding the risks and
        benefits of expectant management versus delivery. Which of the fol-
        lowing statement is most accurate for this patient?
        A. Delivery is generally not indicated until after 34 weeks of gestation.
        B. Delivery is generally performed for the benefit of the mother.
        C. Expectant management is associated with a higher rate of mater-
           nal complications.
        D. Control of the blood pressures with antihypertensive agents are
           associated with improved fetal outcome.

ANSWERS

17.1   **B.** The diagnosis of severe preeclampsia is most often made in the pres-
        ence of severe hypertension (systolic blood pressure of > 160 mm Hg
        and diastolic blood pressure > 110 mm Hg) and significant protein-
        uria (> 5 g of urinary protein per 24 h urine collection). By definition,
        the severe hypertension should be persistent and seen on two readings
        6 hours apart. While the presence of significant edema may be pres-
        ent in the severely preeclamptic patient, it is not part of the diagnos-
        tic criteria. The same may be said for decreased fetal movement.

17.2   **C.** The diagnostic criteria for HELLP syndrome include hemolysis,
        elevated liver enzymes, and low platelets. The preeclamptic patient
        with HELLP syndrome may have oliguria and is at risk for a subcap-
        sular liver hematoma, but these are complications of her disease, not
        part of the diagnostic criteria. Eclampsia is, by definition, a seizure in
        a preeclamptic patient.

17.3   **D.** Magnesium sulfate is given for seizure prophylaxis only. It may
        lower the blood pressure slightly but other drugs should be used to
        treat severe hypertension. Magnesium sulfate therapy frequently
        reduces urinary output; therefore urine production should be closely
        monitored. Magnesium sulfate does not help in reducing peripheral
        edema.

17.4   **B.** Expectant management of the patient with severe preeclampsia only benefits the fetus. There are no maternal benefits, only a higher risk of maternal complications. Expectant management should only be considered for the fetus less than 34 weeks' gestation. Most authorities feel that after 34 weeks of gestation there are few benefits to further delay. While expectant management may reduce the risk of some complications of prematurity to the fetus, there is no guarantee that complications related to prematurity will not occur.

Clinical Pearls

See US Preventive Services Task Force Study Quality levels of evidence in Case 1

➤ Severe preeclampsia by proteinuria alone is not an indication for delivery (Level II-2).

➤ Eclampsia may be seen only in patients who slighted elevated blood pressures (Level III).

➤ Magnesium sulfate is not a CNS depressant for the mother or the fetus (Level II-1).

➤ A persistent headache and abdominal pain are clinical signs of worsening disease (Level III).

➤ Urine dipstick testing for protein has a poor predictive value and a high false-positive rate (Level II-2).

➤ Calcium gluconate 1 g IV should be given to reverse toxicity symptoms of magnesium sulfate (Level II-1).

➤ Methergine for control of postpartum bleeding/hemorrhage is contraindicated in the preeclamptic patient (Level III).

➤ The use of antenatal corticosteroids may result in a temporary improvement in abnormal laboratory values of HELLP syndrome (Level II-2).

REFERENCES

1. American College of Obstetricians and Gynecologists. Diagnosis and management of preeclampsia and eclampsia, *ACOG Practice Bulletin, No. 33.* 2002;33.
2. Sibai BM. Diagnosis and management of gestational hypertension and preeclampsia. *Obstet Gynecol.* 2003;102:181.
3. Williams W J. Complications resulting directly from pregnancy. In: *Obstetrics.* New York and London: D. Appleton and Co.; 1903:455-466.
4. Sibia B, Dekker G, Kupferminc M. Preeclampsia. *Lancet.* 2005;365:785-799.
5. Barton J, Sibai B. Prediction and prevention of recurrent preeclampsia. *Obstet Gynecol.* 2008; 112:359-372.

6. Sibai M. Imitators of Severe Pre-eclampsia. *Semin Periantol.* 2009;33:196-205.
7. Royal College of Obstetricians and Gynaecologists. The Management of Severe Pre-eclampsia/Eclampsia. Guideline No.10 (A), March 2006.
8. Gabbe SG, Niebyl JR, Simpson JL. Preeclampsia. In: *Obstetrics: Normal and Problem Pregnancies.* 5th ed. New York, NY: Churchill Livingstone; 2007:866-890.
9. Bombrys AE, Barton JR, Hable M, Sibai BM. Expectant management of severe preeclampsia at 27 0/7 to 33 6/7 weeks' gestation: maternal and perinatal outcomes according to gestational age by weeks at onset of expectant management. *Am Journ Perinatol.* 2009;26:441-446.
10. Sibai BM, El-Nazer A, Gonzalez-Ruiz AR. Severe preeclampsia-eclampsia in young primigravid women: subsequent pregnancy outcome and remote prognosis. *Am J Obstet Gynecol.* 1986;155:1011.
11. Weinstein L. Preeclampsia-eclampsia with hemolysis, elevated liver enzymes, and thrombocytopenia. *Obstet Gynecol.* 1985;66:657.
12. Pritchard JA, Weisman R J, Ratnoff OD, et al. Intravascular hemolysis, thrombocytopenia and other hematologic abnormalities associated with severe toxemia of pregnancy. *N Engl J Med.* 1954;250:87.
13. Martin JN, Rinehart B, May WL, et al. The spectrum of severe preeclampsia: comparative analysis by HELLP syndrome classification. *Am J Obstet Gynecol.* 1999;180:1373.
14. Van Pampus MG, Wolf H, Mayruhu G, et al. Long-term follow-up in patients with a history of (H)ELLP syndrome. *Hypertens Pregnancy.* 2001;20:15.
15. Hauth JC, Ewell MG, Levine RJ, et al. Pregnancy outcomes in healthy nulliparas who developed hypertension. *Obstet Gynecol* 2000;95(1):24-8.
16. Buchbinder A, Sibai, Caritis S, et al. Adverse perinatal outcomes are signifcantly higher in severe gestational hypertension than in mild preeclampsia. *Am J Obstet Gynecol* 2002;186(1):66-71.
17. Hnat MD, Sibai BM, Caritis S, et al. Perinatal outcome in women with recurrent preeclampisa compared wtih women who developed preeclampsia as nulliparas. *Am J Obstet Gynecol* 2003;189(1):244.

Case 18

A 22-year-old woman presents to the emergency department after experiencing a tonic-clonic seizure witnessed by her husband at home. She is postictal and unable to give a history. Her husband states that she has a history of epilepsy, and has not had a seizure for over 3 years. She currently takes phenytoin (Dilantin) 300 mg daily and an oral contraceptive. He is not certain when her last menstrual period occurred.

An IV is started, and labs are drawn. As the patient becomes more responsive, she states that she has been taking her medications regularly, and her LMP was over 3 months ago. She states that this pattern is not unusual for her since starting low-dose oral contraceptive pills (OCPs) 6 months ago. Blood pressure is 90/60 mm Hg, pulse is 88, and respirations are 16 per minute. Labs show normal electrolytes, glucose, calcium, and magnesium, a borderline therapeutic level of phenytoin, and a positive urine pregnancy test. Urinalysis reveals trace protein and no WBCs or RBCs. Pelvic examination reveals a 14-week sized uterus with fetal heart tones present.

➤ What is the most likely diagnosis?

➤ What is your next step?

➤ What are potential complications of the patient's disorder?

ANSWERS TO CASE 18:
Epilepsy in Pregnancy

Summary: This is a 22-year-old woman with an epileptic seizure who takes low-dose OCPs and phenytoin, which may reduce the effectiveness of OCPs by increasing liver metabolism. She is 14 weeks pregnant and has continued phenytoin during the first trimester, which increases the risk of adverse effects to the fetus.

➤ **Most likely diagnosis:** Epileptic seizure in pregnancy.

➤ **Next step:** Rule out eclampsia, space occupying brain lesions, trauma, infection, electrolyte or glucose abnormalities, intracranial bleeding, and toxins or drug exposure; evaluate the fetus for anomalies from phenytoin exposure; adjust and monitor her antiepileptic drugs (AED).

➤ **Potential complications:** Maternal risk with recurrent seizures with subtherapeutic medication levels; adverse effects on the fetus from AED exposure in first trimester.

ANALYSIS

Objectives

1. Recognize the differential diagnosis of convulsions in pregnancy.
2. Be familiar with the evaluation and management of pregnant patients with a history of epilepsy.
3. Learn about appropriate drug therapy for epilepsy and the potential adverse effects on the fetus.
4. Recognize pregnancy complications associated with epilepsy.

Considerations

Seizures in pregnancy may be the result of eclampsia after 20 weeks or in the presence of a molar pregnancy in any trimester. New-onset seizures may be the result of an intracranial hemorrhage, space occupying lesion, CNS infection, trauma, or toxin or drug exposure. Women with a history of idiopathic epilepsy who seize during pregnancy may have subtherapeutic drug levels and should be advised to increase their dose with careful serum monitoring of levels. Fetal effects of antiepileptic drugs may be significant, and should be sought by ultrasound and maternal serum screening.

APPROACH TO
Epilepsy in Pregnancy

A pregnant patient with new-onset seizures requires a much different evaluation than the one with a history of epilepsy. New-onset seizures after 20 weeks' gestation should always considered to be the result of eclampsia and treated accordingly unless a thorough workup reveals another etiology. While a molar pregnancy prior to 20 weeks' gestation has been associated with preeclampsia in early pregnancy, an intrauterine fetus makes eclampsia prior to 20 weeks' gestation unlikely and another etiology should be sought. Acquired seizures may result from trauma, infection, metabolic disorders, drug or toxin exposure, intracranial hemorrhage, or space occupying lesion. The evaluation for new-onset seizures in pregnancy should include a history for evidence of trauma, drug usage (including cocaine) and toxin exposure, observation for signs of CNS infection or localizing neurologic signs, evaluation of the WBC count, measurement of electrolytes, calcium and magnesium, and glucose, lumbar puncture (LP) for evidence of infection or blood, EEG, and intracranial imaging for signs of bleeding or space-occupying lesion. If eclampsia is suspected, magnesium sulfate is administered and consideration for delivery is discussed with the patient. If no obvious etiology for the seizure is found or the patient has a history of epilepsy, consideration for therapy with AED should occur. Epilepsy in pregnancy with appropriate therapy usually results in a successful pregnancy and healthy neonate.

Effect of Pregnancy on Epilepsy

Nausea and vomiting, insufficient sleep, an expanding plasma volume, and a reduction in plasma proteins which attach and transport AEDs in the blood may all lead to a reduction in serum levels of AEDs and an increased incidence of seizures in pregnancy. Clearance of most of the AEDs increases during pregnancy, and returns to prepregnancy levels by 2 to 3 months postpartum. One notable exception is lamotrigine clearance, which increases dramatically up to 230% above baseline during pregnancy, and returns to prepregnancy levels within a few weeks of birth. Up to 33% of pregnant women will experience an increase in seizure frequency during pregnancy, while 7% to 25% report a decrease, and 50% to 83% report no change. Sleep deprivation or noncompliance may play a role in up to 70% of the increase of seizures in some patients during pregnancy, and the patient should be informed about the importance of compulsive drug maintenance.

Effect of Epilepsy on Pregnancy

Although it is difficult to separate the influence of AEDs from the background risk of maternal epilepsy to the fetus, children of women with epilepsy during pregnancy have an increased risk of mental deficiency that has been reported as high as 6% in some studies. However, while children of mothers with epilepsy have an increased risk of developmental delay, children of fathers with epilepsy do not show that same increased risk, and women with epilepsy who do not take AEDs during pregnancy have no increase in behavioral deficits compared to matched controls. It is clear that women with epilepsy who also take AEDs have an increased risk of fetal anomalies, including IUGR, major and minor malformations, cognitive disorders, microcephaly, and infant mortality, all encompassed in the term "fetal anticonvulsant syndrome" which has been associated with most of the currently prescribed AEDs. IUGR affects 7% to 10% of pregnancies of epileptic women on AEDs, and polytherapy seems to be an even more potent cause of reduced fetal growth. Minor anomalies including distal digital and nail hypoplasias and midline craniofacial anomalies occur in 6% to 20% of infants of epileptic mothers, a 2.5-fold increase compared to the general pregnant population.

Major malformations occur in 4% to 7% of infants of epileptic mothers and include congenital heart defects (ASD, VSD, PDA, pulmonary stenosis, coarctation of the aorta, and tetralogy of Fallot), cleft lip/palate, urogenital disorders (commonly glandular hypospadias), and neural tube defects (NTDs). In a cohort comparison investigating prescribing practices during two different time periods, the older cohort (1972-1979) had more women taking phenobarbital, primidone, and phenytoin while the newer cohort (1981-1985) saw women being prescribed more monotherapy with valproic acid or carbamazepine. The older series resulted in more infants with congenital heart defects, facial clefts, developmental retardation, and minor anomalies while the newer series saw an increased rate of neural tube defects and glandular hypospadias. While the risks of major anomalies vary by AED, multiple studies confirm the greatest risk occurs in the presence of polytherapy, with rates as high as 25% when four or more AEDs are taken during pregnancy. Other studies report malformation rates of 6.5% with monotherapy for epilepsy compared to 15.6% with polytherapy.

Generalized tonic-clonic seizures during pregnancy have been associated with maternal and fetal hypoxia and acidosis, and fetal intracranial hemorrhage has been reported after a single generalized tonic-clonic seizure.

The effect of nonconvulsive seizures increase the mother's risk of trauma with resultant fetal injury or abruptio placenta. Although concerns have been raised about other obstetric complications resulting from maternal epilepsy, a recent large study from India evaluating a number of common pregnancy complications found only spontaneous abortion, anemia, ovarian cysts, fibroids, and peripartum seizures were more common in epileptic women when compared to a nonepileptic control group.

Effect of AEDs on the Fetus

Antiepileptic drug therapy may have a major impact on fetal development, and a thorough preconception discussion with patients who have epilepsy and who are contemplating pregnancy is critical. Taking a patient off all AEDs prior to conception is usually not feasible, and should be based on the same criteria as in nonpregnant situations. Supplemental folic acid 4 mg daily should be prescribed preconceptionally and during the antepartum period to minimize the risk of birth defects. Monotherapy at the lowest dose that prevents seizures should be the goal.

Antepartum Management

Preconception counseling, supplemental folic acid 4 mg daily, and monotherapy at the lowest dose that prevents seizures should be the practitioner's goal. The frequency of monitoring serum levels of AEDs varies with the individual patient's response, and with the level of protein binding of the AED. A recent review article by Patsalos et al in 2008 contains protein binding rates and other important information regarding therapeutic drug monitoring of AEDs.

In general, free serum levels of AED should be followed when the AED is highly or moderately protein bound, and total levels are adequate with minimal protein binding. A baseline level prior to pregnancy when the patient is seizure-free with repeat levels at least each trimester and within 4 weeks of the EDC may be adequate for most patients, although monthly levels should be considered for patients with widely fluctuating serum levels of AED. Maternal serum screening for NTDs at the appropriate time in gestation, and detailed anatomic ultrasound for anomalies associated with AEDs should be performed by 20 weeks of gestation.

While many experts recommend supplemental vitamin K administration 10 mg po daily to pregnant women taking AEDs from 36 weeks until delivery to minimize the chance of hemorrhagic complications in the newborn due to vitamin K deficiency, a recent literature review found inadequate evidence to recommend routine administration of vitamin K during that gestational period.

Intrapartum Management

Labor and delivery is usually uneventful and results in a successful vaginal delivery in the majority of women with epilepsy. Being npo and sleep deprived for extended periods of time predisposes women in labor to a lower seizure threshold, and when generalized tonic-clonic seizures occur during labor, they should be treated promptly and aggressively. The drug meperidine may reduce the seizure threshold and should be avoided when possible during labor. Convulsions in labor may be treated acutely with lorazepam or diazepam intravenously.

Postpartum Management

Most AED levels gradually increase after delivery and plateau around 10 weeks postpartum with the notable exception of lamotrigine which increases immediately and plateaus within 2 to 3 weeks of delivery. These changes necessitate close monitoring of drug levels to avoid toxicity from the increased doses commonly used during pregnancy. Although most AEDs are found in breast milk, breast-feeding is not contraindicated for any of the AEDs used in pregnancy. Sleep deprivation may increase the incidence of seizures in some postpartum individuals.

Comprehension Questions

18.1 A 22-year-old G1P0 woman has witnessed a tonic-clonic seizure. She is 19 weeks' gestation. The obstetrician believes that eclampsia is a possible etiology of convulsions in this instance. Which of the following is most likely to be present?
A. Abnormal appearing fetus on ultrasound
B. Hypertension
C. Headaches
D. Proteinuria
E. Lower extremity edema

18.2 The antiepileptic drugs valproic acid and carbamazepine are associated with an increased risk of which of the following?
A. Hydrops fetalis
B. Multiple gestation
C. Neural tube defects
D. Preterm labor
E. Renal agenesis

18.3 A common minor anomaly in the fetus of a woman with epilepsy is which of the following?
A. Midline craniofacial defects
B. Polydactyly
C. Pyloric stenosis
D. Renal pyelectasis
E. Equinovarus

18.4 Intrapartum convulsions may be treated acutely with intravenously administered which of the following?
A. Diazepam
B. Phenobarbital
C. Valproic acid
D. Carbamazepine
E. Lamotrigine

ANSWERS

18.1   **A.** Unless a molar pregnancy is present, eclampsia occurs only after 20 weeks' gestation so the presence of a normal appearing fetus allows the physician to exclude eclampsia as the etiology of seizures prior to 20 weeks' gestation.

18.2   **C.** Valproic acid and carbamazepine are associated with an increased incidence of neural tube defects, and supplemental folic acid should be offered preconceptionally to women who must continue those drugs in early pregnancy.

18.3   **A.** Midline facial clefts are one of the most common minor anomalies associated with AEDs used in early pregnancy.

18.4   **A.** Acutely during labor, intravenous lorazepam or diazepam may be used to treat generalized convulsions.

Clinical Pearls

See US Preventive Services Task Force Study Quality levels of evidence in Case 1

➤ Most women with epilepsy have a normal and uncomplicated pregnancy (Level II-2).

➤ Because of increased liver metabolism generated by many of the AEDs, unanticipated pregnancy is more likely in women on those AEDs taking oral contraceptives (Level II-2).

➤ Epileptic patients require more intense monitoring of serum levels of AEDs and increasing doses of their medication up to delivery (Level II-1).

➤ Fetal effects of AEDs include IUGR, neural tube defects (primarily valproic acid and carbamazepine), and midline craniofacial defects and congenital heart defects (phenytoin and phenobarbital) (Level II-2).

➤ Monotherapy with AEDs has been associated with fewer fetal effects than polytherapy (Level II-2).

➤ Patients who take AEDs during the first trimester should be offered maternal serum screening and detailed fetal ultrasound prior to 20 weeks' gestation to observe for fetal anomalies that may result from the AEDs (Level III).

➤ Supplemental vitamin K during the last month of pregnancy may be associated with fewer episodes of neonatal hemorrhagic complications (Level III).

REFERENCES

1. Arpino C, Brescianini S, Robert E, et al. Teratogenic effects of antiepileptic drugs: use of an international database on malformations and drug exposure (MADRE). *Epilepsia.* 2000;41:1436-1443.
2. Holmes LB, Rosenberger PB, Harvey EA, Khoshbin S, Ryan L. Intelligence and physical features of children of women with epilepsy. *Teratology.* 2000;61:196-202.
3. Kaaja E, Kaaja R, Hiilesmaa V. Major malformations in offspring of women with epilepsy. *Neurology.* 2003;60:575-579.
4. Lindhout D, Meinardi H, Meijer J, Nau H. Antiepileptic drugs and teratogenesis in two consecutive cohorts: changes in prescription policy paralleled by changes in pattern of malformations. *Neurology.* 1992;42(Suppl 5):94-110.
5. Meador KJ, Zupanc ML. Neurodevelopmental outcomes of children born to mothers with epilepsy. *Cleve Clin J Med.* 2004;71(Suppl 2):38S-40S.
6. Minkoff H, Schaffer R, Delke I, Grunevaum A. Diagnosis of intracranial hemorrhage in utero after a maternal seizure. *Obstet Gynecol.* 1985;65(Suppl):22S-24S.
7. Patsalos PN, Berry DJ, Bourgeois Blaise JD, et al. Antiepileptic drugs—best practice guidelines for therapeutic drug monitoring: a position paper by the subcommission on therapeutic drug monitoring, ILAE Commission on Therapeutic Strategies. *Epilepsia.* 2008;49(7):1239-1276.
8. Pennell PB. Pregnancy in women who have epilepsy. *Neurol Clin.* 2004;22:799-820.
9. Pennell PB, Newport DJ, Stowe ZN, Helmers SL, Montgomery JQ, Henry TR. The impact of pregnancy and childbirth on the metabolism of lamotrigine. *Neurology.* 2004;62:292-295.
10. Thomas SV, Sindhu K, Ajaykumar B, Sulekha Devi PB, Sujamol J. et al. Maternal and obstetric outcome of women with epilepsy. *Seizure.* 2009 Apr;18(3):163-166.
11. Wide K, Winbladh B, Tomson T, Kallen B. Body dimensions of infants exposed to antiepileptic drugs in utero: observations spanning 25 years. *Epilepsia.* 2000;41:854-861.
12. Yasasmit W, Chaithongwongwatthana S, Tolosa JE. Prenatal vitamin K1 administration in epileptic women to prevent neonatal hemorrhage: is it effective? *J Reprod Med.* 2006 June;51(6):463-466.
13. Yerby MS. Quality of life, epilepsy advances, and the evolving role of anticonvulsants in women with epilepsy. *Neurology.* 2000;55:21-31.

Case 19

A 30-year-old G2P0020 presents to the office for preconception counseling secondary to an 8-year history of diabetes mellitus. She regularly
sees an internist who manages her diabetes and general medical care.
She has been treated with multiple oral hypoglycemic medications in
order to achieve appropriate glycemic control. Her current regimen
includes glyburide which she has taken for the past year and metformin
which was added 6 months prior to improve her level of glycemic control. She denies hypertension, retinopathy, and renal disease. Her
obstetric history is significant for two first trimester pregnancy losses
occurring 1 and 3 years prior. The patient and her husband are contemplating a pregnancy; however she is concerned about her risk of pregnancy loss and other potential effects of diabetes on her pregnancy.

➤ What is the next step in evaluating this patient?

➤ What are potential maternal complications of diabetes mellitus in
  pregnancy?

➤ What are potential fetal complications?

➤ How would you counsel this patient in terms of pregnancy planning?

➤ How would you manage her if she became pregnant?

ANSWERS TO CASE 19:
Pregestational Diabetes

Summary: An essential nulliparous with a personal history of diabetes and multiple pregnancy losses presents for preconception counseling.

> **First step in evaluating this patient:** A detailed history and physical examination including baseline laboratory testing should be completed to assess the severity of her disease. A conversation should be had stressing the importance of effective contraception to ensure that conception does not occur until diabetic control is optimized.

> **Potential maternal complications of diabetes mellitus in pregnancy:** Women with diabetes who become pregnant often experience less stable glycemic control. They are also at increased risk of chronic hypertension, preeclampsia, diabetic retinopathy, and cesarean delivery.

> **Potential fetal complications:** Diabetics with suboptimal glycemic control have higher rates of pregnancy loss birth defects, preterm delivery, disturbances in fetal growth, and stillbirth.

> **Counselling this patient in terms of pregnancy planning:** The patient should be counseled that she should optimize her diabetic control prior to conception. A glycosylated hemoglobin level (HbA_{1c}) less than 7% is recommended in order to obtain neonatal morbidity and mortality rates similar to the general population.

> **Management plan in case of pregnancy:** She should receive frequent physician visits in order to monitor glycemic control. She should receive ophthalmologic evaluations every trimester and during the postpartum period. She should receive a detailed anatomy ultrasound and potentially a fetal echocardiogram during the second trimester. Fetal surveillance should be achieved with antenatal testing and serial growth ultrasounds. If glycemic control is optimal, delivery should occur between 39 and 40 weeks' gestation. Women with suboptimal control should be delivered prior to 39 weeks after fetal lung maturity is confirmed.

ANALYSIS

Objectives

1. Describe the effect of pregestational diabetes on the pregnancy.
2. Describe the management of pregestational diabetes.
3. List the complications that may occur to a pregestational diabetic during pregnancy.

Considerations

Diabetes affects approximately 8 million women annually and complicates approximately 1% of all pregnancies. Pregestational diabetes accounts for approximately 10% of insulin resistance encountered in pregnant women with the larger share being owed to gestational diabetes[1] (Level III).

The most important aspects of managing women with diabetes who become pregnant should occur prior to conception. These women should be thoroughly educated on the impact of pregnancy on their disease and disease management in addition to the effect that diabetes may have on their baby. Women with suboptimal diabetic control should be counseled in terms of appropriate contraception in order to ensure that conception occurs only after appropriate control has been established.

Preconception counseling should include a detailed history and physical examination in order to assess the severity of their disease as well as their level of glycemic control. Initial laboratory tests should include measurements of glycosylated hemoglobin (HbA_{1c}), thyroid-stimulating hormone (TSH), screening for creatinine clearance and urinary protein excretion, complete blood count, and a blood chemistry screen[2,3] (Level III). The purpose of these laboratory tests are twofold, first of all it is important to assess the baseline health status and severity of disease prior to pregnancy in order to make plans regarding timing of pregnancy and appropriate surveillance. Second, women with chronic health condition such as diabetes are at risk of other comorbid conditions which may affect maternal and neonatal outcome. All pregestational diabetics should have ophthalmologic examinations prior to and during pregnancy. The frequency of surveillance can be based on the degree of retinopathy. Those with chronic conditions such as hypertension and hypercholesterolemia should receive appropriate evaluations such as ECG and echocardiograms with cardiology consultations as appropriate. Medications which are contraindicated during pregnancy such as angiotensin converting enzyme inhibitors (ACE-I) should be discontinued prior to conception. Oral hypoglycemic agents can be discontinued during the first trimester if glycemic control is optimal based on HbA_{1C}. Insulin treatment can be started based on glucose monitoring. Alternatively, if the patient's glycemic control is suboptimal on oral hypoglycemic agents, she can be switched to insulin immediately.

APPROACH TO
Pregestational Diabetes

The previously used **White classification** was devised to classify diabetes based on the duration of disease and the presence or absence of end-stage organ disease. One of the main utilities of this system was that it assisted physicians in predicting risk of perinatal loss and serious morbidity. As neonatal and maternal prognosis has greatly improved, this system has proven to be less useful. The classification system that most physicians currently use classifies insulin resistance based on whether the physiology is due to β-cell dysfunction resulting in an absolute insulin deficiency as is seen in type 1 diabetes or due to insulin resistance and relative insulin deficiency as is seen in type 2 diabetes[2,4] (Level III). Additional information should be provided concerning diabetic complications. This classification scheme relates outcomes to the degree of metabolic control and thus better directs treatment modalities.

Maternal Effects

Physiologic changes of pregnancy affect the degree of insulin resistance resulting in a need to adjust insulin dosing as pregnancy progresses. The primary fuel source for the fetus is glucose, therefore there are mechanisms in place to ensure that this source is readily available. The placenta produces diabetogenic hormones such as growth hormone, corticotrophin-releasing hormone, human placental lactogen, and progesterone which create an insulin resistant state[3] (Level III). As a result there is postprandial hyperglycemia providing a ready supply for the fetus. In a nondiabetic woman, there is a responsive up-regulation of insulin production by β-cells which restores maternal glycemic levels[2,3,5] (Level II-2, III). In a woman with diabetes, this does not occur, either due to β-cell dysfunction or lack of β-cell reserve resulting in persistent hyperglycemia.

End-organ damage is a major concern in all patients with diabetes; however, there are considerations which are specific to pregnancy. **Diabetic retinopathy is the leading cause of blindness in reproductive age women**[6] (Level II-2). Retinal vasculopathy should be considered in all pregnant women with long-standing diabetes as the progression of diabetic retinopathy is accelerated during pregnancy. The severity of retinopathy and duration of diabetes influence progression of retinopathy during pregnancy. Rapid changes in glucose control are associated with worsening retinopathy; for this reason, it is preferred that control be achieved prior to pregnancy in a gradual manner[1-3,7,8] (Level III, II-2). Women with diabetes should receive baseline screens prior to pregnancy with follow-up evaluations approximately every trimester and again during the post-partum period. Laser photocoagulation during pregnancy may be performed as needed in order to improve maternal symptoms and to decrease the progression of vasculopathy and subsequent vision loss.

While pregnancy does not appear to accelerate renal damage in women with minimal preexisting disease, it is not uncommon to document a transient worsening in creatinine clearance and protein excretion. **Diabetic nephropathy accounts for 40% of all end-stage renal disease.** Although pregnancy is not believed to alter the overall course of this complication, women with pre-existing renal damage defined by creatinine levels greater than 1.4 mg/dL, microalbuminuria or proteinuria may experience a worsening of renal pathology and also experience hypertensive disorders at higher rates[2] (Level III).

Hypertensive disorders are a major complication of women with diabetes who become pregnant. Often times it is hypertension and not diabetes which leads to morbidity and subsequent iatrogenic preterm delivery. This includes chronic hypertension as well as preeclampsia. Approximately 10% to 20% of women with diabetes will experience hypertensive disease related to pregnancy[9] (Level II-2). This percentage is increased in women with preexisting renal dysfunction; as 40% of women with mild preexisting nephropathy and nearly 50% with significant disease will experience pregnancy-related hypertensive disease[9] (Level II-2), **women with diabetic retinopathy and chronic hypertension experience rates of preeclampsia as high as 60%**[2,3] (Level III).

Neonatal Effects

Women with diabetes who become pregnant experience higher rates of fetal wastage which appears to be related to the degree of glycemic control. This includes higher rates of first-trimester losses as well as increased rates of stillbirth in later trimesters[2,3] (Level III).

Fetal overgrowth or macrosomia is commonly associated with poor maternal glycemic control. This is due to increased adiposity manifested by an increase in both size and number of fat cells which has been documented in babies born to mothers with diabetes[1,10] (Level II-2, III). Fetal macrosomia is associated with increased rates of maternal and neonatal birth trauma and higher rates of neonatal ICU admissions.

Care should also be taken to monitor for fetal growth restriction in women with long-standing diabetes. Women with underlying vascular and/or renal disease experience increased rates of fetal growth restriction. It is important to monitor fetal growth and to tailor antenatal surveillance based on findings. In our center, we obtain fetal growth ultrasounds at 32 weeks and again before delivery (36-38 wk gestational) in order to make decisions regarding route of delivery.

Babies born to mothers with suboptimal glycemic control experience increased rates of congenital anomalies[8] (Level III). These include cardiac malformations, skeletal dysplasias, and CNS complications. The rate of anomalies appears to be related to the degree of glycemic control. Women with HbA_{1c} less than 7% prior to conception experience rates similar to nondiabetic women. However, increasingly poorer glycemic control leads to an increase in congenital anomalies. **Women with a HbA_{1c} greater than 10% experience rates of congenital anomalies as high as 20% to 25%.** Therefore, a detailed anatomy ultrasound is recommended for all diabetics. It is our practice to obtain fetal echocardiograms in all patients with a HbA_{1c} greater than 8%.

Medical Management

Antibody-free human insulin is the gold standard for glycemic control during pregnancy; however, the use of insulin analogs may present a better option for the overall health of the patient. Benefits on insulin analogs include elimination of antibody formation seen with the use of natural insulin as well as better efficacy profiles which result in higher peak insulin concentrations in less time with a shorter duration of action[1,5,7,8] (Level II-2, III).

The goal of insulin therapy is to provide coverage for meal-derived glucose loads, to control between-meal glucose levels, and to maintain overnight blood glucose levels during fasting. There are a number of viable options for insulin formulations which are useful, however, certain physiologic changes of pregnancy such as fasting hypoglycemia and postprandial hyperglycemia make intermediate and ultrafast-acting formulations more practical[5] (Level II-2).

Neutral protamine hagedorn (NPH) is intermediate-acting and is the basal insulin of choice as it has more predictability. Use of rapid-acting insulin such as aspart (Novolog) or lispro (Humalog) allows for tighter control and individualized meal titrations on insulin[11] (Level I). Further, by using insulin with a shorter half-life such as Humalog and Novolog we decrease the frequency of hypoglycemic episodes which occur during times of fasting. Preprandial regular insulin also has good coverage of meals; however, postprandial hypoglycemia can develop 2 to 4 hours after meals requiring snacks to oppose this side effect. Glargine (Lantus) has not been studied adequately for use in pregnancy. Single dosing and prolonged action profile increase the risk of nocturnal hypoglycemia as well as undertreatment during the day (Table 19–1).

Open-loop continuous subcutaneous insulin infusion pump therapy is another option for a select group of motivated patients. Use of an insulin pump necessitates 6 to 8 capillary glucose measurements daily for insulin titration. Basal rates are usually 1 U/h, representing 50% to 60% of daily insulin dose. Prior to initiating pump therapy, patients must be thoroughly screened and made aware of the commitment which is necessary to achieve adequate management of their disease[12] (Level I).

Weisz et al looked at the benefits of measuring 1-hour versus 2-hour postprandial glucose levels and found no difference in efficacy. Due to a factor of

Table 19–1 INSULIN TYPES AND PHARMACOKINETICS

INSULIN TYPE	PEAK ACTION (h)	TOTAL DURATION OF ACTION (h)
NPH	4	8
Lispro (Humalog)	1	2
Aspart (Novolog)	1	2
Regular	2	4
Glargine (Lantus)	5	24

convenience most practitioners opt for 1-hour measurements to guide therapy[13] (Level II-2). De Veciana et al looked at preprandial versus postprandial glucose measurements. They found that in the group where postprandial measurements were used there was a better control evident by lower HbA_{1c} levels at delivery, as well as less neonatal hypoglycemia, less neonatal macrosomia, and fewer large for gestational age (LGA) infants[14] (Level II-2). The fourth International Workshop on Gestational Diabetes recommended that fasting as well as postprandial measurements be used to guide therapy[1] (Level III).

It is important to individualize the insulin regimen for each patient taking into account daily activities and meal schedules to provide adequate coverage. Fasting targets should be less than 105 mg/dL and 1-hour postprandial targets should be less than 140 mg/dL. As pregnancy progresses insulin requirements change. In general, during the first trimester insulin requirements are calculated at 0.7 to 0.8 U/kg/d, during the second trimester 0.8 to 1.0 U/kg/d, and during the third trimester 0.9 to 1.2 U/kg/d[1,15] (level II-2, III). In order to initiate insulin therapy it is necessary to calculate the estimated total daily insulin requirements using the above guidelines. Approximately two-thirds of the total insulin should be allotted for daytime coverage, of which approximately two-thirds of this coverage should be achieved with an intermediate-acting formulation such as NPH insulin and one-third of coverage should be achieved using a rapid-acting formulation such as lispro insulin. Approximately one-third of the total daily insulin requirements should be allocated for evening and nighttime coverage; this should be divided equally between intermediate and rapid-acting formulations. Patients should be monitored with fasting and postprandial levels in order to titrate insulin dosing[1,13,15] (Level II-2, III).

Glycemic control is also important during labor and delivery. Infants born with neonatal hypoglycemia are 2 to 3.5 times more likely to have neurodevelopmental delay at 18 months to 7 years of age. Insulin therapy should be titrated to achieve and maintain glucose levels between 80 and 110 mg/dL[16] (Level III). This can be accomplished with insulin infusions or with subcutaneous injections.

Although insulin is the gold standard for glycemic control during pregnancy, oral hypoglycemic medications may present an additional option in some patients. In many cases they are more easily accepted by patients as they eliminate or at least limit the need for injections. Both glyburide as well as metformin have shown promising results in women with gestational diabetes and polycystic ovarian syndrome (PCOS), respectively[17,18] (Level I). However, it is unclear if this data can be applied to women with pregestational diabetes. The American College of Obstetrics and Gynecology recommendations states that "the use of all oral agents for control of type 2 diabetes mellitus during pregnancy should be limited and individualized until data regarding the safety and efficacy of these drugs becomes available"[1] (Level III).

Fetal Surveillance and Delivery

Women requiring insulin therapy for diabetes and those with additional comorbid conditions who do not require insulin should undergo increased surveillance to improve neonatal outcome[19,20] (Level II-2). Early ultrasound evaluations are useful to provide accurate dating, while anatomy surveys performed between 18 to 20 weeks' gestation are important to evaluate for congenital anomalies. In addition, ultrasound evaluations should be performed during the third trimester to assess for signs of fetal hyperglycemia including fetal overgrowth and polyhydramnios[1] (Level III).

Antenatal testing should begin no later than 32 weeks' gestation and may be accomplished at least weekly with fetal non-stress tests or biophysical profile evaluations. Decisions regarding timing of delivery should be based on level of control and maternal and neonatal morbidity. However, generally delivery should occur between 39 to 40 weeks in women with good control. Deliveries occurring prior to 39 weeks should consider documentation of fetal lung maturity via amniocentesis[1,20] (Level II-2, III). Route of delivery should be based on the estimated fetal weight (EFW) by ultrasound and most would agree that elective cesarean delivery should be discussed and offered to diabetics with EFW of greater than 4500 g due to the potential for shoulder dystocia.

Diabetic Emergencies

Diabetic ketoacidosis (DKA) presents a medical emergency which may be more difficult to diagnose during pregnancy. This is due to the fact that during pregnancy it occurs at lower blood glucose levels and its onset may be more rapid than in the nonpregnant state[2,3] (Level III). Precipitating factors include emesis, infection, noncompliance or unrecognized new onset of diabetes, pump failure, and maternal steroid use. Signs and symptoms are similar to those in the nonpregnancy state, however, they also may mimic normal symptoms of pregnancy. These include polyuria, polyphagia, polydipsia, weight loss, weakness and signs of dehydration, nausea/vomiting, abdominal pain, and intercurrent illnesses.

DKA occurs more commonly during the second and third trimesters. Although its prevalence is higher in patients with type 1 diabetes, it may also occur in patients with type 2 diabetes or gestational diabetes. Laboratory findings include hyperglycemia greater than 200 to 250 mg/dL, acidosis defined as an arterial pH less than 7.35, anion gap greater than 12 mEq/L, bicarbonate less than 15 mEq/L, and positive serum ketones[2,3] (Level III).

Aggressive and early resuscitation is the key to effective management of DKA. Fluid replacement should begin with 1 to 2 L of isotonic saline during the first hour followed by 300 to 500 mL/h of normal saline. As glucose levels approach 250 mg/dL, 5% dextrose may be added. Insulin therapy should also be initiated as soon as the diagnosis is made. An appropriate loading dose of regular insulin is 0.2 to 0.4 U/kg regular insulin followed by continuous insulin infusion of 6 to 10 U/h. When glucose levels approach 200 to 250 mg/dL, the insulin infusion rate may be decreased to 1 to 2 U/h[1-3] (Level III).

Electrolyte replacement should be provided as needed. If serum potassium is elevated, potassium replacement should be provided at 20 mEq/h after urine output is established. If serum potassium is below normal, replacement should be initiated immediately at the above rate. Serum magnesium and phosphorus levels should be evaluated and provided as needed. Careful monitoring should be continued at least 12 to 24 hours after resolution of laboratory derangements[1-3] (Level III).

Comprehension Questions

19.1   A 36-year-old G2P1001 presents for her initial prenatal visit at 6 weeks' gestation. She has a long-standing history of type 2 diabetes mellitus which is managed with oral hypoglycemic medications. Initial laboratory test reveals a HbA_{1c} of 10%. The patient is very motivated to have a successful outcome and asks for information concerning management of her pregnancy. Which of the following surveillance tools is not indicated for this patient?

A. Serial umbilical Doppler measurements starting at 32 weeks' gestation.

B. Fetal echocardiogram at approximately 20 weeks' gestation.

C. Antenatal testing with either non-stress test or biophysical profile starting at 32 weeks.

D. Initiation of insulin therapy with titration guided by fasting and postprandial glucose measurements.

E. Detail anatomy survey at 18 to 20 weeks' gestation.

19.2   A 21-year-old G1P0 woman at 11 weeks' gestation is seen in the emergency center complaining of nausea, vomiting, abdominal pain, and fatigue. The patient is a known diabetic since age 12 years, and has been in good control. On examination, her BP is 90/60 mm Hg, HR 120 beats per minute, and RR 28 per minute. The arterial blood gas reveals a pH of 7.28, pO_2 of 100 mm Hg, pCO_2 of 22 mm Hg, and bicarbonate level of 12 mEq/L. Which of the following is the best management of this patient?

A. Administer 2 L of normal saline intravenously.

B. Infuse two ampules of bicarbonate IV.

C. Obtain a spiral CT scan.

D. Obtain a gallbladder ultrasound examination.

ANSWERS

19.1   **A.** Serial Doppler measurements are not indicated in this patient as Doppler studies have only been shown to be informative in cases of growth restriction. Doppler studies are not routinely used for surveillance of other high-risk pregnancies. This patient should undergo a detailed anatomy survey including a fetal echocardiogram due to her elevated HbA_{1c} measurement which increases her risk of structural anomalies including but not limited to cardiac defects. As her glycemic control is suboptimal on oral medications, insulin therapy should be initiated and titrated based on fasting and postprandial values. Finally, women managed with insulin should receive antenatal testing beginning at least by 32 weeks' gestation.

19.2   **A.** This patient likely has diabetic ketoacidosis. Pregnancy will often cause diabetes to become more difficult to control. The pH is acidotic, whereas the normal pH in pregnancy is slightly alkalotic. Together with the low bicarbonate level, this is consistent with an anion gap metabolic acidosis. The patient's oxygenation is good, and thus, a pulmonary embolus is not suspected. The pCO_2 is lower than the normal 28 mm Hg seen in pregnancy, which is indicative of partial respiratory compensation. The blood sugar is likely to be elevated. The cornerstones of management of DKA include IV fluid hydration, insulin intravenous drip to control the blood sugars and correct the acidosis, correction of metabolic abnormalities such as hypokalemia, hypophosphatemia, or hypomagnesemia, and addressing the etiological factor. A gallbladder ultrasound may be indicated; however, the first priority is volume repletion.

Clinical Pearls

See US Preventive Services Task Force Study Quality levels of evidence in Case 1

➤ Diabetic retinopathy may accelerate during pregnancy and thus women should be followed with ophthalmology evaluations prior to conception, every trimester, and at 3 to 6 months postpartum (Level II-3).

➤ Although diabetic nephropathy generally does not generally worsen with pregnancy, women with preexisting moderate to severe nephropathy may experience a worsening of their renal disease (Level III).

➤ Preeclampsia rates may be as high as 50% in some women with diabetes (Level II-2).

➤ HbA$_{1c}$ levels less than 7% prior to conception is associated with neonatal morbidity rates comparable to the general population (Level II-3).

➤ HbA$_{1c}$ levels greater than 11.2% prior to conception are associated with neonatal morbidity rates as high as 25% (Level II-3).

➤ Postprandial glucose measurements are better than preprandial measurement in order to improve neonatal outcomes (Level II-1).

➤ DKA occurs more rapidly and at lower serum glucose levels during pregnancy compared to outside of pregnancy (Level III).

➤ Pregestational diabetics should be recommended delivery at 39 weeks with earlier delivery (after mature amniocentesis) if suboptimal control (Level III).

CONTROVERSIES

- Management of women with pregestational diabetes with oral hypoglycemic medications. ACOG position is that their use in patients with type 2 diabetes mellitus should be limited and individualized until more data are available.
- Patients in whom the estimated fetal weight exceeds 4500 g should be offered cesarean delivery in order to decrease risk of traumatic delivery.

REFERENCES

1. ACOG Practice Bulletin. Clinical Management Guidelines for Obstetrician-Gynecologists. Number 60, March 2005. Pregestational diabetes mellitus. *Obstet Gynecol.* 2005;105:675-685 (Level III).
2. Metzger BE, Phelps RL, Dooley SL. The mother in pregnancies complicated by diabetes mellitus. In: Porte D SR, Baron A, eds. *Ellenberg and Rifkin's Diabetes Mellitus.* New York, NY: The McGraw-Hill Companies Inc.; 2003 (Level III).
3. Moore TR CP. Diabetes in pregnancy. In: Creasy RK RR, Iams JD, Lockwood CJ, Moore TR, eds. *Creasy and Resnik's Maternal-Fetal Medicine, Principles and Practice.* Philadelphia, PA: Saunder Elsevier; 2009 (Level III).
4. Diagnosis and classification of diabetes mellitus. *Diabetes Care.* 2006;29 (Suppl 1): 43S-48S (Level III).

5. Mello G, Parretti E, Mecacci F, Pratesi M, Lucchetti R, Scarselli G. Excursion of daily glucose profiles in pregnant women with IDDM: relationship with perinatal outcome. *J Perinat Med.* 1997;25:488-497 (Level II-2).
6. Rosenn B, Miodovnik M, Kranias G, et al. Progression of diabetic retinopathy in pregnancy: association with hypertension in pregnancy. *Am J Obstet Gynecol.* 1992;166:1214-1218 (Level II-2).
   154 women with insulin dependent diabetes were followed prospectively with serial ophthalmologic evaluations during pregnancy and postpartum to evaluate for progression of retinopathic complications. The investigators found that progression of disease was associated with rapid glycemic changes in early pregnancy and with the presence of hypertensive disorders.
7. Boinpally T, Jovanovic L. Management of type 2 diabetes and gestational diabetes in pregnancy. *Mt Sinai J Med.* 2009;76:269-280 (Level III).
8. Kinsley B. Achieving better outcomes in pregnancies complicated by type 1 and type 2 diabetes mellitus. *Clin Ther.* 2007;29 Suppl D:153S-160S (Level III).
9. Combs CA, Rosenn B, Kitzmiller JL, Khoury JC, Wheeler BC, Miodovnik M. Early-pregnancy proteinuria in diabetes related to preeclampsia. *Obstet Gynecol.* 1993;82:802-807 (Level II-2).
10. Wong SF, Lee-Tannock A, Amaraddio D, Chan FY, McIntyre HD. Fetal growth patterns in fetuses of women with pregestational diabetes mellitus. *Ultrasound Obstet Gynecol.* 2006;28:934-938 (Level II-2).
11. Perriello G, Pampanelli S, Porcellati F, et al. Insulin aspart improves meal time glycemic control in patients with type 2 diabetes: a randomized, stratified, double-blind and cross-over trial. *Diabet Med.* 2005;22:606-611 (Level I).
    A multicenter randomized control trial was conducted to compare efficacy of regular human insulin and insulin aspart in pregnant women with type 2 diabetes. The investigators found that women treated with insulin aspart had better glycemic control and more favorable insulin profiles.
12. Doyle EA, Weinzimer SA, Steffen AT, Ahern JA, Vincent M, Tamborlane WV. A randomized, prospective trial comparing the efficacy of continuous subcutaneous insulin infusion with multiple daily injections using insulin glargine. *Diabetes Care.* 2004;27:1554-1558 (Level I).
13. Weisz B, Shrim A, Homko CJ, Schiff E, Epstein GS, Sivan E. One hour versus two hours postprandial glucose measurement in gestational diabetes: a prospective study. *J Perinatol.* 2005;25:241-244 (Level II-2).
14. de Veciana M, Major CA, Morgan MA, et al. Postprandial versus preprandial blood glucose monitoring in women with gestational diabetes mellitus requiring insulin therapy. *N Engl J Med.* 1995;333:1237-1241 (Level II-2).
15. Langer O, Anyaegbunam A, Brustman L, Guidetti D, Levy J, Mazze R. Pregestational diabetes: insulin requirements throughout pregnancy. *Am J Obstet Gynecol.* 1988;159:616-621 (Level II-2).
    To evaluate insulin requirements during pregnancy 103 women with pregestational diabetes were monitored. The investigators found that insulin requirements were triphasic and that overall requirements were higher in all gestations for women with type 2 diabetes compared to type 1 diabetes.
16. Garber AJ, Moghissi ES, Bransome ED, Jr., et al. American College of Endocrinology position statement on inpatient diabetes and metabolic control. *Endocr Pract.* 2004;10 (Suppl 2):4-9 (Level III).

17. Langer O, Conway DL, Berkus MD, Xenakis EM, Gonzales O. A comparison of glyburide and insulin in women with gestational diabetes mellitus. *N Engl J Med.* 2000;343:1134-1138 (Level I).

18. Rowan JA, Hague WM, Gao W, Battin MR, Moore MP. Metformin versus insulin for the treatment of gestational diabetes. *N Engl J Med.* 2008;358:2003-2015 (Level I).

19. Barrett JM, Salyer SL, Boehm FH. The nonstress test: an evaluation of 1000 patients. *Am J Obstet Gynecol.* 1981;141:153-157 (Level II-2).

20. Graves CR. Antepartum fetal surveillance and timing of delivery in the pregnancy complicated by diabetes mellitus. *Clin Obstet Gynecol.* 2007;50:1007-1013 (Level II-2).

21. Kjos SL, Leung A, Henry OA, Victor MR, Paul RH, Medearis AL. Antepartum surveillance in diabetic pregnancies: predictors of fetal distress in labor. *Am J Obstet Gynecol.* 1995;173:1532-1539 (Level II-2).

Case 20

A 28-year-old G2P1001 at 26⁵/₇ weeks presents to your office following completion of her 1-hour glucose screening. The 1-hour glucose measurement result was 165 mg/dL. This pregnancy has been unremarkable thus far and she has no significant obstetric or medical history. She is of Hispanic descent and her BMI is 35 kg/m². She screened negative for gestational diabetes mellitus (GDM) during her prior pregnancy, however, that pregnancy was significant for the delivery of a term female infant weighing 10 and 3 oz (4.7 kg)

➤ What is the next step in management of this patient?

➤ What risk factors does this patient have for gestational diabetes mellitus?

➤ What are treatment options for women with gestational diabetes mellitus?

➤ What are potential fetal implications for babies born to mothers with gestational diabetes?

➤ What are potential maternal implications following a pregnancy complicated by gestational diabetes?

ANSWERS TO CASE 20:
Gestational Diabetes

Summary: A multiparous woman presents with an abnormal glucose screening test result.

➤ **Next step in management of this patient:** She should complete a 3-hour oral glucose tolerance test.

➤ **Risk factors this patient have for gestational diabetes mellitus:** This patient possesses multiple risk factors for developing gestational diabetes including age greater than 25 years, belonging to an ethnic group with an increased risk for the development of type 2 diabetes, obesity, and prior macrosomic infant.

➤ **Treatment options for women with gestational diabetes mellitus:** While insulin therapy is the gold standard for diabetes therapy, the use of glyburide, an oral hypoglycemic agent, has been found to be effective in select patients.

➤ **Potential fetal implications for babies born to mothers with gestational diabetes:** Infants born to mothers with gestational diabetes are at risk of fetal overgrowth. Recent studies suggest that there is increased risk of long-term chronic health problems in these infants such as early onset diabetes, hyperlipidemia, and obesity.

➤ **Potential maternal long-term implications following a pregnancy complicated by gestational diabetes:** Women who develop gestational diabetes mellitus are at increased risk of developing type 2 diabetes during the years following their pregnancy. These risks may be reduced with interventions such as maternal weight loss through diet and exercise.

ANALYSIS

Objectives

1. List the risk factors for gestational diabetes.
2. Describe the complications of gestational diabetes.
3. Describe the diagnosis and management of GDM.

Considerations

Gestational diabetes mellitus (GDM) is defined as carbohydrate intolerance first recognized during pregnancy. This represents both new-onset glucose intolerance as well as previously undiagnosed pregestational diabetes mellitus. Gestational diabetes complicates approximately 2% to 6% of all gestations in the United States although certain racial and ethnic groups do experience rates which are significantly higher. Ethnic groups that are considered to be at high risk for the development of GDM include persons of Hispanic heritage, persons of African descent, native Americans, southeast Asians, Pacific Islanders, and indigenous Australians[1,2] (Level III).

This patient has an increased risk for developing GDM due to her ethnic background, obese status, age greater than 25 years, and history of giving birth to a macrosomic infant. If GDM is confirmed she would need to be counseled that there is an increased risk of maternal and neonatal morbidity which is related to the degree of insulin resistance. Neonatal morbidity includes increased rates of macrosomia defined as greater than 90% for gestational age, increased risk of birth trauma, and increased neonatal admissions due to metabolic derangements such as hypoglycemia, hyperbilirubinemia, and hypocalcemia[1] (Level III). We also know that infants born to mothers with GDM experience increased rates of childhood obesity and chronic health complications including early-onset type 2 diabetes mellitus, hyperlipidemia, and obesity[3] (Level II-2).

Maternal morbidity includes increased cesarean delivery rates, increased rates of pregnancy associated hypertensive disorders, and an increased risk of developing type 2 diabetes mellitus in the years following the pregnancy. The risk of developing type 2 diabetes is as high as 70% in the years following a gestation complicated by GDM[1] (Level III).

The next step in the management of this patient is a 3-hour oral glucose tolerance test (OGTT). She should be instructed to return to the office while fasting following a period of at least 3 days of an unrestricted carbohydrate diet. After obtaining a fasting glucose measurement, a standard 100 g glucose load is given followed by plasma glucose measurements taken hourly for 3 hours. If two or more glucose measurements are abnormal, she meets the criteria for GDM. Insulin therapy or oral glyburide are treatment options for glycemic control during pregnancy if diet control is unsuccessful.

APPROACH TO

Gestational Diabetes

Screening for GDM

There has been much debate regarding the utility of screening and the best modality which should be used to screen individuals. Selective screening based on risk factors would reduce number of women requiring screening by 10% to 15%, however, it would fail to identify one-third to one-half of affected individuals[4,5] (Level II-2). For this reason the American College of Obstetricians and Gynecologists (ACOG) supports universal screening in all persons except those deemed to be at low risk. This includes women less than 25 years of age, women belonging to an ethnic group with a low prevalence of diabetes, women with body mass index less than 25, and women with no first-degree relative with diabetes[2] (Level III).

In our practice we screen all patients by risk factors during the first prenatal visit. Patient's deemed to be at high risk for developing GDM undergo *early* screening. Women who screen positive are triaged appropriately and those who screen negative are rescreened at 24 to 28 weeks with the general population of patients. Risk factors which trigger early diagnostic testing includes but is not limited to maternal obesity defined as maternal weight greater than 120% ideal body weight, first-degree relatives with diabetes, maternal polycystic ovarian syndrome, or a prior pregnancy complicated by gestational diabetes, fetal macrosomia, or unexplained fetal or neonatal demise[6] (Level III).

A two-step approach has been recommended in order to identify women with GDM. The first step involves a 50 g 1-hour screening test, and the second step utilizes a 100 g 3-hour diagnostic test for those women identified via the initial screening test.

The **1-hour OGTT** can be completed at any time of day without the need for an overnight fast. Women are given a 50 g glucose load and plasma glucose levels are measured 1 hour after completion of the load. It is appropriate to use either 140 mg/dL or 130 mg/dL as a positive result for the 1-hour screening test. Use of the 140 mg/dL value identifies 14% to 18% of women who will require the diagnostic testing with 80% sensitivity. Use of the 130 mg/dL value identifies 20% to 25% of women who will require the diagnostic testing with 90% sensitivity[6,7] (Level III).

Diagnosis

The gold standard for the diagnosis of GDM is the 100 g, **3-hour OGTT**. The 3-hour OGTT is reserved for women with positive screening results. This test should be completed following an overnight fast. Patients are instructed to adhere to an unrestricted diet prior to the administration of the test with at least 150 g of carbohydrates per day for at least 3 days prior to the test. The purpose of carbohydrate loading is to avoid carbohydrate depletion which could increase the risk of false-positive results. Fasting plasma glucose levels are measured prior to the consumption of a standardized 100 g glucose load. Following completion of the load blood plasma glucose levels should be measured at 1, 2, and 3-hour intervals. A positive result is characterized by at least two abnormal values. There are two sets of values which are used to interpret 3-hour OGTT result: Carpenter and Coustan criteria and the National Diabetes Data Group (NDDG). Values described by Carpenter and Coustan for fasting, 1-, 2-, and 3-hour measurements are as follows, 95, 180, 155, and 140 mg/dL. Corresponding NDDG values are 105, 190, 165, and 145 mg/dL. Use of the Carpenter and Coustan criteria is associated with an additional

50% detection rate of women at risk of similar morbidity as are women in the less stringent NDDG identified population. For this reason, the Fourth International Workshop Conference on GDM advocated the use of Carpenter and Coustan, although both set of criteria are acceptable[8] (Level III).

The World Health Organization supports the use of a **2-hour 75 g** diagnostic test utilizing values concurrent with fasting, 1- and 2-hour values set for the 3-hour OGTT. A positive result requires at least two abnormal values. The American Diabetes Association recognizes this as an acceptable option although at this time the 100 g test is generally used in the United States[8] (Level III).

Recently completed, the **hyperglycemia and adverse pregnancy outcome (HAPO)** trial looked at maternal and fetal implications of maternal hyperglycemia less than that which is diagnostic for diabetes. The HAPO trial utilized a one-step diagnostic process with a 75 g 2-hour test. They found a linear relationship between maternal glucose levels and adverse outcomes, even at glucose concentrations below those that are usually diagnostic of GDM. The results of this study are likely to alter not only classification criteria for GDM but are also likely to modify treatment modalities[9] (Level I).

Therapeutic Interventions

Medical nutrition therapy is the first line of therapy in the treatment of women with GDM. The ultimate goal for medical nutrition therapy is to achieve euglycemia without inducing ketosis[2,10,11] (Level I, III). Once the diagnosis of GDM has been made, the woman should receive counseling from a registered dietician or other knowledgeable persons. Recommended diets should aim to decrease total fat intake and to incorporate complex carbohydrates and foods with high fiber content. Good carbohydrates should comprise approximately 35% to 40% of daily caloric intake with protein and fats equally accounting for the rest of the daily diet. Women with BMI within normal limits should have a target goal of 30 kcal/kg/d. This goal should be reduced to 25 kcal/kg/d for obese patients and 20 kcal/kg/d for morbidly obese patients. Patients should be counseled to maintain active lifestyle as exercise has been found to improve insulin sensitivity[2,12] (Level III).

Women being treated with medical nutrition therapy should be followed closely with the goal of maintaining fasting glucose levels less than 105 mg/dL and 1-hour glucose levels less than 140 mg/dL. McFarland et al published an observational study in order to determine the length of time needed to achieve good glucose control. They found that fasting glucose levels strongly correlated with success of medical nutrition therapy. They found that women with fasting levels greater than 95 mg/dL did not significantly improve glycemic control after 1 week, while women with fasting levels less than 95 mg/dL continued to show improvement after 2 weeks[13] (Level II-2). For this reason most clinicians advocate 2 weeks for attempting dietary therapy prior to initiating alternative therapies.

Carbohydrate metabolism is very different during pregnancy due to the influence of pregnancy associated hormones such as growth hormones, corticotrophin-releasing hormone, human placental lactogen, and progesterone. **During pregnancy women experience postprandial hyperglycemia and fasting hypoglycemia** in order to provide adequate glucose for the fetus[14] (Level III). These factors make some insulin formulations more appropriate for use in pregnancy. **Antibody-free human insulin is the gold standard** for glycemic control during pregnancy, however, a number of insulin analogs have shown promise in the treatment of women with GDM[10] (Level III). In our practice we generally use intermediate acting NPH for basal glucose management and insulin lispro, an ultrafast-acting formulation, for postprandial coverage.

Insulin has been traditionally the standard for treatment in those who have failed medical nutrition therapy because it achieves glucose control without the risk of insulin transfer across the placenta. However, emerging evidence in recent years has resulted in a growing acceptance of the use of oral agents in the treatment of GDM. The use of oral hypoglycemic medications offers less invasive alternatives to some women with GDM, allowing them to avoid insulin injections. Perhaps the most well-studied agent available currently is glyburide, a second-generation sulfonylurea. **Glyburide** is an insulin secretagogue which acts by stimulating insulin secretion after meals. There appears to be little or no placental transfer decreasing concerns of possible fetal effects. Glyburide has been shown in randomized controlled trials to be comparable to insulin in terms of efficacy with similar obstetric and neonatal outcomes with significantly fewer episodes of hypoglycemia[15,16] (Level I, III). In Langer's trial, the "glyburide failure rate" was approximately 18%[15] (Level I). The peak effect is single dosing preferably 1 hour before meals is recommended with a maximum of 20 mg per day.

The use of **metformin** has primarily been evaluated in patients with polycystic ovarian syndrome and type 2 diabetes as means of improving insulin resistance. Ovulation induction and possible reductions in first-trimester losses have been reported with the use of metformin. Although the efficacy of metformin appears comparable to insulin therapy[11] (Level I), the level of placental transfer brings into question possible fetal implications. Further studies documenting the safety of metformin for the treatment of gestational diabetes are needed before its use can be supported[11,17] (Level I, III).

Fetal Surveillance and Delivery

Women requiring pharmacologic therapy for GDM and those with additional comorbid conditions who do not require medical therapy should undergo increased surveillance to improve neonatal outcome. Early ultrasound evaluations are useful to provide accurate dating, and anatomy surveys performed between 18 and 20 weeks' gestation are important to evaluate for congenital anomalies. Gestational diabetes mellitus is not associated with the structural anomalies seen in gestations complicated by pregestational diabetes, although it is reasonable to consider these complications for those women diagnosed early in pregnancy who may represent undiagnosed type 2 diabetes. Ultrasound evaluations should be performed during the third trimester to assess for signs of fetal hyperglycemia including fetal overgrowth and polyhydramnios[2,8] (Level III). A number of studies have looked into the utility of third-trimester ultrasound measurements to assist in decisions regarding therapy. Kjos et al found that in women with GDM and fasting hyperglycemia, use of ultrasound measurements in addition to glucose measurements were able to identify women who did not require insulin therapy without increasing morbidity[18] (Level I).

Antenatal testing should begin no later than 32 weeks' gestation in women requiring insulin or oral hypoglycemic therapy. Women treated with diet therapy alone may wait for testing to begin at 38 weeks. Antenatal surveillance should be carried out at least weekly with fetal non-stress tests or biophysical profile evaluations[19] (Level III). Decisions regarding timing of delivery should be based on level of control and maternal and neonatal morbidity. However, generally delivery should occur between 39 and 40 weeks in women with good control pharmacologic therapy. If delivery prior to 39 weeks is undertaken due to suboptimal glycemic control, documentation of fetal lung maturity via amniocentesis should be considered[20] (Level II-2). Route of delivery should be based on the estimated fetal weight (EFW) by ultrasound and most would agree that elective cesarean delivery should be discussed and offered to diabetics with EFW of greater than 4500 g due to the potential for shoulder dystocia.

Postpartum Management

All women diagnosed with GDM should be screened for overt diabetes mellitus during the postpartum period. The Fifth International Workshop-Conference on Gestational Diabetes Mellitus advocates the use of a 75 g oral glucose tolerance test at least 6 weeks postpartum[21] (Level III). Fasting glucose levels greater than 126 mg/dL or 2 hour values greater than 200 mg/dL are diagnostic for diabetes mellitus[2] (Level III). Patients meeting these criteria should be referred to an internist for continued care.

Contraception options are very important to consider in this population as we know that recurrent pregnancies in a woman with GDM increase her risk for overt diabetes mellitus[22] (Level III). **Contraception options with low-dose combinations of estrogen and progesterone do not appear to increase the risk of developing type 2 diabetes.** This includes oral contraceptive pills, vaginal ring inserts, and transdermal delivery systems. In contrast, progestin-only pills and depot progesterone preparations have been associated with impairment of carbohydrate metabolism and increased progression to type 2 diabetes in some populations. For this reason they should be reserved for patients who are not candidates for alternative methods. For women considering more long-term contraception, intrauterine devices are a good option. Both copper

IUD devices and levonorgestrel IUD devices may be used with good safety profiles[18,23,24] (Level I, II-2, III).

Breast-feeding should be encouraged for both infant and maternal benefits. The data are inconclusive regarding the association between breast-feeding and type 2 diabetes[25] (Level III). There is, however, data which show that women who breast-feed for extended periods of time experience a greater decrease in weight, which may decrease their risk of developing type 2 diabetes[26] (Level III). In terms of neonatal effects, breast-feeding has been associated with decreased risk of childhood obesity and the development of diabetes mellitus compared to formula-fed infants[27,28] (Level II-2).

Comprehension Questions

20.1   A 32-year-old G3P2002 Caucasian female presents for prenatal care at 9 weeks' gestation. Her obstetrical history is significant for GDM with her last pregnancy only ending in a term delivery of a 7 lb (3 kg) infant. She was not screened postpartum and denies any medical complications. Her BMI is 29 kg/m². When would you consider screening for GDM?

       A. 9 weeks
       B. 16 weeks
       C. 28 weeks
       D. 6 weeks postpartum

20.2   A 35-year-old woman at 29 weeks' gestation is diagnosed with gestational diabetes. She is placed on a 2200 cal ADA diet. Her blood sugars over the next 2 weeks are as follows:

       Fasting: 110 mg/dL; 105 mg/dL; 107 mg/dL; 113 mg/dL; 109 mg/dL
       2 hour after breakfast: 124 mg/dL; 136 mg/dL; 122 mg/dL; 140 mg/dL
       2 hours after lunch: 139 mg/dL; 144 mg/dL; 123 mg/dL; 111 mg/dL
       2 hours after dinner: 130 mg/dL; 143 mg/dL; 132 mg/dL; 125 mg/dL

       Which of the following is the best management of this patient at this time?

       A. Initiation of insulin subcutaneously.
       B. Continue diet and monitor blood sugars for 1 week more.
       C. Admission to the hospital for intravenous insulin therapy.
       D. Fetal ultrasound, and if EFW is 2000 g or greater then delivery.

ANSWERS

20.1   **A.** This patient should be screened for GDM without delay. A history of GDM increases the risk of this patient having GDM this pregnancy as well as type 2 diabetes mellitus. A 3-hour 100 mg OGTT should be ordered. If she meets criteria for GDM, she is likely to have pregestational diabetes given her early gestational age and should be counseled and managed accordingly. If she does not meet criteria for GDM then repeat testing should be performed at 24 to 28 weeks.

20.2   **A.** With the fasting glucose levels higher than target of 90 to 100 mg/dL and 2-hour postprandial levels exceeding targets of 120 mg/dL, despite 2 weeks of diet, then pharmacologic therapy should be started. Insulin is appropriate, although an oral hypoglycemic agent is also acceptable.

Clinical Pearls

See US Preventive Services Task Force Study Quality levels of evidence in Case 1

➤ Risks factors for GDM include maternal obesity defined as maternal weight greater than 120% ideal body weight, first-degree relatives with diabetes, maternal polycystic ovarian syndrome, or a prior pregnancy complicated by gestational diabetes, fetal macrosomia, or unexplained fetal or neonatal demise. In addition certain ethnic groups experience higher rates of GDM: persons of Hispanic heritage, persons of African descent, native Americans, southeast Asians, Pacific Islanders, and indigenous Australian persons (Level III).

➤ All women with GDM should be screened for overt diabetes during the postpartum period. Glyburide crosses the placenta and is considered a safe alternative to insulin for treatment of GDM (Level III).

➤ Antenatal testing should be initiated by 32 weeks for patients with GDM not managed by diet alone. Patients managed with diet should begin antenatal testing at 38 weeks (Level III).

➤ It is important to counsel women with GDM regarding contraception choices. Although low-dose combination options are preferred over progestin-only options, they are preferred over no therapy at all. Following a pregnancy complicated by GDM, each subsequent gestation increases her risk of developing type 2 diabetes mellitus (Level II-3).

CONTROVERSIES

- Carpenter and Coustan diagnostic criteria for the 3-hour 100 g OGTT is recommended by the Fourth and Fifth International Workshop-Conference of GDM and endorsed by ACOG; however, these expert bodies recognize that other alternative tests are acceptable.
- Further data in pregnancy are needed before the use of metformin for the treatment of GDM can be recommended.

REFERENCES

1. Hollander, MH, Paarlberg KM, Huisjes AJ. Gestational diabetes: a review of the current literature and guidelines. *Obstet Gynecol Surv.* 2007;62(2):125-136 (Level III).
2. ACOG Practice Bulletin. Clinical management guidelines for obstetrician-gynecologists. Number 30, September 2001. *Obstet Gynecol.* 2001;98(3):525-538 (Level III).
3. Catalano PM, Farrel K, Thomas A, et al. Perinatal risk factors for childhood obesity and metabolic dysregulation. *Am J Clin Nutr.* 2009;90(5):1301-1313 (level II-2).
4. Minsart AF, Lescrainier JP, Vokaer A. Selective versus universal screening for gestational diabetes mellitus: an evaluation of Naylor's model. *Gynecol Obstet Invest.* 2009;68(3):154-159 (Level II-2).
   This study compared the ability of selective versus universal screening to effectively identify women with GDM. It was found that selective screening allowed 15% of women to avoid laboratory testing, however, 50% of women who would have screened positive were missed.
5. Coustan DR, Nelson C, Carpenter MW, et al. Maternal age and screening for gestational diabetes: a population-based study. *Obstet Gynecol.* 1989;73(4):557-561 (Level II-2).
6. Hanna FW, Peters JR. Screening for gestational diabetes; past, present and future. *Diabet Med.* 2002;19(5):351-358 (Level III).
7. Ben-Haroush A, Yogev Y, Hod M. Epidemiology of gestational diabetes mellitus and its association with Type 2 diabetes. *Diabet Med.* 2004;21(2):103-113 (Level III).
8. Metzger BE, Phelps PR, Dooley SL. The mother in pregnancies complicated by diabetes mellitus. In: Porte D, Robert S, Baron A, eds. *Ellenberg and Rifkin's Diabetes Mellitus.* 6th ed. New York, NY: The McGraw-Hill Companies Inc.; 2003 (Level III).
9. Metzger BE, Lowe LP, Dyer AR et al. Hyperglycemia and adverse pregnancy outcomes. *N Engl J Med.* 2008;358(19):1991-2002 (Level I).
   Pregnant women with hyperglycemia not diagnostic for diabetes were evaluated to explore the association between hyperglycemia and adverse pregnancy outcome. This study included 25,505 pregnant women from 15 different centers in 9 countries. The investigators found that there was a strong continuous association between mild maternal hyperglycemia and obstetric morbidity including an increase in cesarean delivery, neonatal macrosomia, and neonatal hypoglycemia.
10. Langer O, Hod M. Management of gestational diabetes mellitus. *Obstet Gynecol Clin North Am.* 1996;23(1): 137-159 (Level III).
11. Moore LE, Briery CM, Clokey D et al. Metformin and insulin in the management of gestational diabetes mellitus: preliminary results of a comparison. *J Reprod Med.* 2007;52(11):1011-1015 (Level I).

12. Langer O. Management of gestational diabetes: pharmacologic treatment options and glycemic control. *Endocrinol Metab Clin North Am.* 2006;35(1):53-78, vi (Level III).

13. McFarland MB, Langer O, Conway DL, Berkus MD. Dietary therapy for gestational diabetes: how long is enough? *Obstet Gynecol.* 1999;93(6):978-982 (Level II-2).
    This study evaluated the length of time needed for dietary therapy to achieve good glycemic control. Investigators treated women with GDM for 4 weeks while monitoring blood glucose levels. The investigators found that fasting blood glucose levels were most predictive in terms of success with diet alone and that women with fasting levels less than or equal to 95 mg/dL were the best candidates for dietary therapy. They found that while women with fasting levels greater than 95 mg/dL improved in their control only up to 1 week, women with levels less than or equal to 95 mg/dL continued to show improvement up to 2 weeks. They recommended that women be treated with dietary therapy for at least 2 weeks before insulin is instituted.

14. Lapolla A, Dalfra MG, Fedele D. Insulin therapy in pregnancy complicated by diabetes: are insulin analogs a new tool? *Diabetes Metab Res Rev.* 2005;21(3):241-252 (Level III).

15. Langer O, Conway DL, Berkus MD, Xenakis EM, Gonzalez O. A comparison of glyburide and insulin in women with gestational diabetes mellitus. *N Engl J Med.* 2000;343(16):1134-1138 (Level I).
    A randomized controlled trial of 404 women with GDM between 11 and 33 weeks' gestation comparing glyburide and insulin therapies. Compared to 63% of women on insulin, 86% of women on glyburide reached targets. The rate of hypoglycemia was 2% for the women on glyburide compared to 20% for the women on insulin. There was a 4% failure rate for the women on glyburide. There was negligible placental transfer of glyburide. Neonatal outcomes were similar between the two groups. The investigators concluded that glyburide was comparable to insulin in the treatment of GDM.

16. Nicholson W, Bolen S, Witkop CT, Neale D, Wilson L, Bass E. Benefits and risks of oral diabetes agents compared with insulin in women with gestational diabetes: a systematic review. *Obstet Gynecol.* 2009;113(1):193-205 (Level III).

17. Coustan DR, Pharmacological management of gestational diabetes: an overview. *Diabetes Care.* 2007;30(Suppl 2): 206S-208S (Level III).

18. Kjos SL, Schaefer-Graf U, Sardesi S. A randomized controlled trial using glycemic plus fetal ultrasound parameters versus glycemic parameters to determine insulin therapy in gestational diabetes with fasting hyperglycemia. *Diabetes Care.* 2001;24(11):1904-1910 (Level I).
    A randomized controlled trial to compare treatment of GDM based on maternal glucose versus relaxed glucose criteria and fetal abdomen circumference. The investigators found that using fetal parameters allowed 38% of women to avoid insulin therapy with no significant difference in neonatal outcome.

19. Landon MB, Gabbe SG. Antepartum fetal surveillance in gestational diabetes mellitus. *Diabetes.* 1985;34(Suppl 2):50-54 (Level III).
    This study evaluated an antenatal surveillance protocol for women with GDM. A total of 97 women; 69 controlled with diet only and 28 treated with insulin. Hypertension was also seen in 21.6% of the women. Antenatal surveillance consisted of maternal activity assessment, clinical estimation of fetal weight, non-stress tests, and urinary estriol levels. Out of six women, four with hypertension required interventions. Sixteen infants, six of whom were identified in the antepartum period, were greater than 4000 g at delivery. No perinatal deaths occurred. The investigators concluded that outpatient management was effective in monitoring women with GDM.

20. Kjos SL, Leung A, Henry OA, Victor MR, Paul RH, Medearis AL. Antepartum surveillance in diabetic pregnancies: predictors of fetal distress in labor. *Am J Obstet Gynecol.* 1995;173(5):1532-1539 (Level II-2).
21. Metzger BE, Buchanan TA, Coustan DR, et al. Summary and recommendations of the Fifth International Workshop-Conference on Gestational Diabetes Mellitus. *Diabetes Care.* 2007;30(Suppl 2):251S-260S (Level III).
22. Kjos SL, Peters RK, Xiang A, Schaefer U, Buchanan TA. Hormonal choices after gestational diabetes. Subsequent pregnancy, contraception, and hormone replacement. *Diabetes Care.* 1998;21(Suppl 2): 50B-57B (Level III).
23. Kjos SL, Peters RK, Xiang A, Thomas D, Schaefer U, Buchanan TA. Contraception and the risk of type 2 diabetes mellitus in Latina women with prior gestational diabetes mellitus. *JAMA.* 1998;280(6):533-538 (Level II-2).
24. Kim C. Managing women with gestational diabetes mellitus in the postnatal period. *Diabetes Obes Metab.* 2009 (Level II-2).
25. Gunderson EP. Breast-feeding and diabetes: long-term impact on mothers and their infants. *Curr Diab Rep.* 2008;8(4):279-286 (Level III).
26. Olson CM, Strauderman MS, Hinton PS, Pearson TA. Gestational weight gain and postpartum behaviors associated with weight change from early pregnancy to 1 year postpartum. *Int J Obes Relat Metab Disord.* 2003;27(1):117-127 (Level III).
27. Mayer-Davis EJ, Dubelea D, Lamichhane AP, D'Agostino RB Jr, Liese AD, Thomas J. Breast-feeding and type 2 diabetes in the youth of three ethnic groups: the SEARCH for diabetes in youth case-control study. *Diabetes Care.* 2008;31(3):470-475 (Level II-2).
This study evaluated offspring of women who participated in the Nurses' Health Study II. They found that children aged 9 to 14 who were breast-fed exclusively were less likely to be overweight OR 0.66 (95% CI 0.53-0.82). These findings were independent of maternal BMI or diabetes status.
28. Mayer-Davis EJ, Rifas-Shiman SL, Zhou L, Hu FB, Coliditz GA, William MW. Breast-feeding and risk for childhood obesity: does maternal diabetes or obesity status matter? *Diabetes Care.* 2006;29(10):2231-2237 (Level II-2).

Case 21

A 25-year-old G1P0 woman is seen in your office for a new obstetrical visit. Her last normal menstrual period was 8 weeks ago. She is currently on no medications other than prenatal vitamins. She has noted over the past 3 months weight loss, heat intolerance, and an increase in the number of daily bowel movements. Occasionally, she notices that her heart races. She has a personal history of vitiligo as well as a family history of thyroid disease.

Physical examination reveals her height is 5 ft 3 in, weight is 100 lb (45.3 kg), blood pressure is 133/84 mm Hg, and pulse is 109 bpm. She appears nervous and slightly diaphoretic. She does not exhibit exophthalmos. Her thyroid gland is diffusely enlarged and nontender. Her lungs are clear, and her heart exhibits a 3/6 systolic ejection murmur heard best over the second left intercostal space. The remainder of her examination is unremarkable.

Her initial lab studies are normal except for her TSH which is 0.004 mIU/L (normal 0.5-4.7 mIU/L), and her free T4 which is reported as 5.4 ng/dL (normal 1.2-1.8 ng/dL).

➤ What is the most likely diagnosis?

➤ What is your next step?

➤ What are potential complications of the patient's disorder?

ANSWERS TO CASE 21:
Hyperthyroidism due to Graves Disease

Summary: This is a 25-year-old G1P0 with newly diagnosed hyperthyroidism most likely due to Graves disease who now presents in the first trimester with a hypermetabolic state.

➤ **Most likely diagnosis:** Hyperthyroidism due to Graves disease.

➤ **Next step:** Evaluate patient for Graves disease and thyroid-stimulating immunoglobulins.

➤ **Potential complications:** Maternal thyroid storm; congestive heart failure; spontaneous pregnancy loss; IUGR; preterm labor; fetal demise; preeclampsia; fetal or neonatal hyperthyroidism.

ANALYSIS

Objectives

1. Recognize signs and symptoms consistent with hyperthyroidism.
2. Be able to confirm thyroid disease with laboratory studies.
3. Be able to treat hypo- and hyperthyroidism during pregnancy.
4. Be able to manage acute symptoms of hyperthyroidism during pregnancy.
5. Be able to describe the effects of pregnancy on thyroid disease and of thyroid disease on pregnancy.

Considerations

This is a 25-year-old Caucasian woman G1P0 presenting at 8 weeks' gestation with overt hyperthyroidism. The first priority for the physician is to treat the hypermetabolic state of the patient. Thioamides are the treatment of choice during pregnancy as they have minor side effects and can induce remission in up to 30% of patients. There is a small risk of fetal goiter and hypothyroidism when given during pregnancy. Surgery is reserved for those pregnant women allergic to thioamides. Radioactive iodine is contraindicated during pregnancy.

APPROACH TO
Thyroid Disease in Pregnancy

HYPERTHYROIDISM

Recognition of hyperthyroidism in pregnancy is sometimes difficult due to the hyperdynamic physiological changes in pregnancy. However, unintended weight loss, nervousness, palpitations, tachycardia, or tremor are clinical manifestations that bear evaluation. The diagnosis is established by thyroid function tests, such as TSH and free T4 levels. The immediate treatment includes beta-blocking agents and thioamides.

Table 21–1 TREATMENT FOR HYPERTHYROIDISM

THERAPY	ADVANTAGES	DISADVANTAGES
Thioamides (1-2 y)	• Chance of permanent remission (~30%) • Avoids permanent hypothyroidism • Lower cost • Pregnant women	• Minor side effects: rash, hives, arthralgias, fever, gastrointestinal symptoms • Low risk of agranulocytosis (< 1%) • Risk of fetal goiter and hypothyroidism if pregnant • Frequent physician visits
Radioiodine (I^{131})	• Curative • Most cost effective	• Permanent hypothyroidism • Radiation precautions for several days after treatment; avoid contact with young children and pregnant women • Rare radiation thyroiditis
Surgery	• Rapid, permanent cure • Children/adolescents • Pregnant women allergic to thioamides	• Permanent hypothyroidism • Risk of hypoparathyroidism, recurrent laryngeal nerve damage, and general anesthesia • High cost

Thioamides inhibit thyroid hormone synthesis by reduction of iodine organification and iodotyrosine coupling. Both propylthiouracil (PTU) and methimazole have been used during pregnancy (see Table 21-1), but PTU has been traditionally preferred because of concern regarding reduced transplacental transfer of PTU compared to methimazole. However, recent studies do not confirm this finding. Teratogenic patterns associated with methimazole include aplasia cutis and choanal/esophageal atresia; however, these anomalies do not occur at a higher rate in women on thioamides compared to the general population.

Side effects of thioamides include transient leukopenia (10%); agranulocytosis (0.1%-0.4%); thrombocytopenia, hepatitis, and vasculitis (< 1%) as well as rash, nausea, arthritis, anorexia, fever, and loss of taste or smell (5%). Agranulocytosis usually presents with a fever and sore throat. If a CBC indicates agranulocytosis, the medication should be discontinued. Treatment with another thioamide carries a significant risk of cross-reaction as well.

Initiation of thioamides in a patient with a new diagnosis during pregnancy requires a dose of PTU 100 to 150 mg three times daily or methimazole 10 to 20 mg twice daily. Free T4 levels are used to monitor response to therapy in hyperthyroid patients and should be checked in 4 to 6 weeks. The PTU or methimazole can be adjusted in 50 mg or 10 mg increments, respectively, with a therapeutic range for free T4 of 1.2 to 1.8 ng/dL. The goal of treatment is to maintain the free T4 in the upper normal range using the lowest possible dose in order to protect the fetus from hypothyroidism. The required dose of thioamide during pregnancy can increase up to 50% for patients with a history of hyperthyroidism prior to conception. The patient's TSH should be checked at the initial prenatal visit and every trimester. Medication adjustments, testing intervals, and therapeutic goals for the free T4 are the same as for patients with new-onset disease.

Beta-blockers initially can be used to relieve the adrenergic symptoms of tachycardia, tremor, anxiety, and heat sensitivity by decreasing the maternal heart rate, cardiac output, and myocardial oxygen consumption. Longer-acting agents, such as atenolol and metoprolol 50 to 200 mg/d, are recommended. Beta-blockers are contraindicated in patients with asthma and congestive heart failure and should not be used at the time of delivery due to possible neonatal bradycardia and hypoglycemia.

The most common cause of hyperthyroidism is Graves disease, which occurs in 95% of all cases at all ages. The diagnosis of Graves disease is usually made by the presence of elevated free T4 level or free thyroid index with a suppressed TSH in the absence of a nodular goiter or thyroid mass. The differential diagnosis of hyperthyroidism, in the order of decreasing frequency, includes subacute thyroiditis, painless (silent or postpartum) thyroiditis, toxic multinodular goiter, toxic adenoma (solitary autonomous hot nodule), iodine-induced (iodinated contrast or amiodarone), iatrogenic overreplacement of thyroid hormone, factitious thyrotoxicosis, *struma ovarii* (ovarian teratoma), and gestational trophoblastic disease. The general symptoms of hyperthyroidism include palpitations, weight loss with increased appetite, nervousness, heat intolerance, oligomenorrhea, eye irritation or edema, and frequent stools. The general signs include diffuse goiter, tachycardia, tremor, warm, moist skin, and new-onset atrial fibrillation. Diagnosis during pregnancy is even more difficult because the signs and symptoms of hyperthyroidism may overlap with the hypermetabolic symptoms of pregnancy. Discrete findings with Graves disease include a diffuse, toxic goiter (common in most young women), ophthalmopathy (periorbital edema, proptosis, and lid retraction in only 30%), dermopathy (pretibial myxedema in < 1%), and acropachy (digital clubbing).

The pathogenesis of Graves disease is characterized by an autoimmune process with production of thyroid-stimulating immunoglobins (TSIs) and TSH-binding inhibitory immunoglobulin (TBIIs) that act on the TSH receptor on the thyroid gland to mediate thyroid stimulation or inhibition, respectively. These antibodies, in effect, act as TSH agonists or antagonists, to stimulate or inhibit thyroid growth, iodine trapping, and T4/T3 synthesis. Maternal Graves disease complicates 1 out of every 500 to 1000 pregnancies. The frequency of poor outcomes depends on the severity of maternal thyrotoxicosis with a risk of preterm delivery of 88%, stillbirth of 50%, and risk of congestive heart failure of over 60% in untreated mothers. As a result of transplacental transfer of the TSIs, 1% to 5% of neonates born to mothers with Graves disease have hyperthyroidism, or neonatal Graves disease. Although fetal hyperthyroidism requiring treatment is rare because of these antibodies (< 0.01% of pregnancies), it is possible in any woman with a past or current history of Graves disease. Fetal hyperthyroidism can be associated with IUGR, fetal tachycardia, fetal goiter, fetal hydrops, preterm delivery, and fetal demise. Because TSIs freely cross the placenta and can stimulate the fetal thyroid, these antibodies should be measured by the end of the second trimester in mothers with a current or past history of Graves disease, including those who have undergone treatment with surgery or I[131] or who have had a prior infant with neonatal Graves disease. Close observation of pregnancies with elevated TSI levels or antithyroid drug treatment is recommended with monthly ultrasound after 20 weeks. Those women with negative TSI levels and no medication are not at increased risk of fetal goiter or thyroid disease.

Maternal thyroid storm is a medical emergency characterized by a hypermetabolic state in a woman with uncontrolled hyperthyroidism. Thyroid storm occurs in less than 1% of pregnancies but has a high risk of maternal heart failure. Usually, there is an inciting event, such as infection, cesarean delivery, or labor, which leads to acute onset of fever, tachycardia, altered mental status (restlessness, nervousness, confusion), seizures, nausea, vomiting, diarrhea, and cardiac arrhythmias. Shock, stupor, and coma can ensue without prompt intervention, which includes OB-ICU admission, supportive measures, and acute medical management (see Table 21-2). Therapy includes a standard series of drugs, each of which has a specific role in suppression of thyroid function: PTU or methimazole blocks additional synthesis of thyroid hormone, and PTU also blocks peripheral conversion of T4 to T3. Saturated solutions of potassium iodide or sodium iodide block the release of T4 and T3 from the gland. Dexamethasone decreases thyroid hormone release and peripheral conversion of T4 to T3. Propranolol inhibits the adrenergic effects of excessive thyroid hormone. Phenobarbital can reduce extreme agitation or restlessness and may increase catabolism of thyroid hormone. Fetal surveillance is performed throughout, but intervention for fetal indications should not occur until the mother is stabilized.

Other complications of hyperthyroidism during pregnancy include severe preeclampsia, congestive heart failure, thyroid storm, early pregnancy failure, preterm delivery, fetal growth restriction, intrauterine fetal demise, and fetal thyrotoxicosis due to TSI antibodies in women with Graves disease.

Table 21–2 MANAGEMENT OF THYROID STORM IN PREGNANCY

MEDICATION	ALTERNATIVE	MECHANISM OF ACTION
• **PTU** 600-800 mg po, stat, then 150-200 mg po every 4-6 h.	• Use methimazole rectal suppositories if po intake not possible.	• Blocks T4/T3 synthesis. • Blocks peripheral T4 → T3.
• Start 1-2 h after PTU, saturated solution of **potassium iodine** (SSKI), 2-5 drops po every 8 h, OR	• Sodium iodide, 0.5-1.0 g IV every 8 h, OR • Lugol solution, 8 drops every 6 h, OR • Lithium carbonate, 300 mg orally every 6 h.	• Blocks T4/T3 release.
• **Dexamethasone**, 2 mg IV or IM every 6 h × 4 doses.		• Blocks T4/T3 synthesis. • Blocks peripheral T4 → T3.
• **Propranolol**, 20-80 mg po every 4-6 h, OR propranolol, 1-2 mg IV every 5 min for a total of 6 mg, then 1-10 mg IV every 4 h.	• If patient has history of severe bronchospasm. • Reserpine, 1-5 mg IM every 4-6 h. • Guanethidine, 1 mg/kg po every 12 h. • Diltiazem, 60 mg po every 6-8 h.	• Beta-blocker inhibits adrenergic effects of excess T4/T3.
• **Phenobarbital**, 30-60 mg po every 6-8 h PRN extreme restlessness.		• Reduces agitation. • May increase T4/T3 catabolism.

Data from Thyroid Disease in Pregnancy. ACOG Practice Bulletin No. 37. Washington DC: American College of Obstetricians and Gynecologists; August, 2002.

Hypothyroidism in Pregnancy

Overt hypothyroidism occurs in 1 to 3 out of every 1000 pregnancies. Transient hypothyroidism occurs in up to 6% of postpartum women while congenital hypothyroidism, or cretinism, affects 1 out of 4000 newborns. Most causes of hypothyroidism result from a primary thyroid defect. Hypothalamic dysfunction is a much less frequent etiology. The most common causes in pregnancy and postpartum are Hashimoto thyroiditis (chronic thyroiditis or chronic autoimmune thyroiditis), subacute thyroiditis, thyroidectomy, radioactive iodine ablation, and iodine deficiency. In developed countries Hashimoto thyroiditis is the most common etiology and is characterized by the production of antithyroid antibodies, including antimicrosomal, antithyroglobulin, and antiperoxidase (TPO) antibodies. Worldwide, iodine deficiency is the leading cause of primary hypothyroidism. Secondary, or central, hypothyroidism results from defects at the level of the pituitary (TSH deficiency) or hypothalamus (TRH deficiency) as well as generalized thyroid hormone resistance. Types of pituitary disease include Sheehan syndrome, pituitary macroadenoma, or pituitary surgery. Hypothalamic disease includes lymphocytic hypophysitis or history of hypophysectomy.

The clinical manifestations of hypothyroidism include somatic changes (fatigue, dry skin, alopecia, cold intolerance, constipation, myalgias, carpel tunnel syndrome, weight gain of 5 to 10 kg, prolonged relaxation phase of the deep tendon reflexes); cognitive and mood changes (impaired memory, depression, slowed thinking, irritability); and reproductive changes or issues (menorrhagia, amenorrhea, infertility, precocious or delayed puberty). Hypothyroidism is characterized by vague, nonspecific signs and symptoms with insidious onset, which can be confused with the normal complaints of pregnancy. Maternal complications of hypothyroidism include early pregnancy failure, preeclampsia, abruptio placenta, nonreassuring fetal heart rate tracing, low birth weight due to prematurity, an increased rate of cesarean delivery, and postpartum hemorrhage. However, adequate treatment greatly reduces the risk of a poor obstetrical outcome. Congenital complications include cretinism due to iodine deficiency, which can lead to IUGR, mental retardation, and neuropsychologic deficits.

The diagnosis of overt hypothyroidism is based on serum TSH elevation. The serum-free T4 level distinguishes between overt and subclinical hypothyroidism as the free T4 should be low, or suppressed, in overt disease while the free T4 level remains normal in subclinical hypothyroidism. The diagnosis of overt secondary hypothyroidism is made in the presence of low serum TSH and low serum-free T4.

Treatment for overt hypothyroidism in pregnancy is levothyroxine, the prohormone of thyroxine (T4), which is converted to active T3 in the peripheral tissues. Levothyroxine has a long half-life of 1 week, which allows once-a-day dosing. Average dose requirements are 1.6 to 1.8 µg/kg/d. Initiation of levothyroxine in a patient with a new diagnosis during pregnancy requires a dose of 0.1 to 0.2 mg/kg/d or 100 to 125 μg per day. Serum TSH levels are used to monitor response to therapy in hypothyroid patients and should be checked in 4 to 6 weeks. Levothyroxine can be adjusted in 25 to 50 μg increments with a therapeutic range for TSH of 0.5 to 2.5 mU/L. The goal of treatment is to maintain the TSH in the upper normal range using the lowest possible dose in order to protect the fetus from hypothyroidism. The required dose of levothyroxine can increase up to 50% for patients with a history of hypothyroidism prior to conception. The patient's TSH should be checked at the initial prenatal visit and every trimester. Medication adjustments, testing intervals, and therapeutic goals for TSH are the same as for patients with new-onset disease.

Physiologic Changes in Thyroid Function during Pregnancy

Multiple physiologic changes occur in thyroid function during pregnancy. Moderate thyroid enlargement develops due to pregnancy, hormone-induced glandular hyperplasia, and hypervascularity (see Table 21-3). Major changes in thyroid function tests are the result of an estrogen-mediated increase in thyroid-binding globulin (TBG), the major transport protein for thyroid hormone. As TBG increases, total T4, total T3, and free thyroid index increase as more thyroid hormone is bound to TBG. However, the serum levels of free T4 and free T3, the unbound active thyroid hormones, remain the same during pregnancy as do serum TSH levels. The resin T3 uptake (RT3U) decreases during pregnancy. In addition, thyroid stimulation occurs due to a "spillover" effect by hCG, especially in the first trimester. Iodine availability declines as maternal renal clearance increases and with additional losses to the fetus and placenta.

Pregnancy also affects thyroid function test results in disease states. In pregnant patients with hyperthyroidism, serum TSH decreases, free T4 increases, free thyroid index increases, total T4 increases, total T3 increases or remains unchanged, and the resin T3 uptake increases. In pregnant patients with hypothyroidism, serum TSH increases, free T4 decreases, free thyroid index decreases, total T4 decreases, total T3 decreases or remains unchanged, and the resin T3 uptake decreases.

Thyroid Function and the Fetus

The fetal thyroid begins to concentrate iodine at 10 to 12 weeks' gestation with control by fetal pituitary TSH at 20 weeks' gestation. Fetal serum TSH, TBG, free T4, and free T3 reach adult levels at 36 weeks gestation. The placenta does not allow transfer of TSH, but TRH, iodine, and TSI do cross the placental barrier. Small amounts of PTU and methimazole also cross, as well as T4 and T3, which prevent the stigmata of congenital hypothyroidism at birth.

Table 21–3 PREGNANCY-ASSOCIATED PHYSIOLOGIC CHANGES IN THYROID FUNCTION

MATERNAL STATUS	TSH	FT4	FTI	TOTAL T4	TOTAL T3	RT3U
Euthyroid Pregnancy[a]	No change	No change	No change	Increased	Increased	Decreased
Hyperthyroid[b]	Decreased	Increased	Increased	Increased	Increased or no change	Increased
Hypothyroid[b]	Increased	Decreased	Decreased	Decreased	Decreased or no change	Decreased

[a]Findings as compared to nonpregnant state
[b]Findings as compared to pregnancy euthyroid state
TSH—thyroid stimulating hormone
Total T4—total thyroxine
Total T3—total triiodothyronine (T3)
RT3U—resin T3 uptake
FT4—free thyroxine (T4)

Comprehension Questions

21.1 During pregnancy, the preferred method of assessing the dosage of antithyroid drug needed to keep a patient with Graves disease in remission is to monitor which of the following?
A. TSH level
B. TSI level
C. Total T4 levels
D. Free T4 levels
E. The fetal thyroid with ultrasonography

21.2   A 30-year-old patient at 32 weeks' gestation presents to labor and
       delivery with onset of preterm contractions. Her cervical examination
       is 3 cm and 80% effaced with bulging membranes, and she is contract-
       ing every 2 to 3 minutes on external tocometry. She has a history of
       Graves disease and is on PTU 200 mg t.i.d, but it is uncertain if she
       has been compliant with therapy. She becomes febrile with a temper-
       ature of 103°C and tachycardic with heart rate of 124 beats per
       minute. She seems very anxious and agitated and wants to walk
       around her room. Thyroid function studies are obtained but the results
       won't be available for several hours. The next most appropriate step in
       management includes all of the following EXCEPT:
       A. Amniocentesis
       B. Betamethasone administration
       C. Emergent cesarean delivery
       D. Propylthiouracil 600 to 800 mg orally stat
       E. ICU admission

21.3   Neonatal Graves disease is associated with which maternal autoim-
       mune antibody production?
       A. Thyroid-stimulating immunoglobin (TSI)
       B. Antimicrosomal antibodies
       C. Antithyroglobulin antibodies
       D. Antiperoxidase (TPO) antibodies
       E. Antinuclear antibodies

21.4   Hyperthyroidism in pregnancy is associated with all of the following
       maternal and fetal complications EXCEPT:
       A. Preeclampsia
       B. IUGR
       C. Thyroid storm
       D. IUFD
       E. Venothromboembolic events

ANSWERS

21.1   **D.** During pregnancy, the preferred method of assessing the dosage of antithyroid drug needed to keep a patient with Graves disease in remission is to monitor the free T4 levels. Free T4 levels are used to monitor response to therapy in hyperthyroid patients and should be checked in 4 to 6 weeks. The PTU or methimazole can be adjusted in 50 mg or 10 mg increments, respectively, with a therapeutic range for free T4 of 1.2 to 1.8 ng/dL. The goal of treatment is to maintain the free T4 in the upper normal range using the lowest possible dose in order to protect the fetus from hypothyroidism. TSH levels are used to measure response to levothyroxine therapy in hypothyroidism. Thyroid-stimulating immunoglobin (TSI) levels are measured in women with Graves disease to determine possible risk for fetal or neonatal Graves disease. Total T4 levels increase during pregnancy due to estrogen-mediated increases in thyroglobulin binding protein (TBG), but the free T4 levels remain unchanged in normal pregnancy. Fetal thyroid surveillance with ultrasonography is not recommended for detection of fetal goiter in gravid women with Graves disease, and it is not used for monitoring drug therapy response in hyperthyroidism.

21.2   **C.** This patient with hyperthyroidism appears to be in preterm labor. It is not clear if she has concomitant chorioamnionitis and/or maternal thyroid storm given her fever and tachycardia. Her altered mental status points toward the diagnosis of thyroid storm, but both diagnoses are possible. Given the fact that her thyroid function studies won't be resulted immediately, the presumption is uncontrolled thyrotoxicosis and PTU administration would be indicated. Intrauterine infection would be ruled out with amniocentesis. Betamethasone for fetal pulmonary lung maturation is reasonable given prematurity less than 34 weeks' gestation. Even ICU admission could be indicated given the catastrophic nature of possible thyroid storm and need for high-acuity care. However, maternal stabilization is necessitated before delivery unless fetal indications outweigh the maternal risks.

21.3   **A.** In developed countries Hashimoto thyroiditis is the most common etiology of primary hypothyroidism and is characterized by the production of antithyroid antibodies, including antimicrosomal, antithyroglobulin, and antiperoxidase (TPO) antibodies. While these antibodies may be detected in maternal Graves disease, it is the production of thyroid-stimulating immunoglobin (TSI), which crosses the placenta and impacts the fetus. Specifically, thyroid-stimulating immunoglobin (TSI) and TSH-binding inhibitory immunoglobulin (TBII) act as TSH agonists or antagonists on the TSH receptor on the thyroid gland and mediate thyroid stimulation or inhibition, respectively, of thyroid growth, iodine trapping, and T4/T3 synthesis. Maternal Graves disease complicates 1 out of every 500 to 1000 pregnancies. One to 5% of neonates born to mothers with Graves disease have hyperthyroidism, or neonatal Graves disease, as a result of transplacental transfer of TSI. Although fetal hyperthyroidism requiring treatment is rare (< 0.01% of pregnancies), it is possible in any woman with a past or current history of Graves disease.

21.4   **E.** Untreated hyperthyroidism in pregnancy is associated with many maternal and fetal complications; however, hypercoagulability is not one of them. Women with hyperthyroidism in pregnancy are not at increased risk for deep venous thrombosis or pulmonary embolism.

Clinical Pearls

See US Preventive Services Task Force Study Quality levels of evidence in Case 1

➤ An increase in thyroid-binding globulin early in pregnancy causes a rise in total T3 and total T4 but does not affect free T3 or T4 levels (Level II-3).
➤ hCG levels in early pregnancy may transiently decrease maternal TSH levels (Level II-3).
➤ Signs of hypo- and hyperthyroidism may be confused with normal changes occurring in pregnancy (Level III).
➤ Women with a history of Graves disease (treated or untreated) should have TSI levels measured in the second trimester so those with positive levels may have more intense fetal monitoring (Level III).

REFERENCES

1. Thyroid Disease in Pregnancy. ACOG Practice Bulletin No. 37. Washington DC: American College of Obstetricians and Gynecologists; August, 2002.
2. Casey BM, Leveno KJ. Thyroid disease in pregnancy. Clinical expert series. *Obstet Gynecol.* 2006;108:1238-1292.
3. Neal DM, Cootauco AC, Burrow G. Thyroid disease in pregnancy. *Clin Perinatol.* 2007;34: 543-557.

Case 22

A 36-year-old African American woman, G4P3003, presents to OB triage at 38 weeks' gestation complaining of painful contractions, vaginal bleeding, and decreased fetal movement. Her prenatal course was complicated by chronic hypertension treated with labetalol 300 mg twice a day. Vital signs at presentation are: BP 116/60 mm Hg, temperature 98°F, pulse 116 bpm, RR 16 breaths/minute. The external monitor shows a baseline fetal heart rate of 120 beats per minute with minimal variability and no accelerations. Contractions are occurring every 1 to 2 minutes. Abdominal examination reveals a firm, tender fundus. The cervix is dilated to 5 cm and completely effaced, with the fetal head at −2 station. Fifty cubic centimeters of blood is removed from the vaginal vault. The patient is transferred from triage to labor and delivery where the nurse reports difficulty finding fetal heart tones. Ultrasound at the bedside confirms the absence of fetal heart activity. There is 100 cc of blood on the bed liner. A Foley catheter is inserted and the bladder is emptied of 50 cc of dark urine. Hemoglobin and hematocrit are not yet available. The patient is given a fluid bolus of 1 L of lactated Ringer and complains of pelvic pressure. Shortly thereafter a stillborn infant is delivered vaginally, the placenta follows immediately and estimated blood loss is 2 L. There has been no urine output since the bladder was catheterized.

➤ What is the most likely cause of anuria following placental abruption?

➤ What is your next step?

➤ What are the short-term and long-term consequences of this patient's diagnosis?

ANSWER TO CASE 22:

Acute Kidney Injury

Summary: This is a 36-year-old G4P3003 at term with frequent contractions, vaginal bleeding, tachycardia, uterine tenderness, and fetal death. This presentation is attributable to abruption of the placenta. After delivery, the patient is hypovolemic and virtually anuric.

➤ **Most likely cause of anuria following placental abruption:** Sudden severe volume depletion from hemorrhage, leading to decreased renal blood flow (ischemia).

➤ **Next step:** Immediate volume replacement with typed and screened or O–(do not wait for cross match) blood and crystalloid. Check a CBC, complete metabolic profile, a coagulation panel, urinalysis, and toxicology screen. Tape a red-top tube containing 2 to 3 cc of blood to the wall.

➤ **Potential complications:** Acute tubular necrosis, acute cortical necrosis, possible hemodialysis to manage volume overload, acidosis, electrolyte imbalance, or worsening uremia, death.

ANALYSIS

Objectives

1. Recognize the most common causes of acute kidney injury (AKI) in the obstetric patient.
2. Learn how to prevent acute renal failure caused by hypovolemia, severe hypertension, and sepsis.
3. Be familiar with the evaluation and management of AKI.

Considerations

This is a multiparous 36-year-old African American woman with chronic hypertension requiring antihypertensive therapy. She initially presented with vaginal bleeding, frequent contractions, tachycardia, and was then discovered to have a fetal demise. The fetal monitor in the triage unit was actually amplifying and displaying the maternal pulse. Abruption severe enough to result in fetal death is associated with disseminated intravascular coagulation (DIC) in 30% of cases which, in turn, will exacerbate blood loss. Acute blood loss accounts for the postpartum anuria noted in this case.

APPROACH TO
Acute Kidney Injury

DEFINITIONS

ACUTE KIDNEY INJURY: An abrupt decline in renal function resulting in an inability to excrete metabolic waste products and maintain fluid, acid-base, and electrolyte balance. (See Table 22–1 for risk, injury, failure, loss, and end stage kidney disease [ESKD]. The acronym for these five stages is RIFLE, which highlights the spectrum of severity encompassed by the term "acute kidney injury.")

ACUTE TUBULAR NECROSIS (ATN): Renal tubule cell damage and death. This is seen at the severe end of the spectrum of acute kidney injury. Muddy brown granular or tubular epithelial cell casts may be found on urinalysis.

ACUTE CORTICAL NECROSIS (ACN): This requires a renal biopsy for diagnosis, but biopsy can miss the diagnosis due to the patchy nature of the disease process. This severe kidney injury can follow a prolonged period of acute tubular necrosis. In the developing world, obstetric emergencies like the placental abruption presented still contribute many cases of cortical necrosis.

TILT TEST: A decrease in systolic pressure of 20 mm Hg or an increase in pulse of 20 beats per minute associated with a change in posture, for example, lying to sitting, sitting to standing, lying to standing (allowing at least 2 min for equilibrium after position change).

CLINICAL APPROACH

For decades the lack of clear, concise, and widely accepted definitions for acute renal failure has made it difficult to compare incidence and outcomes between studies. In 2005, the term acute renal failure was changed to acute kidney injury. At around the same time, the RIFLE criteria (Table 22–1) were proposed to clarify the spectrum of acute kidney injury.[1] The literature search conducted for this review included the terms pregnancy, acute renal failure, acute kidney injury, hemodialysis, and renal replacement therapy. Because the term AKI and the RIFLE criteria have been in use for only a relatively short time, the authors have referenced some of the earlier work on acute renal failure in pregnancy.

The incidence of AKI related to pregnancy varies widely, from just under 1/1000 to 1/20,000.[2,3] It is plausible that the higher figure includes women with serum creatinine levels greater than 0.8 mg/dL while the lower figure is confined to women requiring dialysis. Allowing for this degree of disparity in definition, other factors affecting incidence include study methodology and country of origin (developed or developing). Separate RIFLE criteria have not been applied to pregnant women and, given the 50% increase in glomerular

Table 22–1 THE RIFLE CRITERIA FOR ACUTE KIDNEY INJURY		
	P$_{Cr}$ or GFR Criteria	Urine Output Criteria
RISK	Increased P$_{Cr}$ > 1.5 or GFR decrease > 25%	UO <0.5 mL/kg/h × 6 h
		High Sensitivity
INJURY	Increased P$_{Cr}$ > 2 or GFR decrease > 50%	UO <0.5 mL/kg/h × 12 h
FAILURE	Increased P$_{Cr}$ > 3 GFR decrease 75% or P$_{Cr}$ ≥ 4 mg/dL Acute rise ≥ 0.5 mg/dL	UO < 0.3 mL/kg/h (Oliguria) × 24 h or Anuria × 12 h
LOSS	Persistent AKI = complete loss of kidney function > 4 wk	
		High Specificity
ESKD	End stage kidney disease (> 3 mo)	

GFR = glomerular filtration rate
AKI = acute kidney injury

filtration rate (GFR) during pregnancy, this may be problematic. Over 80% of cases of AKI related to pregnancy are confined to the postpartum period, and thus do not affect the fetus. There may be a distinction between postpartum AKI encountered in the first 48 hours compared to those that are diagnosed 3 or more days postpartum.

Most cases of AKI in pregnancy result from hypertensive disease (preeclampsia, eclampsia, and HELLP syndrome) and hemorrhage (especially placental abruption severe enough to cause the death of the fetus, as in the case presented).[4] Other causes include microangiopathic diseases (HUS and TTP), sepsis, and obstruction. No matter what the cause, it is axiomatic that drugs such as magnesium and gentamicin used commonly by obstetricians require dosage adjustment or discontinuation if severe renal dysfunction is present.

One factor which may contribute to the recent decline in AKI secondary to hypertensive disorders is the early detection and subsequent prompt delivery of women with these disorders. There is no evidence that loop diuretics like furosemide favorably affect the prognosis in AKI and their use is not recommended, particularly when they are used in an attempt to convert oliguric to nonoliguric renal failure.

Before considering general management principles in pregnant or postpartum women, it is important to emphasize that prevention of AKI in the case presented at the start of this chapter is both possible and desirable. More than 40 years ago, obstetricians at Parkland Hospital developed transfusion guidelines for the management of hypovolemia secondary to hemorrhage.[5] These guidelines, referred to as the "30-30 rule," called for transfusion to maintain the woman's hematocrit at or close to 30% and her urine output at ≥ 30 mL/h. If available, whole blood was given, but it is recognized that whole blood is not readily available at many centers, so packed red blood cells +/− fresh frozen plasma may be substituted. A recent publication from Parkland Hospital reported an incidence of ATN of 0.3% (2/659) among women who were transfused with whole blood, compared to 2% (12/593) who received only packed red blood cells (PRBCs).[6] This difference was statistically significant. Finally, whole blood contains considerably more clotting factors than PRBCs. This is important because DIC complicates 30% of cases of placental abruption severe enough to result in fetal death. Using either crystalloid or colloid alone is not recommended for volume replacement. Criteria for hypovolemia include hypotension (systolic blood pressure < 100 mm Hg) unrelated to regional anesthesia, resting tachycardia (pulse > 100 bpm), a positive tilt test (see Definitions), and low urine output (< 30 mL/h). Even if evidence of hypovolemia is lacking, transfusion is indicated if the hematocrit is less than 20% in the setting of hemorrhage.

Other measures used to prevent progression of AKI to ATN include early recognition and treatment of sepsis and avoidance of vasoconstrictors if sepsis is not suspected.

The definition of AKI in Williams Obstetrics[5] is a rapid decrease in the glomerular filtration rate (GFR) over minutes to days. Clinically, creatinine clearance is used to approximate GFR and is calculated as:

$$C_{Cr} = \frac{U_{Cr} \cdot \dot{V}}{P_{Cr}}$$

where urine and plasma creatinine are measured in milligrams per deciliter and $\dot{V}$ = urine flow, in units of milliliters per minute. Classically, the period of urine collection is 24 hours (1440 min). Thus, the $\dot{V}$ term represents the volume of urine excreted (in 24 h) divided by 1440 minutes.

Another important formula in managing women with AKI is the fractional excretion of sodium (FEN). This formula makes use of the general formula for clearance of a substance (see preceding equation) and compares the clearance of sodium to the clearance of creatinine:

$$FE_{Na} = \frac{C_{Na}}{C_{Cr}} = \frac{\dfrac{U_{Na} \cdot \dot{V}}{P_{Na}}}{\dfrac{U_{Cr} \cdot \dot{V}}{P_{Cr}}}$$

Manipulating the right side of the equation and multiplying by 100 yields FE_{Na} as a percent:

$$FE_{Na}(\%) = \frac{U_{Na} \cdot P_{Cr}}{P_{Na} \cdot U_{Cr}} \times 100$$

A FE_{Na} of less than 1% suggests that AKI is due to prerenal causes, often hypovolemia, whereas a FE_{Na} greater than 1% implies that intrinsic renal injury is present. Prior use of diuretics invalidates the FE_{Na} result. The values used in the formula require the determination of both plasma and urine electrolytes.

Diagnostic Evaluation

Evaluation of women suspected of having acute kidney injury is relatively simple and straightforward. Frequent assessment of vital signs (including testing for orthostatic changes), monitoring of urine output hourly if indicated, daily weight determination, and heart and lung examination should be supplemented by hemoglobin and hematocrit, serum and urine electrolytes, urinalysis and, if abruption is suspected, a coagulation panel. Taping a red top tube to the wall, mentioned at the beginning of this chapter, has practical utility. Also called the clot observation test, the important feature is the size of the clot that evolves and persists, not measuring the time it takes to clot. A small, soft, "mushy" clot which later dissolves indicates a high probability of overt hypofibrinogenemia long before a fibrinogen result is returned from the lab. The absolute level of serum creatinine, rate of rise, and weight-based urine output are each incorporated into the RIFLE criteria (Table 22–1).

Management Considerations

Management by the obstetrician of acute kidney injury obviously depends on the severity of the injury. Prompt restoration of circulating volume and appropriate management of preeclampsia, eclampsia, and HELLP syndrome including expeditious delivery are critically important steps. Close observation and supportive care usually suffice for mild to moderate azotemia. Cases complicated by persistent oliguria despite volume resuscitation and resulting in steady increase in serum creatinine to levels beyond 3 to 4 mg/dL (F level in the RIFLE criteria) should prompt nephrology consultation and, in turn, a high likelihood of the need for some type of renal replacement therapy (hemofiltration or hemodialysis). Dialysis for acute kidney injury is most often indicated for worsening uremia. Other indications include volume overload, acidosis, and hyperkalemia.

Finally, there remains a debate about whether postpartum renal failure is a unique clinical entity in some cases. First reported more than 40 years ago and regarded as idiopathic, postpartum renal failure (PPRF) was differentiated from renal failure secondary to obstetric complications like the one outlined in this chapter. The time of onset, 3 or more days postpartum for the idiopathic type, was felt to be one of the key distinguishing features. A case report from 2008 that would have fulfilled the criteria for idiopathic PPRF instead concluded that renal failure occurred as a result of catastrophic antiphospholipid antibody syndrome.[7] The woman who was the subject of that report was admitted 2 weeks postpartum with a creatinine of 2.4 mg/dL (stage I or F of the RIFLE criteria). Within just a few days she became persistently oliguric, the serum creatinine increased to 5.4 mg/dL, and she was treated with hemodialysis for 24 days in the hospital. Because her kidneys did not recover by the time of discharge, hemodialysis was continued as an outpatient. This suggests that a proportion of PPRF cases may no longer be properly classified as idiopathic.

Comprehension Questions

22.1   With placental abruption severe enough to cause fetal death, what is the incidence of DIC?
       A. 10%
       B. 30%
       C. 50%
       D. 70%

22.2   Most cases of acute kidney injury in pregnancy and the postpartum period are caused by which of the following?
       A. Hypertension and hemorrhage
       B. Sepsis and DIC
       C. HUS and TTP
       D. Acute fatty liver

22.3   The fractional excretion of sodium (FE_{Na}) is expressed in which of the following units?
       A. mg/dL
       B. mL/min
       C. %
       D. mg/min

22.4   An increase in GFR by 50% in normal pregnancy accounts for which of the following facts?
       A. Decreased FE_{Na} in pregnancy
       B. Increase in blood volume by 50%
       C. A slight decrease in pH to 7.37
       D. An upper limit of normal for plasma creatinine of 0.8 mg/dL

ANSWERS

22.1   **B.** DIC complicates 30% of abruptions severe enough to cause fetal death. DIC is most often manifested by overt hypofibrinogenemia.

22.2   **A.** The combination of hypertension and hemorrhage accounts for more than 80% of cases of AKI in pregnancy.

22.3   **C.** FE_{Na} is expressed in %. The urine flow cancels out in numerator and denominator, and so do the units of urine and plasma sodium and creatinine.

22.4   **D.** The upper limit of normal for plasma creatinine is 0.8 mg/dL. The meaning of an increased clearance from blood of a substance like creatinine is that there is a lower than normal amount left in the blood. This fact is very important to the diagnosis of AKI in pregnancy.

Clinical Pearls

See US Preventive Services Task Force Study Quality levels of evidence in Case 1

➤ Normal pregnancy is associated with an increase in GFR and a decline in serum creatinine. Therefore, in pregnancy, a creatinine greater than 0.8 mg/dL is abnormal (Level II-3).

➤ All obstetricians should be able to calculate, interpret, and use clinically the fractional excretion of sodium and the creatinine clearance (Level III).

➤ Magnesium sulfate is excreted primarily (> 95%) by the kidneys. Both oliguria (< 100 cc in 4 h) or elevated creatinine (> 1 mg/dL) necessitate at least careful monitoring of serum magnesium level and possibly dose reduction or discontinuation of the intravenous administration of magnesium sulfate (Level II-3).

➤ Appropriate indications for nephrology consultation have not been codified. However, severe oliguria less than 0.3 mL/kg/h or anuria for 6 to 12 hours, accompanied by rapid rise in serum creatinine suggests the need for consultation. Early initiation of dialysis may hasten recovery (Level II-3).

REFERENCES

1. Ricci Z, Cruz D, Ronco C. The RIFLE criteria and mortality in acute kidney injury: a systematic review. *Kidney Int.* 2008;73:538-546.
2. Gammill HS, Jeyabalan A. Acute renal failure in pregnancy. *Crit Care Med.* 2005;33:372S-384S.
3   Drakeley AJ, Le Roux PA, Anthony J, Penny J. Acute renal failure complicating severe preeclampsia requiring admission to an obstetric intensive care unit. *Am J Obstet Gynecol.* 2002;186:253-256.

4. Silva GB Jr., Monteiro FA, Mota RM, et al. Acute kidney injury requiring dialysis in obstetric patients: a series of 55 cases in Brazil. *Arch Gynecol Obstet.* 2009;279:131-137.

5. Cunningham FG, Leveno KJ, Bloom SL, Hauth JC, Rouse DJ. *Williams Obstetrics.* 23rd ed. New York, NY: McGraw Hill; 2010:1045-1046.

6. Alexander JM, Sarode R, McIntire DD, Burner JD, Leveno KJ. Whole blood in the management of hypovolemia due to obstetric hemorrhage. *Obstet Gynecol.* 2009;113:1320-1326.

7. Magee CC, Coggins MP, Foster CS, Muse VV, Colvin RB. Case 2-2008: A 38-year-old woman with postpartum visual loss, shortness of breath and renal failure. *N Engl J Med.* 2008;358:275-289.

Case 23

A 31-year-old nulligravida presents for preconceptional counseling secondary to a history of pulmonary embolism 7 years ago. She was anticoagulated for 3 months and has not required any further treatment or prophylaxis. As part of her evaluation at that time, she had thrombophilia testing and was found to have antithrombin (AT) deficiency (42%; normal 80%-140%). As a result, her two sisters sought testing and were also identified to have the same thrombophilia. There is no family history of thrombosis or other clotting disorders. She was told by her physician at the time of her pulmonary embolus that she should not conceive. However, she has recently married and is contemplating pregnancy. She is otherwise healthy and is using condoms for contraception.

➤ What is the next step in evaluating this patient?

➤ What are potential maternal complications of AT deficiency in pregnancy?

➤ What are potential fetal complications?

➤ How would you manage the pregnancy of a woman with AT deficiency?

ANSWERS TO CASE 23:

Thrombophilia

Summary: A nulligravida with a personal history of pulmonary embolus and AT deficiency presents for preconceptional counseling. She has no family history of thrombosis.

➤ **Next step in evaluating this patient:** Confirmation that the patient is truly AT deficient and does not have any other inherited or acquired thrombophilias.

➤ **Potential maternal complications of AT deficiency in pregnancy:** Venous thromboembolism and although significantly rarer, arterial thromboses have been reported.

➤ **Potential fetal complication:** Fetal growth restriction, stillbirth, and placental abruption.

➤ **Management plan for a pregnancy in a woman with AT deficiency:** Therapeutic (adjusted-dose) anticoagulation with unfractionated (UH) or low-molecular-weight heparin (LMWH), serial growth ultrasounds.

ANALYSIS

Objectives

1. Recognize maternal and fetal complications of AT deficiency.
2. Understand how to diagnose and treat AT deficiency.
3. Understand whom to screen for inherited thrombophilias.
4. Know which women with thrombophilias are candidates for treatment during pregnancy.

Considerations

Antithrombin (AT; initially designated antithrombin III) is a plasma protease inhibitor that is able to neutralize all proteases of the intrinsic coagulation pathway, including thrombin, factors XIIa, XIa, Xa, and IXa. Of the heritable thrombophilias, AT deficiency is the most uncommon with a prevalence of 1 in 5000; however, it is also the most thrombogenic with a 70% to 90% lifetime risk of thromboembolism. It is usually inherited in an autosomal dominant fashion, and two major types of inherited AT deficiency exist. Type I AT deficiency, the most common type, is characterized by low levels of both antigen and activity. In type II AT deficiency, there is a specific defect within the

AT protein itself, which leads to markedly decreased functional activity with essentially no effect on antigenic levels. Type II AT deficiency is further sub-classified based on the actual site of the mutation, such as a defect at the heparin-binding site or a defect at the thrombin-binding site. This subclassi-fication scheme further affects risk of thromboembolic events, with the type II heparin-binding site variant having the least clinical significance.

Because of the low prevalence of AT deficiency, it is only present in 1% of patients who present with a thrombotic event (Figure 23–1). This patient's AT deficiency was detected after she suffered a pulmonary embolism. Similar to this patient, 42% of those with AT deficiency suffer an initial thrombotic event spontaneously, while the remaining cases occur in the presence of an

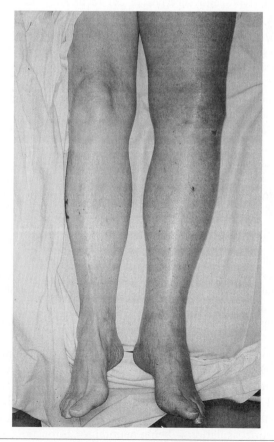

Figure 23–1. A patient with classic findings of left lower extremity DVT with swelling, erythema, pain, and tenderness. *(Reproduced, with permission, from Knoop KJ, Stack LB, Storrow AB, et al. Atlas of Emergency Medicine. 3rd ed. New York, NY: McGraw-Hill; 2010:336. Photo contributor: Kevin J. Knoop, MD, MS.).*

additional risk factor such as pregnancy, oral contraceptive use, surgery, or trauma. Additional common sites of thrombosis are the deep veins of the leg, the iliofemoral veins, and the mesenteric veins. Arterial thrombosis has been reported, but does not seem to be characteristic of AT deficiency.

The first step in evaluating this patient is confirmation of her AT deficiency. Erroneous diagnoses of hereditary AT deficiency can occur. For instance, acute thrombosis, heparin therapy, sepsis, disseminated intravascular coagulation (DIC), oral contraceptives, and other acquired conditions such as liver disease can lead to decreased AT levels. There is also some controversy as to whether oral anticoagulation can falsely increase plasma AT concentrations into a normal range. Thus, optimally, repeat testing should be performed at least 2 weeks after completion of anticoagulation therapy for the acute thrombotic event, and an AT-factor Xa assay that measures AT activity will detect all types and subtypes of AT deficiency. Levels of AT are unchanged in pregnancy.

Once the diagnosis of AT deficiency is confirmed, preconceptional consultation should include a discussion regarding the additive effect of pregnancy on hypercoagulability The potential complications that may arise during pregnancy because of AT deficiency should also be reviewed. Although the data on thrombophilia and adverse pregnancy outcomes are heterogeneous, it appears that among the hereditary thrombophilias, AT deficiency appears to have the highest risk of stillbirth. Similarly, retrospective data also suggest that there is an increased risk for fetal growth restriction and placental abruption, and serial growth ultrasounds should be performed.

While the absolute risk of developing thromboembolism in pregnancy is low in the setting of AT deficiency, the relative risk is at least 250-fold greater when compared to that of controls without a known thrombophilia. Thus, in this patient with a "higher-risk" thrombophilia and a personal prior history of venous thromboembolism, therapeutic anticoagulation during pregnancy and the postpartum period is not unreasonable. Both unfractionated heparin (UH) and low-molecular-weight heparin (LMWH) are appropriate choices. With UH, subcutaneous administration three times a day should be prescribed, with an activated partial thromboplastin time (aPTT) trough of 1.5 to 2 times the mean control aPTT. Enoxaparin, one of the more frequently prescribed LMWHs, can be given subcutaneously twice daily (1 mg/kg) in order to account for increased renal clearance and larger volume of distribution during pregnancy. With LMWH, peak anti-factor Xa levels should be drawn 4 hours after administration of a dose with a goal of approximately 0.5 to 1.0 IU/mL. Either aPTT or anti-factor Xa levels should also be checked serially depending on which anticoagulant is used to ensure that therapeutic anticoagulation is being maintained throughout pregnancy. A platelet count should be checked prior to initiating anticoagulation, and serial assessment of platelet counts should be performed for an additional 3 weeks thereafter to ensure that the patient is not developing heparin-induced thrombocytopenia (HIT) which may occur in 2% of those treated. While the extent of therapeutic doses of UH or LMWH on bone mineral density is unclear, consideration should be given to an additional 500 mg of calcium supplementation daily.

APPROACH TO
Thrombophilia

In general, inherited thrombophilias in pregnancy increase the risk of thrombosis in either the maternal, fetal, or placental venous systems. AT deficiency, as well as protein C and protein S deficiencies, are less common causes of genetic thrombophilias with prevalence 0.2% to 0.5% and 0.08%, respectively and they are inherited in an autosomal dominant fashion. In contrast, mutations of the factor V Leiden (FVL) gene, the prothrombin G20210A mutation (PTGM), and hyperhomocysteinemia secondary to homozygosity for the MTHFR mutation (TT genotype) are more common genetic causes of thrombophilia, with hetero- or homozygous gene status affecting the degree of hypercoagulability. The prevalence is 5% to 9%, 2% to 3%, and 11% in white European population for FVL, PTGM, and MTHFR (TT genotype), respectively. Higher risk thrombophilias include AT deficiency, homozygotes for either FVL or PTGM, or compound heterozygotes with one copy of the FVL mutation and one copy of the PTGM. While protein C deficiency, protein S deficiency, and heterozygosity for FVL or PTGM are considered lower risk thrombophilias, personal and family history are important considerations in ascertaining thrombogenic risk.

Indications for Thrombophilia

Routine screening for inherited thrombophilias should not be performed. Testing should be performed in women with a personal history of thrombosis. There is controversy surrounding whether individuals with a strong family history of thromboembolism should be tested. Consideration to testing these patients should be given, especially if family members suffered from thrombosis earlier in life and in the absence of any associated risk factors (eg, oral contraceptives, trauma, etc.). There is even more uncertainty regarding testing in the setting of prior adverse pregnancy outcomes, but in the absence of substantial evidence in favor of testing for inherited thrombophilias, the American College of Obstetricians and Gynecologists (ACOG) recommends discussing the implications of testing and positive test results for an inherited thrombophilia on management. Of note, ACOG suggests that patients with a history of thrombosis, recurrent fetal loss, early/severe preeclampsia, or severe unexplained fetal growth restriction be tested for antiphospholipid antibodies.[1]

Thrombophilia and Pregnancy Outcome

From an obstetrical standpoint, inherited thrombophilias have been associated with an increased risk for various adverse pregnancy outcomes. However, findings are often conflicting. For instance, with regard to inherited thrombophilia and early pregnancy loss, a recent meta-analysis of 31 studies concluded that presence of the PTGM or FVL mutation increases the risk of early (< 13 weeks) recurrent (≥ 2) fetal loss approximately twofold, whereas there did not appear to be an association between protein C deficiency, protein S deficiency, AT deficiency, and MTHFR.[2] In contrast, a subsequent cohort study performed by Roque and colleagues found that the presence of thrombophilia appeared protective of recurrent early pregnancy loss, decreasing the risk by approximately 50%[3] (Level II-2). Early pregnancy is associated with a low oxygen environment and decreased flow through uteroplacental circulation.[4,5] Thus, oxygen may actually be harmful to early pregnancy and maternal thrombophilias may paradoxically be helpful during this time in gestation.

The association between inherited thrombophilias and late fetal loss appears to be stronger, although the definition of late varies between studies. The same cohort study by Roque found that the presence of an inherited thrombophilia carries at least a threefold risk of late fetal loss, which the authors defined as loss after 14 weeks' gestation. Similarly, a retrospective cohort analysis from data gathered by the European Prospective Cohort on Thrombophilia (EPCOT) demonstrated that the risk for stillbirth after 28 weeks' gestation was significantly greater in women with a heritable thrombophilia such as AT and protein C and S deficiency. Moreover, these results were more pronounced in those with AT deficiency and combined defects[6] (Level II-2).

Other potentially related obstetrical complications in the setting of inherited thrombophilia include abruption, intrauterine fetal growth restriction, and preeclampsia. For the most part, when the thrombophilias are examined individually, there are varying conclusions surrounding its association with these specific adverse pregnancy outcomes. However, when taken as a group, the presence of thrombophilia appears associated with placental abruption, and one study also found that this risk increased as the number of maternal thrombophilias increased.[3,7] With regard to preeclampsia and fetal growth restriction, the relationship with thrombophilia is less clear, with certain studies demonstrating no link but others finding an association only in the setting of specific thrombophilias[7,8] (Level II-2). Thus, without clear evidence of an association between thrombophilia and preeclampsia or fetal growth restriction, it is not unreasonable to consider intermittent growth ultrasounds, especially in the setting of a more thrombogenic thrombophilia.

Management Recommendations

Thrombogenic potential varies with the specific thrombophilia. Those with high-risk thrombophilias such as AT deficiency, homozygosity for either FVL or PTGM, or compound heterozygotes for FVL and PTGM require some degree of anticoagulation in pregnancy. ACOG recommends adjusted-dose anticoagulation in these patients.[1] For patients who are incidentally found to be carriers of inherited thrombophilia such as heterozygotes for FVL or PTGM, treatment guidelines are based primarily on expert opinion. Many recommend low-dose prophylaxis in these patients who do not have a history of thrombosis but have a strong family history of idiopathic thrombosis or adverse pregnancy outcome. It is even less clear whether women who are incidental heterozygotes but lack personal, or family history of thrombosis or are without a history of adverse pregnancy outcome would benefit from anticoagulation. Consensus is also lacking regarding whether patients with a history of thrombosis who are afflicted with either protein C or protein S deficiency should receive low-dose or adjusted-dose anticoagulation in pregnancy.

Appropriate adjusted-dose anticoagulation regimens in pregnancy are described earlier. Low-dose prophylaxis can be achieved with UH in increasing doses each trimester (eg, 5000 U q12h in the first trimester, 7500 U q12h in the second trimester, and 10,000 U q12h in the third trimester). Similarly, LMWH is also appropriate, and as an example, enoxaparin 40 mg can be given q 12 hours. The recommendation to administer twice daily enoxaparin in pregnancy is based on pharmacologic data demonstrating that the pharmacokinetics of enoxaparin are significantly different during pregnancy than in the same cohort when nonpregnant, although outcome data are lacking at this point[9] (Level II-3). A platelet count should be checked prior to initiating anticoagulation therapy and every week thereafter for an additional 3 weeks to observe for any evidence of HIT. While more common in patients receiving UH, LMWH may cross-react with the heparin/platelet factor IV antibodies and should not be used in women who have previously developed HIT. Consideration should also be given to additional calcium supplementation to women who are on either UH or LMWH during pregnancy.

Comprehension Questions

23.1   A 28-year-old G3P0030 presents at 7 weeks' gestation. Her history is significant for a three prior miscarriages, ranging from 8 weeks' to 11 weeks' gestation. Which test is most indicated?

    A. Lupus anticoagulant
    B. Antithrombin-factor Xa assay
    C. Protein S activity assay
    D. Serum beta-hCG

23.2   A 30-year-old nulligravida recently suffered from a deep vein thrombosis and was diagnosed with homozygosity for the prothrombin gene G20210A mutation. What anticoagulation regimen would you recommend for her in pregnancy?

    A. No anticoagulation
    B. Warfarin
    C. Low-dose LMWH
    D. Adjusted-dose LMWH

ANSWERS

23.1   **A.** Recurrent pregnancy loss is an indication for testing for antiphospholipid syndrome, an acquired thrombophilia.

23.2   **D.** Homozygosity for prothrombin gene *G20210* mutation is considered to be in the high-risk category of inherited thrombophilias. With a personal history of thrombosis and a high-risk thrombophilia this patient should be treated with adjusted-dose LMWH.

Clinical Pearls

See US Preventive Services Task Force Study Quality levels of evidence in Case 1

➤ Women with a personal history (and possibly a strong family history) of thrombosis should be tested for inherited and acquired thrombophilias (Level II-3).

➤ Individuals with adverse pregnancy outcomes such as recurrent miscarriage, stillbirth, early/severe preeclampsia, and severe unexplained fetal growth restriction should be tested for acquired thrombophilias. Further discussion and consideration of implications is warranted regarding testing for heritable thrombophilias (Level III).

➤ Protein S free and total levels are normally decreased by 60% to 70% in normal pregnancy (Level II-2).

➤ Thrombophilias with more thrombogenic potential such as AT deficiency, homozygosity for FVL mutation or PTGM, or compound heterozygosity for FVL/PTGM require adjusted-dose anticoagulation (Level II-2).

➤ Platelet counts should be assessed prior to starting anticoagulation and serially for the next 3 weeks to ensure no evidence of HIT (Level III).

CONTROVERSIES

- The extent of the association between inherited thrombophilias and early recurrent pregnancy loss, severe preeclampsia, and fetal growth restriction remains uncertain.
- It is unknown whether low-dose or adjusted-dose anticoagulation should be administered to individuals with a history of thrombosis who are identified with protein C or protein S deficiency.
- The effects of adjusted-dose anticoagulation on bone mineral density and its potential response to calcium supplementation are unknown.

REFERENCES

1. Thromboembolism in Pregnancy. ACOG Practice Bulletin No. 19; 2000.

2. Rey E, Kahn SR, David M, Shrier I. Thrombophilic disorders and fetal loss: a meta-analysis. *Lancet.* 2003;361:901.
   Meta-analysis of 31 prospective and retrospective observational studies, which found that FVL and PTGM were associated with a two-to threefold increase in both early recurrent pregnancy loss and late, nonrecurrent fetal loss.

3. Roque H, Paidas MJ, Funai EF, Kuczynski E, Lockwood CJ. Maternal thrombophilias are not associated with early pregnancy loss. *Thromb Haemost.* 2004;91:290.
   This retrospective cohort study found that the presence of one or more thrombophilias decreased the risk of recurrent early pregnancy loss (< 10 wk) by approximately one-half. The authors comment on the biologic plausibility of this finding as low oxygen tension is normally present in early pregnancy.

4. Rodesch F, Simon P, Donner C, Jauniaux E. Oxygen measurements in endometrial and trophoblastic tissues during early pregnancy. *Obstet Gynecol.* 1992 Aug;80(2):283-285.

5. Watson AL, Skepper JN, Jauniaux E, Burton GJ. Susceptibility of human placental syncytiotrophoblastic mitochondria to oxygen-mediated damage in relation to gestational age. *J Clin Endocrinol Metab.* 1998 May;83(5):1697-1705.

6. Preston FE, Rosendaal FR, Walker ID, et al. Increased fetal loss in women with heritable thrombophilia. *Lancet.* 1996;348:913.
   These authors analyzed the frequencies of miscarriage, which they defined as loss at or before 28 weeks gestation, and stillbirth, which was loss after 28 weeks gestation. They found that the risk of fetal loss overall was about one-third greater in women with an inherited thrombophilia, although when subcategorized, the association was stronger between stillbirth and thrombophilia.

7. Kupferminc MJ, Eldor A, Steinman N, et al. Increased frequency of genetic thrombophilia in women with complications of pregnancy. *N Engl J Med.* 1999;340:9.
   The authors performed a case-control analysis of 110 women who had an adverse pregnancy outcome such as severe preeclampsia, placental abruption, fetal growth restriction, and stillbirth and tested them for inherited thrombophilias in comparison to a control population.

8. Infante-Rivard C, Rivard GE, Yotov WV, et al. Absence of association of thrombophilia polymorphisms with intrauterine growth restriction. *N Engl J Med.* 2002;347:19.
   This case-control study demonstrated that the risk of fetal growth restriction was not increased among women with a thrombophilia.

9. Casele H, Laifer SA, Woelkers DA, Venkataramanan R. Changes in the pharmacokinetics of the low-molecular-weight heparin enoxaparin sodium during pregnancy. *Am J Obstet Gynecol.* 1999;181:1113.
   Subjects requiring prophylactic doses of enoxaparin sodium were tested in early pregnancy, in late pregnancy, and in the nonpregnant state for anti-factor Xa activity. These authors found that the area under the plasma activity versus time curve was significantly lower in pregnancy than in the postpartum state, suggesting that the pharmacokinetics of enoxaparin in pregnancy may reach more steady-states with twice-daily dosing.

Case 24

A 22-year-old primigravida is seen in your office at 32 weeks' gestation for a routine prenatal visit. Her gestational age was calculated by her last normal menstrual period which agreed with an ultrasound at 8 weeks' gestation. Her pregnancy has been uneventful to date, although she has continued to smoke 1 pack or more of cigarettes daily. She relates normal fetal movement and no uterine contractions.

Physical examination reveals her height to be 5 ft 6 in, her weight to be 118 lb (53.5 kg), and her blood pressure to be 90/60 mm Hg. She has gained 10 lb (4.5 kg) since becoming pregnant. Her fundal height is 26 cm. On ultrasound, you note an estimated fetal weight of 900 g with an elevated head circumference (HC) to abdominal circumference (AC) ratio, and an amniotic fluid index (AFI) that is at the fifth percentile.

➤ What is the most likely diagnosis?

➤ What is your next step?

➤ What are potential complications of the patient's disorder?

ANSWERS TO CASE 24:
Intrauterine Growth Restriction (IUGR)

Summary: This is a 22-year-old woman at 32 weeks' gestation who continues to smoke cigarettes during pregnancy with poor weight gain and a growth-restricted fetus by ultrasound.

> **Most likely diagnosis:** Intrauterine growth restriction (IUGR).

> **Next step:** Evaluate fetal well-being.

> **Potential complications:** Preterm birth; fetal stress; intrauterine demise.

ANALYSIS

Objectives

1. List risk factors for IUGR.
2. Understand signs in pregnancy that may indicate a growth-restricted fetus.
3. Be able to evaluate a patient with suspected IUGR.
4. Develop a plan of management for patient whose fetus is growth-restricted.

Considerations

This gravida has multiple risks for a fetus with IUGR: She is underweight (body-mass index [BMI] = 17.4 prior to pregnancy), has had poor pregnancy weight gain (10 lb [4.5 kg]), and is a smoker.

There are many risk factors for IUGR, which may be divided into three broad categories: maternal, uterine/placental, and fetal (see Table 24–1).

Maternal factors include hypertension (HTN), cardiac disease, respiratory diseases, renal disease, anemia, toxic habits, and malnutrition. HTN—whether antecedent to pregnancy or first appearing during pregnancy—places the fetus at risk for IUGR. Cardiac and respiratory diseases may impact oxygenation; poor maternal oxygenation is associated with IUGR. Gravidas with severe anemia are at increased risk of having a fetus with IUGR. Toxic habits, such as drug and tobacco use, are potentially the most modifiable risk factors for IUGR. Evidence suggests that advanced maternal age (AMA) is a risk for IUGR.

Uterine/placental factors include abruptio, placenta previa, and infection. Abruptio is more common in women with HTN, as well as in those who smoke. Cocaine use is a risk factor for abruption. Toxoplasmosis, herpes, and parvovirus have all been associated with IUGR. Early-onset IUGR (< 20 wk) is associated with cytomegalovirus.

Table 24–1 ETIOLOGIES OF IUGR

Maternal factors:
- HTN
- Renal disease
- Cardiac and respiratory disease
- Underweight and/or poor pregnancy weight gain
- Anemia
- Toxic habits: cocaine, tobacco

Uterine/placental factors:
- Abruptio placenta
- Placenta previa
- Infection

Fetal factors:
- Multiple gestation
- Aneuploidy
- Syndromes
- Structural malformations
- Infection

Fetal factors include multiple pregnancy, aneuploidy, structural malformations, and infection. Multiple gestations are at increased risk of IUGR. Aneuploid fetuses—trisomy 13, trisomy 18, trisomy 21—are typically smaller than their euploid siblings. Many syndromes are associated with IUGR, including Russel-Silver syndrome, Bloom syndrome, and cretinism (hypothyroidism). Fetal structural malformations, such as gastroschisis or omphalocele, place the fetus at risk for IUGR. As noted above, infection is also associated with IUGR.

APPROACH TO
IUGR

The definition of IUGR is a matter of some debate. Some authors suggest a cutoff of the third percentile (2 SD below the mean) to define IUGR. Others have proposed using the fifth percentile. The most commonly used definition is a **birthweight less than the 10th percentile** for gestational age (GA).

The American College of Obstetricians and Gynecologists (ACOG) Practice Bulletin 12 (January, 2000) acknowledges "confusion in terminology," since by definition 10% of infants in a population will have birth weight less than the 10th percentile. This bulletin notes that while defining a pathologic condition using a 10th percentile cutoff makes statistical sense, it may not be clinically relevant.

The clinical challenge of greatest relevance: distinguishing the small-but-healthy fetus from the one who is compromised. Bernstein and Gabbe elegantly **define the IUGR fetus as one who suffers morbidity and/or mortality associated with the failure to reach growth potential.** This is in contrast to a fetus that is constitutionally small.

Early insults to fetal growth are thought to more commonly manifest as symmetric IUGR. Symmetric IUGR may be caused by aneuploidy or early transplacental infection. On the other hand, asymmetric IUGR describes a pattern with a relatively smaller abdominal circumference in comparison to the fetal head circumference, and is thought to reflect a more recent insult to fetal growth. An example of this type of situation occurs in association with hypertension developing late in the pregnancy. The patterns may ultimately merge in the setting of long-standing complications, such as preexisting hypertension.

The excess morbidity and mortality in the setting of IUGR is significant. An early study of infants born between 38 and 42 weeks with a birthweight between 1500 and 2500 g found that **perinatal morbidity and mortality were up to 30 times greater than that seen in infants born between the 10th and 90th percentile.** Expert commentary on this study offered the following perspective: "An infant with a weight of 1250 g at 38 to 42 weeks' gestation has a greater perinatal mortality risk than one born of similar weight at 32 weeks."

Some of the neonatal morbidities associated with IUGR include increased meconium aspiration, necrotizing enterocolitis, hypoglycemia, respiratory distress, hypothermia, and thrombocytopenia.

It has been suggested that IUGR has long-term consequences, beyond those seen in the immediate postnatal period. The Barker hypothesis states that undernutrition during fetal life—a time of great developmental plasticity—increases the risk of adult-onset coronary artery disease, type II diabetes, stroke, and HTN. This increased morbidity is thought to be secondary to the allocation of energy to one trait (such as brain growth) at the expense of allocation to traits such as tissue repair processes.

Screening

In this case, the patient's lagging fundal height prompted an ultrasound, which revealed an estimated fetal weight (EFW) of 900 g. This EFW is below the third percentile for GA.

The diagnosis of IUGR using fundal height has several limitations. Maternal size, parity, ethnic group, and bladder volume can all impact the measurement. Fundal height performs best when done by the same examiner. The accuracy of the test is limited, with observational studies reporting IUGR detection rates ranging from 28% to 86%. Fundal height is probably a reasonable screen for low-risk pregnancies. A lagging fundal height should prompt further evaluation with ultrasound.

The major limitation to ultrasound is that the predictive value of the test depends upon the prevalence of IUGR in the population being analyzed. Estimates of fetal weight that incorporate the following seem to provide the most accurate assessment of fetal weight: AC, biparietal diameter (BPD), and femur length (FL). In diagnosing IUGR, the AC is the most sensitive of these parameters. The small abdominal circumference is secondary to depletion of abdominal adipose tissue, and decreased hepatic size due to reduced glycogen storage. Most studies report reduced AC as the most sensitive single morphometric indicator of IUGR.

A key factor in the utilization of ultrasound: the time interval between measurements. The time interval between measurements has a major impact on the false-positive rate. Overutilization of ultrasound can be hazardous, as a false-positive diagnosis may lead to iatrogenic harm, that is, un-indicated preterm delivery. Mongelli et al describe the following false-positive rates for IUGR depending upon the frequency of ultrasound evaluation:

- 1-week interval—31% false-positive diagnosis of IUGR
- 2-week interval—17% false-positive diagnosis of IUGR
- 4-week interval—3% false-positive diagnosis of IUGR

Most authors suggest waiting a minimum of 2 weeks between growth scans.

Once a diagnosis of IUGR is suspected, the clinical challenge becomes distinguishing the small and sick (IUGR) fetus from the one who is small but healthy. Several tools help make this distinction: clinical history and risk factors, the amniotic fluid index, and Doppler studies.

A detailed history and physical should unearth any factors that would increase the risk of a pathologically small fetus (see Table 24-2). In the sample

Table 24–2 EVALUATION OF IUGR

Evaluation of IUGR:
- Detailed history and physical.
- Close attention to current blood pressure and blood pressure trend.
- Detailed fetal anatomic survey.
- Amniocentesis—the specific tests will depend upon the GA.
  - Karyotype: Increased risk of aneuploidy in the setting of IUGR.
  - Infectious workup: Some authors have questioned the yield of an infectious workup in the setting of IUGR, would consider most strongly if IUGR presents prior to mid-gestation (cytomegalovirus).
  - Fetal lung maturity studies: Will depend upon the GA at presentation.
- Modified or complete BPP.
- Umbilical artery Doppler studies.
- Antenatal corticosteroids if less than 34 weeks GA.

Decision for inpatient or outpatient monitoring will depend upon the clinical circumstances.

patient, for example, the low BMI, poor weight gain, and smoking all point toward a pathologically—rather than constitutionally—small fetus.

Pay attention to any first or second-trimester screening results, as aneuploidy is associated with IUGR. **Amniocentesis is often indicated**, although this will depend on the GA at presentation. While infection is associated with IUGR, the yield of an infectious workup after midgestation is low, and some authors argue that the cost is not justified unless other signs suggest infection as the etiology for IUGR.

Decreased AFI is associated with IUGR, and may be the earliest pathologic sign detected on ultrasound. Decreased perfusion of fetal kidneys and decreased urine output explain the low AFI. **In general, pregnancies with the most severe oligohydramnios have the highest perinatal mortality rate, incidence of anomalies, and incidence of IUGR.** There is a positive correlation between the maximum vertical pocket (MVP) of amniotic fluid and the incidence of IUGR.

- MVP > 2 cm: 6% incidence of IUGR
- MVP between 1 and 2 cm: 20% incidence of IUGR
- MVP < 1 cm: 39% incidence of IUGR

At the other extreme, polyhydramnios and IUGR has been dubbed an "ominous combination." This combination is associated with a high rate of structural and chromosomal anomalies.

Doppler studies have proven a powerful tool in the evaluation of a suspected IUGR fetus. Increased resistance in the placental circulation manifests as increased Doppler blood flow indices in the umbilical arteries. This finding has been demonstrated by many investigators in both animal and human models.

By signaling an underlying pathology, the utilization of umbilical artery Doppler flow measurements improves clinical outcomes. Numerous trials confirm that **the use of Doppler flow measurements can significantly reduce both perinatal death and unnecessary induction of labor** (iatrogenic preterm birth of the small-but-healthy fetus). Absence or reversal of end-diastolic flow (AEDF, REDF) in the umbilical artery is suggestive of poor fetal condition. Conversely, normal flow is rarely associated with significant morbidity.

In a retrospective review of greater than 500 singletons with a diagnosis of IUGR, the mean GA at delivery correlated with Doppler studies:

- Normal Doppler studies: 37 weeks at delivery
- AEDF: 31 weeks at delivery
- REDF: 29 weeks at delivery

Similarly, the perinatal mortality increases as Doppler indices worsen:

- Normal Doppler studies: 1.3% perinatal mortality rate
- AEDF: 25% perinatal mortality rate
- REDF: 54% mortality rate

Some investigators advocate the addition of **venous** Doppler studies in evaluating the fetus with suspected IUGR. Abnormal Dopplers in the venous circulation (ductus venosus, umbilical vein) put the IUGR fetus at even greater risk of mortality. Many clinicians consider delivery *before* venous abnormalities develop.

Treatment

Treatment of the fetus with suspected IUGR will depend upon the clinical circumstances, particularly the GA. A physical examination—with close attention to blood pressure—will help guide management. Fetal anatomic survey and assessment of amniotic fluid are critical. Gravidas at less than 34 weeks GA should **receive a course of antenatal corticosteroids**. The decision for inpatient or outpatient management is difficult to generalize. Doppler studies are very useful. Antenatal testing with BPP or modified BPP—along with a repeat growth scan in 2 to 4 weeks—is suggested.

Timing of delivery is based primarily on expert opinion, and will depend on the clinical circumstances. In general, most authorities advise delivery of the term or near-term fetus with IUGR in the following settings:

- Hypertension
- Absence of growth over a 2 to 4 week window
- Nonreassuring fetal testing
- Absent or reversal of end-diastolic flow on Doppler studies

In the gravida remote from term, normal Doppler studies are reassuring. AEDF will often trigger delivery, and REDF will almost always mandate delivery. Very close monitoring is required in those situations.

Comprehension Questions

24.1   A patient with chronic hypertension (CHTN) is being followed in the third trimester with growth scans, given the increased risk for IUGR. Which of the following intervals between ultrasound evaluations balances the sensitivity and specificity of the test?
A. Daily ultrasound for EFW
B. Weekly ultrasound for EFW
C. Ultrasound for EFW every 4 weeks
D. Ultrasound for EFW every 8 weeks

24.2   In which circumstance are umbilical artery Doppler studies **not** indicated, based on current evidence:

  A. Further evaluation of a well-dated pregnancy (sure LMP consistent with an 8-week sonogram) noted to have symmetric IUGR.

  B. Further evaluation of a gravida with late entry into prenatal care (LMP given as a 2-week range, no first or second-trimester sonographic dating), but with strong clinical suspicion for IUGR (patient has CHTN and has a history of a growth-restricted newborn).

  C. Further evaluation of a healthy patient seen for lagging fundal height with an EFW at the 30th percentile for GA, normal AFI.

  D. Further evaluation of a patient seen for lagging fundal height with an EFW at the 30th percentile for GA, AFI of 4 cm.

24.3   A healthy P1 at 32 weeks' of gestation has a fundal height of 27 cm. She is 58 in tall and has a BMI of 21 kg/m^2. The father of the baby is 64 in tall. The EFW of 1600 g is just below the 10th percentile for age. How would you proceed?

  A. Repeat ultrasound in 3 weeks.

  B. Perform umbilical artery Doppler studies.

  C. Perform middle cerebral artery Doppler studies.

  D. Deliver without further evaluation.

24.4   A previously healthy P1 has a lagging fundal height at 35 weeks. Ultrasound reveals an EFW of 2000 g, which is below the 10th percentile for GA. She received a course of antenatal corticosteroids at 29 weeks for threatened preterm birth. Which of the following should prompt delivery?

  A. An AFI of 3 cm, no single pocket measuring greater than 2 cm

  B. History of childhood asthma

  C. History of preeclampsia in her first pregnancy

  D. Threatened preterm birth in this pregnancy

ANSWERS

24.1   **C.** The accuracy of ultrasound in detecting IUGR depends upon the prevalence of IUGR in the population being evaluated. Even in gravidas with HTN—a population with increased incidence of IUGR—the sensitivity of ultrasound decreases if the test is performed too frequently. When serial ultrasounds are performed, attention should be paid to the individual fetal curve. An otherwise uncomplicated pregnancy with a fetus who is consistently growing at the 10th percentile is less worrisome than a fetus who abruptly falls from the 50th to the 10th percentile for GA.

24.2   **C.** Umbilical artery Doppler studies have been most extensively evaluated in the setting of IUGR. Aside from their use in the management of IUGR, Dopplers may have a role in identifying patients with idiopathic oligohydramnios who are at increased risk of adverse outcome. However, in this fetus with an appropriate EFW and normal amount of amniotic fluid, the utility of Doppler studies has not been demonstrated.

24.3   **B.** Given that both the parents are of small stature, this fetus is likely constitutionally—not pathologically—small. However, further reassurance is needed before simply scheduling an ultrasound in 3 weeks. Attention should be paid to the mother's medical history and habits, as well as her blood pressure. Ask the patient about fetal movement. Assess the amount of amniotic fluid, as well as the fetal anatomy.

Note the size of the various growth parameters. Growth restriction that spares the BPD/HC—sometimes referred to as asymmetrical IUGR—may be more worrisome than a symmetrically small fetus.

Doppler studies of the umbilical artery are particularly useful in this setting; they suggest that the fetus is likely constitutionally small. Doppler studies of the middle cerebral artery are most commonly used in the setting of suspected fetal anemia. Delivery without further evaluation is not advised.

24.4   **A.** Remember that the combination of IUGR and oligohydramnios is associated with a high rate of perinatal mortality. In this near-term gravida who has received a course of corticosteroids, delivery is advised.

Clinical Pearls

See US Preventive Services Task Force Study Quality levels of evidence in Case 1

➤ Estimates of fetal weight that incorporate the AC, FL, and BPD/HC most accurately assess fetal weight (Level II-2).

➤ While ultrasound is a component in the diagnosis of IUGR, it should not be used indiscriminately. The time interval between measurements has a major impact on the false-positive rate (Level II-3).

➤ Delivery is typically indicated when IUGR is coupled with oligohydramnios (Level III).

➤ Umbilical artery Dopplers is a powerful tool in distinguishing the constitutionally small fetus from the pathologically small fetus. The use of Dopplers has been shown to significantly reduce perinatal death and unnecessary induction of labor (Level I).

➤ Timing of delivery is based primarily on expert opinion, and will depend on the clinical circumstances. Hypertension, the absence of growth over a 2 to 4 week period, and nonreassuring testing typically trigger delivery. AEDF will often trigger delivery, and REDF will almost always mandate delivery (Level III).

REFERENCES

1. Barker DJ. The developmental origins of well-being. *Philos Trans R Soc Lond B Biol Sci.* 2004 Sep 29;359(1449):1359-1366.
2. Baschat AA. Arterial and venous Doppler in the diagnosis and management of early onset fetal growth restriction. *Early Hum Dev.* 2005 Nov;81(11):877-887.
3. Carroll BC, Bruner JP. Umbilical artery Doppler velocimetry in pregnancies complicated by oligohydramnios. *J Reprod Med.* 2000 Jul;45(7):562-566.
4. Chamberlain PF, Manning FA, Morrison I, Harman CR, Lange IR. Ultrasound evaluation of amniotic fluid volume. The relationship of marginal and decreased amniotic fluid volumes to perinatal outcome. *Am J Obstet Gynecol.* 1984 Oct 1; 150(3):245-249.
   A landmark paper that described perinatal outcome in gravidas with oligohydramnios, with and without IUGR.
5. Miller J, Turan S, Baschat AA. Fetal growth restriction. *Semin Perinatol.* 2008 Aug;32(4):274-280.
   An excellent, recent review on IUGR. Baschat has published widely on the use of Doppler in pregnancy.
6. Mongelli M, Elk S, Tambyrajia R. Screening for fetal growth restriction: a mathematical model of the effect of time interval and ultrasound error. *Obstet Gynecol* 1998;92(6):908-12.
7. Odegård RA, Vatten LJ, Nilsen ST, Salvesen KA, Austgulen R. Preeclampsia and fetal growth. *Obstet Gynecol.* 2000 Dec;96(6):950-955.
8. Odibo AO, Nelson D, Stamilio DM, Sehdev HM, Macones GA. Advanced maternal age is an independent risk factor for IUGR. *Am J Perinatol.* 2006 Jul;23(5):325-328.
9. Ott WJ. Diagnosis of IUGR: comparison of ultrasound parameters. *Am J Perinatol.* 2002 Apr;19(3):133-137.
10. Owen P, Maharaj S, Khan KS, Howie PW. Interval between fetal measurements in predicting growth restriction. *Obstet Gynecol.* 2001 Apr;97(4):499-504.
11. Resnik R. IUGR. *Obstet Gynecol.* 2002 Mar;99(3):490-496.
    An excellent review article on IUGR, with practical advice on management.
12. Soregaroli M, Bonera R, Danti L, et al. Prognostic role of umbilical artery Doppler velocimetry in growth-restricted fetuses. *J Matern Fetal Neonatal Med.* 2002 Mar;11(3):199-203.
13. Williams RL, Creasy RK, Cunningham GC, Hawes WE, Norris FD, Tashiro M. Fetal growth and perinatal viability in California. *Obstet Gynecol.* 1982 May; 59(5):624-632.
    One of the early articles to describe the influence of IUGR on increased mortality.

Case 25

A 26-year-old primigravida at 12 weeks' gestation is seen in your office for her second prenatal visit. In reviewing her labs, you note that her blood type is O+ and she has anti-Kell antibodies at a titer of 1:32. She reminds you that when she was 18 years of age, she was involved in a serious auto accident in which she suffered a splenic laceration. She requires 8 units of packed red blood cells transfusion and a splenectomy. She denies any prior pregnancies or other medical complications, and says she has received the Pneumovax vaccination. The remainder of her labs and her physical examination today are unremarkable.

➤ What is the most likely diagnosis?

➤ What is your next step?

➤ What are potential complications of the patient's disorder?

ANSWERS TO CASE 25:

Kell Alloimmunization

Summary: This is a 26-year-old primigravida at 12 weeks' gestation with a history of blood transfusion in the past, and antibodies to the Kell antigen at a 1:32 titer.

➤ **Most likely diagnosis:** Kell isoimmunization.

➤ **Next step:** Develop plan for monitoring pregnancy with Kell isoimmunization, starting with paternal zygosity, and if the fetus is at risk for anemia then ultrasound monitoring.

➤ **Potential complications:** Fetal anemia, hydrops, intrauterine demise, preeclampsia, preterm birth.

ANALYSIS

Objectives

1. Understand the risk of isoimmunization with blood transfusions.
2. Be able to describe the titer above which further monitoring should be done in pregnancy.
3. Develop a plan for monitoring a patient who is Rh isoimmunized.
4. Understand indications for preterm delivery with Rh isoimmunization.

Considerations

This is a 26-year-old primigravida at 12 weeks' gestation with a history of blood transfusion and antibodies to the Kell antigen. The first step in the management of this case is to perform paternal zygosity testing for the Kell antigen in order to determine if the fetus is at risk for alloimmunization. The Kell blood group is the most common of the minor RBC antibodies and the K antigen is present in 9% of Caucasian blood donors. Genotype frequencies in Caucasians are: KK (0.2%), Kk (8.7%), kk (91.1%). If the father is homozygous for the K antigen (KK), the fetus will be at risk for alloimmunization since the only "allele" the father can pass to the fetus will be K. If the father of the fetus is genotype Kk, then an amniocentesis can be done (with an attempt to avoid the placenta) to determine the fetal genotype and whether or not the fetus is at risk. Chorionic villus sampling CVS should be avoided since this can result in fetomaternal hemorrhage and an amnestic response in maternal antibody titer, therefore potentially worsening the disease. If the father of the fetus has the genotype kk, then the fetus is not at risk and no further testing is needed. Paternal blood should be sent with the amniotic fluid so that paternal gene rearrangement or paternity is not a potential source of laboratory error.

Since the patient was sensitized after a transfusion, there is a 91% chance that the baby's father is Kell-negative (kk), thus the fetus will be Kell-negative and will be unaffected by maternal antibodies. If the fetus is K+ then the fetus is at risk for anemia as a result of the maternal antibodies against the Kell antigen. These antibodies cross the placenta and cause hemolysis of the fetal red cells as they do in Rh (D) alloimmunization. However, unlike Rh alloimmunization, the Kell antibodies have a second mechanism by which they cause fetal anemia, anti-Kell antibody-mediated suppression of erythropoiesis at the progenitor cell level. The anemia by this mechanism is through decreased fetal red cell production. For this reason, the titer of anti-Kell antibody in maternal serum and the amniotic fluid bilirubin level do not correlate well with the degree of fetal anemia.

As in Rh (D) alloimmunization, there is a critical maternal antibody titer that, once reached, indicates the fetus could be affected. Most laboratories use a critical titer for anti-D antibodies of 1:16 as a cut off (each laboratory should establish their own critical titer). In cases of Kell sensitization, the critical titer is lower, usually 1:8, because severe fetal anemia can occur at lower antibody titers than in cases of Rh (D) alloimmunization. Once the critical titer is reached, antenatal testing should begin. Of importance, if the patient has had a prior child affected by alloimmunization, then titers do not need to be followed, but rather, antenatal testing is begun at 18 weeks. If the critical titer is not reached, then titers can be repeated monthly until 24 weeks and then every 2 weeks until delivery.

APPROACH TO
Kell Alloimmunization

Once it is established that the fetus is at risk for anemia, ultrasound becomes the primary screening tool for the majority of the pregnancy. An ultrasound should also be done early in the pregnancy in order to correctly assign the gestational age. This is of paramount importance since all of our normative values to screen for fetal anemia are in respect to the gestational age of the fetus.

The Doppler assessment of the fetal middle cerebral artery (MCA) peak systolic velocity (PSV) has come forward as the best noninvasive tool for fetal anemia screening. This test is founded on the principle that the anemic fetus preserves oxygen delivery to the brain by increasing cerebral flow. The sensitivity of increased MCA-PSV (above 1.5 multiples of the median [MoMs]) for the prediction of moderate or severe anemia is approximately 100%, either in the presence or absence of hydrops, with a false-positive rate of 12%. The optimal screening interval has not yet been determined; however, cases have been missed when more than 2 weeks elapse between Doppler studies. Most physicians are screening for anemia in 1 to 2 weeks intervals.

Doppler assessment of the fetal MCA-PSV is the preferred tool for determination of fetal anemia in Kell sensitized pregnancies since the delta OD 450 value is less accurate in these cases. In Kell sensitized fetuses, suppression of erythropoiesis rather than hemolysis (which generates bilirubin) is the major cause of fetal anemia.

If MCA-PSV is above 1.5 MoMs or delta OD 450 readings are in the lower portion of the Rh (D) affected zone (Queenan curve) or 65% or greater into zone 2 of the Liley curve, then cordocentesis for fetal hematocrit/hemoglobin and confirmation of blood type should be performed to make the diagnosis of fetal anemia. When a cordocentesis is planned, preparations should always be made for possible fetal transfusion.

Screening

Maternal blood type and antibody screen are sent at the first prenatal visit along with the other prenatal labs. If the patient screens positive for an RBC antibody, then the fetus may be at risk for hemolytic disease depending on the titer of antibody detected and whether or not the fetus has the offending antigen. Once the antibody titer reaches the critical value, then antepartum testing is begun.

Treatment

The treatment for fetal anemia is transfusion or delivery depending on the gestational age at which the anemia is detected. If the fetal MCA Dopplers remain below the 1.5 MoM, then delivery can be scheduled at 37 to 38 weeks after an amniocentesis result suggests lung maturity (lecithin-sphingomyelin ratio or lamellar body counts should be used since bilirubin can interfere with the fluorescence depolarization techniques, TDx-FLM). If the MCA Dopplers are found to be above 1.5 MoM, and the patient is not yet 35 weeks, then fetal cordocentesis is done with preparation for possible fetal transfusion. If the MCA Dopplers are greater than 1.5 MoM, and the patient is 35 weeks gestational age or more, then an amniocentesis is done for delta OD 450 and fetal lung maturity; MCA Dopplers can overestimate the possibility of fetal anemia after 35 weeks, therefore, a second test, delta OD 450, is done to screen further for anemia if the Dopplers are abnormal. Recently, administration of phenobarbital (30 mg po three times a day for 10 days) has been found to reduce the need for neonatal exchange transfusion in fetuses with hemolytic disease by enhancing hepatic maturation.

After fetal transfusion, the MCA Dopplers improve immediately. For the subsequent Doppler studies, a value over 1.69 has been used to predict the timing of the next transfusion. The increased peak systolic velocity is thought to be the result of the presence of adult hemoglobin as well as a change in the fetal cerebral circulation due to the differential oxygen binding capacity of these transfused red cells. Some physicians estimate that the hematocrit will drop by 1% per day. The final posttransfusion hematocrit will predict the time of the next transfusion to occur when the hematocrit is expected to be less than 30%.

With all forms of Rh isoimmunization, careful monitoring for preeclampsia is important during the second and third trimesters of pregnancy because of its association with isoimmunization.

Comprehension Questions

25.1   A 29-year-old G3P2 with antibody titers of 1:4 which are stable and not increasing presents to your office at 22 weeks' gestation. She states that in her last pregnancy, her baby was found to be jaundiced and anemic at birth. What is the next best step in the care of this patient?

   A. Continue to follow serial antibody titers and if they are found to be increasing, then start screening with MCA Doppler studies every 2 weeks.

   B. Start screening for anemia right away with MCA Dopplers every 2 weeks.

   C. Reassure the mother that since the baby did not need a transfusion this fetus will not be at risk.

   D. Start serial amniocentesis for delta OD 450 at 35 weeks.

25.2   Which of the following fetuses (A-D) is most likely to have a normal hemoglobin level?

   A. A Caucasian patient who was transfused 10 units of packed RBCs after a car accident that was found to have anti-Kell antibodies of 1:16 at her first prenatal visit.

   B. A patient with + Kell antibodies of 1:64 and a delta OD 450 in the "unaffected zone" of the Queenan curve.

   C. A fetus with ascites and pleural effusions in a patient with RBC alloimmunization in a prior pregnancy.

   D. Fetus with a MCA Doppler of over 1.5 MoM and an anti-D antibody titer of 1:32.

25.3   A 29-year-old G1P0 at 11 weeks' gestation is being seen for her fist prenatal visit. Which of the following statements is most accurate regarding tests for isoimmunization?

   A. If the antibody screen is positive, there is strong likelihood of isoimmunization.

   B. If the patient is Rh positive, an antibody screen does not need to be performed.

   C. Antibody screen on paternal blood is important in Rh negative women to determine likelihood of the fetus being affected.

   D. In a patient with a positive antibody screen for Rh antibodies, RhoGAM is not needed.

25.4   In an Rh-isoimmunized patient, which of the following tests for fetal
        lung maturity is unreliable when performed on amniotic fluid?
        A. Lecithin-sphingomyelin ratio (L/S)
        B. TDx or surfactant albumin ratio
        C. Lamellar body count
        D. Phosphatidylglycerol (PG)

ANSWERS

25.1   **B.** This patient has a prior child who was affected by red cell alloim-
        munization; therefore, there is no need to follow antibody titers during
        this pregnancy. The best next step is to start screening every 2 weeks
        with MCA Dopplers for evidence of fetal anemia. When performing
        MCA Dopplers, other ultrasound signs of anemia can be assessed, such
        as signs of cardiac failure (tachycardia, ascites/effusions, skin edema),
        abnormal fetal growth, and polyhydramnios. Amniocentesis for delta
        OD 450 can be done serially if MCA Doppler studies are not available.
        This would replace the MCA Dopplers every 2 weeks for fetal anemia
        screening. In this patient, screening should not be delayed until 35 weeks.
        In patients followed by MCA Dopplers, after 35 weeks there is an
        increase in the false-positive rate so that a positive test should be followed
        by an amniocentesis for delta OD 450, while a negative test would rule
        out the possibility of fetal anemia.

25.2   **A.** All of the above scenarios represent patients with pregnancies at
        risk for possible fetal anemia. The patient "A" is at the lowest risk for
        fetal anemia because she developed antibodies after a trauma which
        resulted in the transfusion of multiple blood products. The chance
        that the father of the baby has the Kell antigen is less than 10% and
        the chance that the father is KK+ is less than 1%. The father, if he
        has the Kell antigen, is more likely to be heterozygous and therefore,
        there is a 50% chance he will not transmit the gene to his offspring,
        so the possibility of fetal anemia is even lower.
            The fetus with the Kell antibodies and "unaffected" zone of the
        Queenan curve is still at risk since the Kell antibody also suppresses red
        blood cell production and does not only cause anemia by hemolysis.
        The bilirubin level in the amniotic fluid can be falsely reassuring in
        these cases because the amniotic fluid will not reflect the decrease in
        red cell production. The fetus in case "C" has other ultrasound evi-
        dence of anemia and a strong clinical history which together would
        prompt the need for a diagnostic test such as a cordocentesis. The final
        scenario in case "D" is the most typical. The patient is followed care-
        fully after her antibody titers increase above the critical level and then
        she has MCA Doppler results which suggest that the fetus is anemic.
        This patient will need a cordocentesis to confirm the diagnosis and
        possible transfusion if the fetal hemoglobin is under 30.

25.3 **D.** If a pregnant woman has a positive antibody screen for Rh, and already has been sensitized, RhoGAM is not indicated, since RhoGAM is used to prevent isoimmunization. The antibody screen only indicates that antibodies against common red blood cell antigens are present in the patient's serum. The titer strength and identification of the antibody help to determine the likelihood of isoimmunization. An antibody screen needs to be performed regardless of the Rh status, since other antigens can cause sensitization such as Kell or Duffy.

25.4 **B.** TDx is performed by light polarization. Bilirubin in the amniotic fluid can falsely elevate the TDx value and give the impression of lung "maturity." The PG and L/S ratios are performed by thin-layer chromatography and are not affected by the presence of bilirubin. The lamellar body count is unaffected by the presence of bilirubin since it is a direct count of lamellar bodies.

Clinical Pearls

See US Preventive Services Task Force Study Quality levels of evidence in Case 1

➤ Phenobarbital (30 mg po three times a day for 10 days) has been found to reduce the need for neonatal exchange transfusion in fetuses with hemolytic disease by enhancing hepatic maturation (Level II-2).

➤ In cases of Kell sensitization, the critical titer is lower, usually 8, because severe fetal anemia can occur at lower antibody titers than in cases of Rh alloimmunization (Level III).

➤ The sensitivity of increased MCA-PSV (above 1.5 multiples of the median [MoMs]) for the prediction of moderate or severe anemia is approximately 100%, either in the presence or absence of hydrops, with a false-positive rate of 12% (Level II-2).

REFERENCES

1. Ashwood, ER. Standards of laboratory practice: evaluation of fetal lung maturity. National Academy of Clinical Biochemistry. *Clin Chem.* 1997;43:211.
2. Daniels G, Hadley A, Green CA. Causes of fetal anemia in hemolytic disease due to anti-K. *Transfusion.* 2003;43:115.
3. Detti L, Oz U, Guney I, et al. Doppler ultrasound velocimetry for timing the second intrauterine transfusion in fetuses with anemia from red cell alloimmunization. *Am J Obstet Gynecol.* 2001;185:1048.
4. Mari G. Middle cerebral artery peak systolic velocity: is it the standard of care for the diagnosis of fetal anemia? *J Ultrasound Med.* 2005;24:697.

5. Mari G, Deter RL, Carpenter RL, et al. Noninvasive diagnosis by Doppler ultra-sonography of fetal anemia due to maternal red-cell alloimmunization. Collaborative group for Doppler assessment of the blood velocity in anemic fetuses. *N Engl J Med.* 2000;342:9.
6. Moise KJ Jr., Carpenter RJ Jr., Chorionic villus sampling for Rh typing: clinical implications [Letter]. *Am J Obstet Gynecol.* 1993;168:108-113.
7. Neerhof MG, Dohnal JC, Ashwood ER, et al. Lamellar body counts: a consensus on protocol. *Obstet Gynecol.* 2001;97:318.
8. van Dongen H, Klumper FJ, Sikkel E, et al. Non-invasive tests to predict fetal anemia in Kell-alloimmunized pregnancies. *Ultrasound Obstet Gynecol.* 2005;25:341.
9. Vaughan JI, Manning M, Warwick RM, et al. Inhibition of erythroid progenitor cells by anti-Kell antibodies in fetal alloimmune anemia. *N Engl J Med.* 1998;338:798.
10. Weinstein L. Irregular antibodies causing hemolytic disease of the newborn: a continuing problem. *Clin Obstet Gynecol.* 1982 Jun;25(2):321-332.

Case 26

A 28-year-old G4P3 at 40 weeks' gestation presents to labor and delivery in active labor and ruptured membranes. Her antenatal course was complicated by diet-controlled gestational diabetes. Her previous three pregnancies ended in vaginal delivery at term with the largest infant weighing 4000 g. She is 5 ft tall and weighs 220 lb. Fundal height was 42 cm, fetal heart tones (FHTs) were normal, and the EFW was 3800 g. The first stage of labor was uneventful, but after just 10 minutes of the second stage, the fetal head delivered and promptly retracted against the vulva (positive turtle sign). Normal traction by the operator did not result in delivery of the anterior shoulder.

➤ What is the most likely diagnosis?

➤ What is your next step?

➤ What are the potential complications for mother and baby in this situation?

ANSWER TO CASE 26:

Shoulder Dystocia

Summary: An obese, parous gestational diabetic was admitted in active labor. Following a very short second stage, the head delivered but the anterior shoulder became impacted behind the symphysis pubis.

➤ **Most likely diagnosis:** Shoulder dystocia.

➤ **Next step:** Initiate a well-planned sequence of maneuvers[1] (see following discussion) designed to accomplish delivery of the infant.

➤ **Potential complications:**
Maternal—third or fourth degree laceration or extension of an episiotomy. Neonatal—fractures of clavicle or humerus, brachial plexus injury, asphyxia, stillbirth.

ANALYSIS

Objectives

1. Be able to recognize the most common risk factors for shoulder dystocia.
2. Appreciate that most risk factors for shoulder dystocia have very low positive predictive value.
3. Develop a personal algorithm for the management of shoulder dystocia.
4. Understand the importance of simulation training, shoulder dystocia drills, and thorough documentation of the event in the patient's medical record.

Considerations

The patient in the case scenario has multiple risk factors for shoulder dystocia including multiparity, obesity, gestational diabetes, and a precipitous second stage of labor. A short second stage may not allow sufficient time for the shoulders of the infant to accommodate to the bony pelvis. Despite the presence of well-recognized individual risk factors for shoulder dystocia, at least 50% of cases have no known risk factors. The most common risk factors for shoulder dystocia are listed in Table 26–1.

In this case, the time between delivery of the head and delivery of the body (head-to-body interval or HBI) is critical since adverse neonatal outcomes correlate with increasing time on the perineum.[2] For obstetricians of widely varying experience, shoulder dystocia represents a true emergency, exemplified by the words of Woods, for whom a secondary but occasionally life-saving maneuver is named: "Very few of our mechanical problems in obstetrics

Table 26–1 RISK FACTORS FOR SHOULDER DYSTOCIA

Macrosomia
Obesity
Diabetes
Postterm pregnancy
Prolonged second stage
Midpelvic instrumental delivery
Precipitous labor
Previous delivery complicated by shoulder dystocia
Weight gain during pregnancy
Multiparity

require emergency treatment. Difficulty in delivery of the shoulders, however, usually comes as a complete surprise. We have no warning, a real emergency exists, and the minutes we have in which to make a safe delivery usually pass much faster than expert help can arrive."[3]

APPROACH TO
Shoulder Dystocia

DEFINITIONS

SHOULDER DYSTOCIA: Failure of normal downward traction to deliver the anterior shoulder. Additional maneuvers therefore become necessary. Some investigators use a head-to-body interval of greater than 1 minute as a definition.[2]

McROBERTS MANEUVER: Flexion of the maternal hips followed by abduction of the thighs, thereby rotating the pubic symphysis cephalad and straightening the lumbosacral angle.

WOODS MANEUVER: Abduction of the posterior shoulder by pressure on its ventral surface to accomplish rotation.[3] The original description of this maneuver included the application of fundal pressure once the shoulders were rotated, but fundal pressure is no longer advocated.

BARNUM MANEUVER: Delivery of the posterior arm, described more than 60 years ago by Barnum. Some authors have recommended assigning this maneuver to a higher priority in the management algorithm for shoulder dystocia.[4]

CLINICAL APPROACH

In the case presented, shoulder dystocia was associated with a very short second stage ("precipitous" delivery). This is one circumstance where it might be indicated to allow a little more time for the shoulders to rotate to the more favorable oblique diameter of the pelvis. In all other shoulder dystocia cases, the practitioner would be well-served to take a few seconds to assess, digitally, whether the anterior shoulder is impacted behind the symphysis and whether the posterior shoulder occupies the sacral hollow. Even though time is critical, as previously mentioned, the time is measured in minutes, not seconds. Excessive anxiety over failure of the shoulders to deliver immediately after the head may actually contribute to rather than resolve problems. The fetal head retracting back toward the perineum (turtle sign) is commonly encountered, see Figure 26–1.

Once the diagnosis of shoulder dystocia is evident, every obstetric provider should initiate a personal algorithm for managing the dystocia. Published evidence does not support the existence of a single "best practice" approach. Therefore, a brief description of several commonly used maneuvers follows, without championing a preferred order of employing these maneuvers.

McRoberts maneuver (see definitions) was described in 1983, but likely used before that.[5] Because it led to delivery without additional maneuvers in

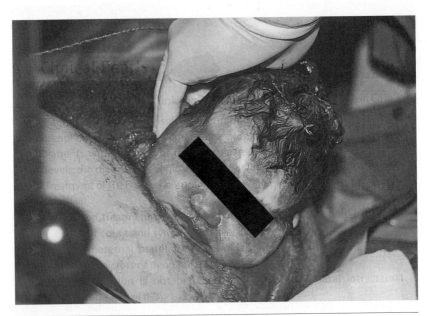

Figure 26–1. Shoulder dystocia with turtle sign. *(Reproduced, with permission, from Knoop KJ, Stack LB, Storrow AB, et al. Atlas of Emergency Medicine. 3rd ed. New York, NY: McGraw-Hill; 2010:259. Photo contributor: William Leninger, MD.)*

a fair number of cases, it was very popular in the decade or two following its description. Evidence that its use lowers the prevalence of brachial plexus injuries is lacking, however. MacKenzie and colleagues[6] reported that of 20 cases of brachial plexus injuries, 19 were managed with the McRoberts maneuver. It must be remembered that once the woman has been placed in McRoberts position, the next step is still traction and that traction may still be excessive. Further, it is not necessary to simultaneously apply suprapubic pressure with McRoberts maneuver. Instead, suprapubic pressure, correctly applied in a direction that leads to adduction of the anterior shoulder should be regarded as a separate intervention in the algorithm.

The Rubin maneuver consists of finger pressure to the anterior or posterior shoulder to produce adduction. This maneuver is designed to reduce the bisacromial diameter of the fetus. It should be combined with oblique traction in the axis of the shoulders rather than direct anteroposterior traction.

The Barnum maneuver involves delivery of the posterior arm of the fetus (see Definitions). At least one group has recommended that this be considered as an initial maneuver, but executing the maneuver is often technically difficult, especially with limited room in the vagina. On occasion, difficulty in delivery may still be encountered after successful delivery of the posterior arm.

The Woods maneuver is no longer performed as it was originally described. Fundal pressure has been eliminated and pressure is sometimes placed on the posterior rather than the anterior aspect of the posterior shoulder (see Figure 26–2). The goal of this maneuver is to move the impacted anterior shoulder from behind the symphysis utilizing the rotational principle of a screw. Thus, the maneuver is sometimes referred to as the Woods screw or the Woods corkscrew maneuver.

Clearly, the maneuvers described above are just a few of the many that have been suggested for managing shoulder dystocia. Other potentially useful maneuvers include the Gaskin (all-fours) maneuver, Zavanelli maneuver, symphysiotomy, intentional clavicular fracture, suprapubic pressure, and the recently described posterior axillary sling traction.[7] Not all of these maneuvers are strongly recommended, and maternal and neonatal complications may be attributable to their use. However, in the worst of dystocias, knowing about these unusual maneuvers and how to perform them may be lifesaving for the infant. Whatever the sequence employed, and whether the sequence is repeated by the same or a more experienced provider, injury to the brachial plexus is not always preventable, nor is it always an indication of improper delivery technique. There is convincing evidence that brachial plexus injury can occur without shoulder dystocia.[8]

The frequency of shoulder dystocia has been reported to be between 2/1000 and 2/100 deliveries. Because it is uncommon, unpredictable, and potentially catastrophic, there has been much emphasis on shoulder dystocia drills and simulation training.[9] Such training fosters recognition of the need to call for help, the importance of teamwork, practice executing the various maneuvers

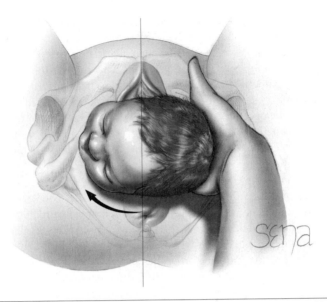

Figure 26–2.   The figure illustrates the modified Woods maneuver. The hand is placed behind the posterior shoulder of the fetus. The shoulder is then rotated progressively 180 degrees in a corkscrew manner so that the impacted anterior shoulder is released. *(Reproduced, with permission, from Cunningham FG, Leveno KJ, Bloom SL, et al. Williams Obstetrics. 23rd ed. New York, NY: McGraw-Hill; 2010.)*

and, perhaps most importantly, facilitates teaching in a controlled rather than an emergency environment. Simulation training also provides an opportunity to practice documentation of delivery-related events[10] (see Table 26–2).

Experience has shown that prevention of shoulder dystocia is not an achievable goal. Therefore, it is incumbent on everyone who delivers babies to optimize their management of this obstetric emergency. Calm execution of a carefully rehearsed personal management algorithm should enable providers to minimize the occurrence of catastrophic outcomes including permanent brachial plexus injury, hypoxic brain injury, and stillbirth resulting from failure to deliver in a reasonable period of time.

Table 26–2 MEDICAL RECORD DOCUMENTATION OF A DELIVERY COMPLICATED BY SHOULDER DYSTOCIA		
DOCUMENTATION		
ROUTINE	BEST PRACTICE	UNIQUE TO SHOULDER DYSTOCIA
Date/time	Cord gases	Classify as shoulder dystocia
Birth weight	Peds presence	Which shoulder anterior
Apgar scores	All providers present	Head-to-body interval
Estimated blood loss		Moving all extremities: Y/N
Type of anesthesia		Name/order of maneuvers
Other items to document for completeness:		
Induction/ augmentation		Length of stage 1
Meconium: Y/N		Length of stage 2
FHR pattern		Height/weight
Diabetes: Y/N		Who did what (who delivered)
Forceps/vacuum/ spontaneous		Site of delivery— LR, OR

Comprehension Questions

26.1 What head-to-body interval has been used to define shoulder dystocia?
A. 25 seconds
B. 1 minute
C. 3 minutes
D. 5 minutes

26.2 Extraction of the posterior arm is known as what maneuver?
A. McRoberts
B. Rubin
C. Barnum
D. Woods

26.3   What percentage of shoulder dystocias are complicated by neonatal brachial plexus injuries?
        A. 5%
        B. 15%
        C. 30%
        D. 50%

ANSWERS

26.1   **B.** The head-to-body interval is 25 seconds in a normal delivery. Shoulder dystocia is defined by some as a head-to-body interval of 1 minute. Deliveries that take 3 to 5 minutes or even longer are associated with increased neonatal adverse outcomes.

26.2   **C.** The McRoberts maneuver involves repositioning the mother. The Rubin maneuver is designed to disimpact the anterior shoulder from behind the symphysis. The Woods maneuver is a rotational maneuver that utilizes the principle of a screw. The Barnum maneuver advocates extraction of the posterior arm of the fetus over the perineum, substituting a smaller diameter for the arrested bisacromial diameter.

26.3   **B.** Although the incidence of brachial plexus injuries varies in different reports, 15% is the best answer among the choices provided. Less than 10% of brachial plexus injuries resulting from shoulder dystocia are permanent.

Clinical Pearls

See US Preventive Services Task Force Study Quality levels of evidence in Case 1

➤ When faced with a shoulder dystocia, call for additional help (Level III).
➤ Although most dystocias are due to obstruction by the bony pelvis, proper maternal position and episiotomy may facilitate delivery (Level III).
➤ Be alert for newly described techniques to add to your personal algorithm for shoulder dystocia management (Level III).
➤ Develop a conviction that you will get the baby out. Injury is preferable to stillbirth (Level III).

REFERENCES

1. Gherman RB, Ouzounian JG, Goodwin TM. Obstetric maneuvers for shoulder dystocia and associated fetal morbidity. *Am J Obstet Gynecol.* 1998;178:1126-1130.
2. Beall MH, Spong C, McKay J, Ross MG. Objective definition of shoulder dystocia: a prospective evaluation. *Am J Obstet Gynecol.* 1998;179(4):934-937.
3. Woods CE. A principle of physics as applicable to shoulder delivery. *Am J Obstet Gynecol.* 1943;45:796-804.
4. Poggi SH, Spong CY, Allen RH. Prioritizing posterior arm delivery during severe shoulder dystocia. *Obstet Gynecol.* 2003;101:1068-1072.
5. Gurewitsch ED. Optimizing shoulder dystocia management to prevent birth injury. *Clin Obstet Gynecol.* 2007;50:592-606.
6. MacKenzie IZ, Shah M, Lean K, Dutton S, Newdick H, Tucker, DE. Management of shoulder dystocia. *Obstet Gynecol.* 2007;110:1059-1068.
7. Cluver CA, Hofmeyr GJ. Posterior axilla sling traction: a technique for intractable shoulder dystocia. *Obstet Gynecol.* 2009;113:486-488.
8. Doumouchtsis SK, Arulkumaran S. Are all brachial plexus injuries caused by shoulder dystocia? *Obstet Gynecol Surv.* 2009 Sep;64(9):615-623.
9. Crofts JF, Fox R, Ellis D, Winter C, Hinshaw K, Draycott TJ. Observations from 450 shoulder dystocia simulations. *Obstet Gynecol.* 2008;112:906-912.
10. Deering S, Poggi S, Hodor J, Macedonia C, Satin AJ. Evaluation of residents' delivery notes after a simulated shoulder dystocia. *Obstet Gynecol.* 2004;104:667-670.

Case 27

A 37-year-old G3P2002 African American female at 38 weeks' gestation presents to labor and delivery complaining of absent fetal movement for 1 day. The nurse is unable to obtain fetal heart tones. The patient has a history of chronic hypertension diagnosed 2 years prior to pregnancy and was previously treated with a diuretic. She discontinued her medication when she found out that she was pregnant and has not required medication during this pregnancy. She had two previous term uncomplicated vaginal deliveries both weighing approximately 7 lb.

Aneuploidy screening, maternal serum alpha-fetoprotein (MSAFP), and anatomy ultrasound at 20 weeks' gestation were within normal limits. She declined amniocentesis for fetal karyotype. Her initial prenatal laboratories are as follows: O Rh-positive, indirect Coombs test negative (ICT), rubella immune, rapid plasma reagin nonreactive (RPR), hepatitis B surface antigen negative (HBsAg), and HIV negative. In addition, urine culture was negative, baseline 24-hour urine protein collection was less than 300 mg, and serum creatinine was 0.6 mg/dL. Her 1 hour 50 g oral glucose challenge was 109 mg/dL, RPR was nonreactive at 28 weeks, and group B streptococcus performed at 35 weeks was also negative. Fetal growth has been followed by ultrasound since 28 weeks with the last ultrasound at 36 weeks showing appropriate fetal growth and amniotic fluid. Fetal surveillance with weekly biophysical profiles (BPP) was initiated at 32 weeks and has been reassuring.

Today she denies contractions, vaginal bleeding, loss of fluid, headache, visual changes, or epigastric pain. Her BP is 138/88 mm Hg, HR 98 beats per minute, weight 225 lb, BMI 36 kg/m^2, and negative protein on urine dip. Her physical examination is within normal limits including a benign abdominal examination. Fundal height is at 37 cm. Her cervical examination is 1 to 2 cm long, −3 station, and posterior. She has 2+ deep tendon reflexes bilaterally. There are no contractions by external tocodynamometer. Bedside this, ultrasound examination confirms absent fetal cardiac activity. Fetal biometry is consistent with 37 weeks' gestation and amniotic fluid index is appropriate. The only additional finding is that of overlapping cranial bones.

➤ What is your next step?

➤ What are potential maternal complications of stillbirth?

ANSWERS TO CASE 27:

Stillbirth

Summary: This is a 37-year-old African American female G3P2002 at 38 weeks' gestation with chronic hypertension and stillbirth.

> ➤ **Next Step:** counsel the patient about the diagnosis of stillbirth and discuss recommendations for evaluation emphasizing the importance of fetal karyotype, fetal autopsy, and placental evaluation.

> ➤ **Potential maternal complications of fetal demise:** Maternal complications with expectant management include infection and maternal coagulopathy. In addition, patients with adverse pregnancy outcome are at higher risk for postpartum blues and depression.

ANALYSIS

Objectives

1. Identify risk factors and causes of stillbirth.
2. Become familiar with the evaluation of stillbirth.
3. Understand management options and recurrence risk of stillbirth.

Considerations

The first priority for the clinician in a patient who complains of decreased or absent fetal movement is to ascertain fetal heart tones. If this is unsuccessful, real-time ultrasonography should be performed to definitively diagnose the presence of a fetus and the absence of fetal cardiac activity. If the physician is inexperienced with ultrasound, the diagnosis should be confirmed by a different examiner with appropriate expertise.

There are numerous risk factors for stillbirth and this patient has four: advanced maternal age, obesity, race, and chronic hypertension. Women greater than 35 years of age at delivery have a twofold risk of stillbirth compared to those that are younger. This patient is also obese based on her body mass index (BMI) of 36 kg/m^2. Obese women have a twofold risk of stillbirth compared to nonobese women. Moreover, stillbirth rates are highest in African Americans compared to other races. Finally, abruptio placentae, superimposed preeclampsia, intrauterine growth restriction, and perinatal death are complications more common in women with chronic hypertension. Even uncomplicated chronic hypertension is associated with increased perinatal death.

When discussing the diagnosis of stillbirth with this patient it is important to convey sensitivity and offer support. In many instances such as this, the cause of stillbirth may not be apparent at the time of diagnosis and, in approximately half of the cases, an identifiable cause of stillbirth may not be known even after appropriate evaluation. It is important to convey this to the patient so that reasonable expectations are set. Once the diagnosis of stillbirth has been made and if the patient is clinically stable, it is appropriate to offer her time alone with her family or friends before further discussion of the evaluation and management. Involvement of religious leaders at any time is an option and should be offered to any patient. It is also important for all health care providers to refer to the baby by name if the patient desires.

A thorough medical and obstetrical history should be obtained. It is also important to obtain a detailed three-generation pedigree and ascertain exposures such as sick contacts or drugs. A physical examination should be performed paying particular attention to evidence of preeclampsia, abruption placentae or evidence of fetal growth restriction. A bedside ultrasound should be performed to evaluate for oligohydramnios, placental abnormalities, and to obtain fetal growth parameters. The presence of fetal scalp edema and overlapping cranial bones (Spalding sign) may indicate fetal demise occurred more than 48 hours ago.

An appropriate evaluation of stillbirth is extremely important. For the patient and her family, ascertaining a cause for the adverse pregnancy outcome can help them to cope with the loss. For the physician, an identifiable cause can be helpful in counseling about the recurrence risk and management in subsequent pregnancies. That said, the patient should be offered fetal autopsy, placental evaluation, and fetal karyotype analysis. Many couples are reluctant to consent to autopsy due to emotional or cultural reasons. It is important to address their specific concerns and educate them regarding the procedure (eg, the face is not touched) and clarify the importance of autopsy. An assessment of fetal-maternal hemorrhage, maternal serology for parvovirus B-19 infection (B19), antiphospholipid syndrome, and toxicology screen is recommended. Additional studies can be performed if indicated and these will be addressed in more detail in the next section.

It is reasonable to offer the patient the opportunity to choose the timing of delivery provided she is clinically stable without evidence of abruption, preeclampsia, infection, or other indications that preclude waiting. The patient may elect immediate induction of labor, await spontaneous labor, or choose an alternate delivery date provided she understands the risks associated with expectant management. After delivery, gross examination of the baby and placenta should be performed and abnormalities noted. The patient should be offered the opportunity to hold her baby and allow for religious ceremonies to be performed if desired. A supportive environment should be provided so that the patient and her family can spend the appropriate time they feel is needed with their baby. A referral to a peer support group, bereavement counselor, or mental health professional should be offered to assist the patient in dealing with grief and depression. The physician should notify the patient of the results from the evaluation in a timely manner and discuss their significance. A copy of the results and excluded diagnoses should also be provided.

APPROACH TO
Stillbirths

Stillbirth is defined as in utero fetal death after 20 weeks' gestation. If gestational age is unknown, a birth weight of $\geq$ 350 to 500 g is used depending on state reporting guidelines.[1] The **stillbirth rate** (number of stillborn neonates/1000 total births, including live births and stillbirths) in the United States has been relatively unchanged over the past 20 years, remaining at approximately 6.2/1000 in 2003 to 2005[2] (Level II-3). Approximately half of all stillbirths are of undetermined cause making it difficult for physicians to optimize management in a subsequent pregnancy.

Risk Factors and Causes

There are very few conditions that can unequivocally be established as directly causing fetal death and many more that have been associated with stillbirth. For example, numerous maternal demographic risk factors have consistently been associated with stillbirth. These include lower socioeconomic status and education level, as well as, lack of prenatal care. Even when controlling for these confounders, significant racial disparities exist between race and pregnancy outcome. The rate of stillbirth in African American women is double that of whites, 11.13 versus 4.79, respectively[2] (Level II-3). Hispanics are also at increased risk of stillbirth compared to whites.

Due to the rise in obesity and delayed childbearing, recent data has become available regarding these maternal characteristics and pregnancy outcome. Obesity defined as prepregnancy BMI greater than 30 kg/m[2] confers a twofold increased risk of stillbirth even in an otherwise uncomplicated pregnancy.[3] In the absence of age-related maternal complications, age alone also confers an increased risk of stillbirth. Fretts and colleagues established an increased odds ratio (OR) for women age 35 to 39 and for those greater than 40 of 1.9 (95% confidence interval [CI] 1.3-2.7) and 2.4 (95% CI 1.3-4.5), respectively[4] (Level II-2). Although less established, maternal stress has also been associated with stillbirth. The underlying mechanisms for why obesity, maternal age, and stress increase the risk of stillbirth have not been well elucidated.

Cocaine and tobacco use during pregnancy also increase the risk of stillbirth, sixfold and twofold, respectively[5] (Level II-2). Interestingly, women who stop smoking in the first trimester decrease their risk of stillbirth to that of nonsmokers[5] (Level II-2). Obesity, smoking, and cocaine use are all modifiable risk factors.

Chromosomal abnormalities are the best studied genetic causes of fetal death and are reported in 6% to 12% of stillbirths[1,6] (Level III). This may very well be an underestimation since genetic testing is not always performed or when it is performed, cell culture may not be successful in up to 50% of cases[7] (Level II-2). **Congenital anomalies account for up to 15% to 20% of stillbirths**[6] (Level III). That said, fetuses with anomalies identified on antenatal sonogram, postmortem examination or those noted to be small for gestational age have a higher rate of chromosomal abnormalities than those without these findings. In the absence of these abnormalities, the risk of aneuploidy is thought to be less than 2%. The most common specific abnormalities include monosomy X (23%), trisomy 21 (23%), trisomy 18 (21%), and trisomy 13 (8%)[6] (Level III). Stillborn infants who have a normal karyotype but have dysmorphic features on autopsy may have genetic conditions not detectable by routine cytogenetic analysis. Autosomal recessive metabolic disorders (eg, hemoglobinopathies, amino acid disorders, glycogen storage diseases) and X-linked disorders (lethal in male fetuses) have also been reported as causes of stillbirth. Confined placental mosaicism in which the fetal karyotype is normal may also be associated with fetal death and intrauterine growth restriction[5] (Level II-2).

Maternal disease contributes to approximately 10% of all stillbirth cases[8] (Level III). Many diseases have been linked to stillbirth with the most common being pregestational diabetes (type 1 and 2) and chronic hypertension. Others include thyroid disease, cardiovascular disease, kidney disease, antiphospholipid syndrome, and systemic lupus erythematosus. In most cases, however, stillbirth occurs only in the setting of overt clinical disease.

Despite improvements in care, pregestational diabetes mellitus (type 1 and 2) have an increased risk of stillbirth, more commonly in the second and third trimesters than those without diabetes. Women with type 2 diabetes mellitus have a 2.5-fold increased risk for stillbirth than nondiabetic women[9] (Level II-2). Maternal comorbidities, fetal anomalies, and growth disorders may play a role in the risk of stillbirth, however, even when controlling for these, the stillbirth risk is increased. The exact factors that account for the increased risk of stillbirth in pregestational diabetics are not fully understood and the glycemic threshold that places them at risk is also not well established. Data suggest that the risk of stillbirth can be reduced in pregestational diabetics by identifying and treating their disease.

Maternal infections comprise approximately 10% to 25% of stillbirth cases in developed countries[8] (Level III). Infection is more common in early cases of stillbirth compared to those occurring at term (19% vs 2% at term)[10] (Level III). Direct infection, placental damage, and systemic maternal illness are all thought to be possible mechanisms. However, the relationship between maternal infection and stillbirth is not always clear since serologic and histologic isolation of a particular organism does not always prove causation. The most common ascending bacterial infections are caused by *Escherichia coli*, group B streptococci, *Ureaplasma urealyticum*, *Mycoplasma hominis* and *Bacteroides* while, *Listeria monocytogenes* can reach the fetus by hematogenous route.

Parvovirus B19 (B19) is the virus with the strongest association with stillbirth. Less than 1% of stillbirths in this country are reported to be due to parvovirus although this may be an underestimation due to the lack of systematic testing[10] (Level III). B19 crosses the placenta attacking both the fetal erythropoietic tissue and myocardium resulting in severe fetal anemia and cardiac damage. This in turn may lead to subsequent nonimmune hydrops and stillbirth if in utero fetal transfusion is not performed. Interestingly, half of all pregnant women in the United States have been exposed to parvovirus and are considered to be immune. Of those who are susceptible, approximately 25% will have acute infection with exposure. Thirty percent of those mothers with acute infection will pass the infection to the fetus. Fetal hydrops or other associated findings occur in only 10% of those affected and stillbirth occurs in about 1% of infected fetuses[10] (Level III). The majority will not result in stillbirth with intrauterine transfusion. The risk of stillbirth is highest when infection occurs at less than 20 weeks gestation.

Cytomegalovirus (CMV) is the most common congenital viral infection. Primary maternal infection during pregnancy occurs in approximately 1% of pregnant women with a 50% risk of transmission to the fetus[10] (Level III). The risk of congenital infection increases with increasing gestational age and is greatest when maternal infection occurs in the third trimester. However, the risk of severity of disease and resulting fetal injury is highest when infection occurs in the first trimester. The presence of maternal antibodies does not confer absolute immunity, therefore pregnant women remain at risk, albeit low, for recurrent infection with fetal infection occurring in only 5% to 10% of cases. Congenital infection is manifested by intrauterine fetal growth, restriction, ventriculomegaly, and intracranial calcifications while neonatal sequelae include central nervous system abnormalities and multiorgan failure. CMV rarely results in fetal death; however, it has been described in case reports. Other viruses less commonly associated with stillbirth include Coxsackie A and B, echoviruses, enterovirus, chickenpox, measles, rubella, mumps, polio, rubeola, herpes simplex virus, and HIV.

Maternal primary infection with the parasite *Toxoplasma gondii* occurs in 1 per 1000 susceptible pregnancies in the United States. Like CMV, the fetus is most likely to be infected if maternal infection occurs in the third trimester; however, fetuses infected in the first trimester are associated with the greatest risk of injury[10] (Level III). Clinical manifestations of infection include ventriculomegaly, increased placental thickness, hepatomegaly, ascites, intracranial calcifications, microcephaly, and hydrocephalus. Stillbirth from *Toxoplasma* occurs in 5% of cases after the first trimester as a result of direct infection from transplacental passage but it is considered to be an uncommon cause of stillbirth overall[8] (Level III). Other organisms such as *Treponema pallidum*,

Borrelia burgdorferi (Lyme disease), *Leptospira interrogans* (leptospirosis), *Plasmodium falciparum* (malaria), *Coxiella burnetii* (Q fever), and *Trypanosoma brucei* (trypanosomiasis) while rare in this country should be considered in those with potential travel exposures.

Antiphospholipid syndrome (APS) is an acquired thrombophilia that is characterized by the presence of at least one clinical feature and at least one laboratory criteria of antiphospholipid antibodies levels (anticardiolipin antibodies, lupus anticoagulant, anti–beta-2 glycoprotein-I). APS has been identified as the cause of pregnancy loss in women with recurrent spontaneous abortion and stillbirth[5] (Level II-2). Anembryonic pregnancy loss has not been associated with antiphospholipid antibodies. The exact mechanism(s) that leads to fetal loss are uncertain but it is hypothesized that thrombosis and inflammation may lead to infarction in the placenta resulting in second or third-trimester fetal deaths. Treatment with heparin or low-molecular-weight heparin and low-dose aspirin may improve obstetrical outcomes in women with APS.

Heritable thrombophilias have been associated with an increased risk of vascular thrombosis and are strongly associated with losses greater than 10 weeks rather than early pregnancy losses although this association is not always consistent across studies. In a meta-analysis of 31 studies, however, only factor V Leiden, prothrombin G20210A gene mutation and protein S deficiency were associated with late nonrecurrent fetal loss after 19 weeks (odds ratio [OR] 3.26, 95% confidence interval [CI] 1.82-5.83, OR 2.30, 95% CI 1.09-4.87, and OR 7.39, 95% CI 1.28-42.63, respectively).[11] Protein C deficiency, antithrombin III, and methylenetetrahydrofolate mutation associated with hyperhomocysteinemia were not associated with pregnancy loss.[11] A retrospective study of a cohort of women participating in The European Prospective Cohort on Thrombophilia (EPCOT) trial demonstrated a slight increased risk of stillbirth in women with combined inherited thrombophilia defects and those with antithrombin deficiency[12] (Level II-2). In contrast, a recent prospective cohort study did not show an association between the factor V Leiden mutation and pregnancy loss[13] (Level II-2). Therefore, the clinician must be cautious in attributing the cause of stillbirth to heritable thrombophilias as most individuals with these thrombophilias will have a normal outcome.

Fetal-maternal hemorrhage (FMH) is reported in 3% to 14% of cases of **stillbirths**[5] (Level II-2). While occult FMH during pregnancy is common, the volume transfused is often very small. Excessive FMH (> 30 mL) occurs in 1 in 1000 deliveries. Acute hemorrhage greater than 40% of fetal blood volume often results in fetal death. Evidence of fetal anemia and tissue hypoxia by autopsy and placental examination support the diagnosis of FMH as a cause of stillbirth. FMH in the absence of placental abruption is a rare cause of stillbirth.

Fetal growth restriction is an important cause of stillbirth with a reported incidence of approximately 4% to 5%[14] (Level III). This estimate is difficult to ascertain due to dating inaccuracies and the use of population-based charts for weight percentiles that may not accurately reflect an individual's inherent growth potential. Available evidence supports the risk of stillbirth increases when fetal weight declines below the 10th percentile for gestational age. The risk of stillbirth is 1.5% and almost 2.5% when estimated fetal weight is less than 10th percentile and less than fifth percentile for gestational age, respectively.[1] Findings consistent with chronic placental dysfunction are seen in cases of stillbirths related to growth restriction.

Stillbirths are often attributed to **umbilical cord or placental abnormalities**. Umbilical cord accidents due to cord occlusion from true knots, nuchal cords, or body cords may be associated with stillbirths, especially those occurring at term. Of note, up to 30% of normal pregnancies may have cord entanglement[8] (Level III). Before attributing cord accident as the cause of stillbirth, it is important to exclude other causes and confirm the presence of cord occlusion and fetal tissue hypoxia. Other placental/umbilical cord abnormalities that can cause stillbirth include placental abruption (10%-20% cases), placental infarction, umbilical cord thrombosis, cord prolapse, velamentous cord insertion, vasa previa, and amniotic band syndrome.

Finally, the risk of stillbirth is increased with **multiple gestations** compared to singletons 0.5%, twins 1.8%, triplets 2.4%, and quadruplet 3.7%[15] (Level II-2). The reason for fetal death may be associated with obstetrical complications which occur more often with multiple gestations such as preeclampsia, intrauterine growth restriction, preterm labor, and placental abruption. Unique complications that may results in stillbirth include twin-twin transfusion syndrome complicating 10% to 15% of monochorionic/diamniotic gestations and cord entanglement complicating approximately half of monoamniotic gestations.

Evaluation

Several classification systems have been proposed to aid in reducing the number of unexplained cases of fetal deaths. No single system has been universally accepted and comparison between systems is difficult. The goal in the evaluation is to focus on individual risk factors, common conditions, and those that may be associated with an increase risk of recurrence.

The optimal evaluation of stillbirth is controversial and primarily based on expert opinion[1,5] (Level II-2). Most would agree that fetal autopsy, gross and microscopic evaluation of the placenta including the membranes and umbilical cord, and fetal karyotype are the most important part of the evaluation (Table 27–1). If the parents decline autopsy, a partial autopsy, photography, whole body x-rays, or postmortem MRI should be offered as they may provide valuable information. Gross examination of the fetus by a pathologist or geneticist can also be useful. Successful culture of fetal cells can be difficult especially with a long interval between fetal death and delivery. To improve the yield of obtaining a reliable karyotype, amniocentesis or chorionic villus sampling can be performed prior to delivery. If the patient declines these invasive

Table 27–1 EVALUATION OF STILLBIRTH

Recommended
- Fetal autopsy
- Placental evaluation
- Fetal karyotype

Generally accepted in addition to recommended
- Antibody screen (if negative on initial prenatal screen, does not require repeat testing)
- Serologic screen for syphilis in high-risk patients
- Screen for fetal-maternal hemorrhage (Kleihauer-Betke or other)
- Toxicology screen
- Parvovirus B19 screen
- Lupus anticoagulant screen
- Anticardiolipin antibodies
- Anti–beta-2 glycoprotein-I

Useful if clinically suspected
- Factor V Leiden mutation
- Prothrombin G20210A mutation
- Protein C, protein S, and antithrombin III deficiency screen

Generally not recommended
- TSH
- HbA_{1c}
- TORCH titers
- Placental cultures

procedures or resources to perform them are lacking, tissues such as placenta, fascia lata, skin from the nape of the neck, and tendons can be collected after delivery for fetal karyotype[5] (Level II-2). The placental sample should consist of 1 cm³ from the fetal surface near the cord insertion (chorionic plate) including the membranes. It is important to avoid placing placental or fetal tissue in formalin as they will not grow in culture. If cell culture for fetal karyotype is unsuccessful, the physician should investigate whether comparative genomic hybridization is available.

Although additional testing is controversial, screening for FMH (eg, Kleihauer-Betke or flow cytometry) is advised as it is a common cause of stillbirth and is inexpensive as well as noninvasive. Ideally, evaluation for FMH should be undertaken before induction of labor because small amounts of fetal blood may enter the maternal circulation with delivery. Antibody screen (indirect Coombs test) to exclude red cell alloimmunization is also recommended. If it was previously performed during pregnancy, repeat testing is unnecessary since sensitization during pregnancy rarely results in stillbirth. Serologic testing for B19 and toxicology screen is also recommended while repeat serologic testing for syphilis can be reserved for high-risk women.

Most authorities would agree that routine testing for APS (lupus anticoagulant, anticardiolipin antibodies, and anti–beta-2 glycoprotein-I) is recommended[1,5] (Level II-2). Testing for heritable thrombophilias is acceptable in cases with severe placental pathology, fetal growth restriction, or a personal or family history of thromboembolic disease. The usefulness of "TORCH titers" (serology for toxoplasmosis, rubella, cytomegalovirus, and herpes simplex) remains debatable and routine testing is not recommended[1,5,8] (Level II-2; Level III). These titers almost never aid in the diagnosis of congenital infection in the absence of autopsy and placental findings of infection. In the absence of data suggesting subclinical disease associated with stillbirth, routine testing for thyroid disease or diabetes in asymptomatic women is unnecessary.

Management

Patients should be given the option of proceeding with delivery at the time of diagnosis although expectant management is reasonable as long as there are no medical indications for immediate delivery. Patients may elect for expectant management to allow them an opportunity to cope with the news or if they desire to avoid induction of labor. Within 2 weeks of the stillbirth 80% to 90% of women will enter labor spontaneously. The risks of expectant management include intrauterine infection and maternal coagulopathy. It is difficult to quantify the risk of coagulopathy because most women elect delivery at the time of diagnosis. Older literature suggests the risk of coagulopathy (due to thromboplastin release from the placenta into the maternal circulation) is approximately 25% after 4 weeks of fetal death[8] (Level III). If the patient opts for expectant management it is important to arrange for weekly outpatient follow-up for assessment of temperature, abdominal pain, bleeding, and labor symptoms. Weekly assessment of complete blood count, platelet count, and fibrinogen are not necessary unless there is clinical suspicion of coagulopathy[8] (Level III).

Delivery options include surgical and medical management depending on the gestational age, experience of the clinician, and patient preference taking into consideration her desire to see the baby. Dilation and evacuation (D&E) is considered equally safe as medical induction in centers where clinicians have the training and expertise to perform this surgical procedure. This surgical approach limits the ability to perform a full fetal autopsy and is generally not performed after 24 weeks' gestation. On the other hand, medical induction of labor can be accomplished at any gestational age with oxytocin, prostaglandins $E_{2\alpha}$ ($PGE_{2\alpha}$) or E_1 (PGE_1) or dilators such as laminaria (osmotic) or Foley bulb (mechanical). Higher doses of prostaglandin E_1 and oxytocin can be used if gestational age is less than 28 weeks[16] (Level II-2). For women with prior documented or suspected low transverse cesarean delivery, the use of prostaglandins is not recommended if the gestational age is greater than 28 weeks. For these women, low-dose oxytocin and transcervical Foley bulb are reasonable alternatives. Cesarean delivery should be reserved for unusual circumstances since there are potential maternal risks with absolutely no fetal benefits.

Recurrence Risk and Subsequent Pregnancy

The reported recurrence risk of stillbirth is 2-to 10-fold, depending on maternal race (higher in African Americans), maternal disease (diabetes, hypertension), and characteristics of the prior stillbirth[17] (Level III). The risk is higher for those with earlier losses (< 24 wk) compared to term stillbirths. Moreover, losses associated with placental insufficiency, abruption or genetic conditions are more likely to recur than due to infection or twinning. Importantly, women with a prior preterm, live birth associated with growth restriction have a stillbirth rate (21.8 per 1000) in a subsequent pregnancy that is higher than those with a prior stillbirth.[1] Women with a prior stillbirth also have an increased risk of fetal growth restriction, abruption, and preterm birth in subsequent pregnancies.

Patients should be counseled prior to subsequent pregnancies to address all modifiable risk factors such as obesity and cocaine and tobacco use. A large meta-analysis suggested an association between perinatal death and interpregnancy interval, with increased risk at short (< 6 mo) and long intervals (> 50 mo).[18] Although waiting 6 months is reasonable for some, maternal age and psychological stability are important considerations. The patient should be encouraged to continue with therapy as well as antidepressant medications as needed.

Management of subsequent pregnancies is individualized and based on whether a cause of fetal death was identified. Interestingly, the decline in stillbirth rates over the past three decades coincides with increased surveillance; however, it remains unclear whether increased surveillance reduces the risk of recurrent stillbirth. Antenatal testing at 32 to 34 weeks is appropriate in healthy women with a history of prior stillbirth.[1] It is reasonable to start fetal surveillance earlier (26-28 wk) if the patient has additional risk factors for stillbirth such as hypertension, renal disease, or fetal growth restriction. Initiating fetal testing several weeks before the gestational age of the prior stillbirth for patients who are very anxious is also acceptable. Fetal surveillance with non-stress test (NST), contraction stress test (CST), biophysical profile (BPP), or modified BPP is appropriate. The reported stillbirth rate (per 1000) within 1 week of a normal test is 1.9, 0.3, 0.8, and 0.8, respectively for NST, CST, BPP, and modified BPP, with a negative predictive value of 99.8% to 99.9%.[19] Trials evaluating fetal kick counting have revealed conflicting results and the effectiveness in preventing stillbirth remains uncertain.

Timing of delivery should be discussed with the couple in advance and factors such as maternal anxiety, cervical status, and cause of prior stillbirth should be considered. If fetal surveillance remains reassuring, and in the absence of other risk factors that may increase the risk of stillbirth, elective induction at 39 weeks is reasonable. If elective delivery is undertaken between 37 and 38 completed weeks, amniocentesis for documentation of fetal lung maturity profile is recommended. Throughout pregnancy, the patient is likely to be anxious and will require ongoing support and reassurance, especially around the time of the prior stillbirth.

Comprehension Questions

27.1   A patient with uncomplicated prenatal care now presents with preeclampsia at 26 weeks, IUGR, and stillbirth. In addition to offering fetal autopsy, genetic evaluation, and placental examination which of the following laboratory tests do you believe would be the next most important to order as a part of this evaluation?
        A. HgA1c
        B. TORCH titers
        C. Lupus anticoagulant, anticardiolipin antibodies, anti–beta-2 glycoprotein-I
        D. Thyroid-stimulating hormone (TSH)

27.2   A 28-year-old woman has recently delivered vaginally and asks about the length of time recommended between delivery and the next pregnancy, because she had read something on the internet about too short a pregnancy interval being associated with stillbirth. Which of the following is the most accurate statement?
        A. There is no proven pregnancy interval associated with stillbirth.
        B. There is an increased risk associated with pregnancy interval shorter than 3 months, but normal risk after this duration.
        C. There is an increased risk associated with pregnancy interval shorter than 6 months, but normal risk after this duration.
        D. There is an increased risk associated with pregnancy interval shorter than 9 months, but normal risk after this duration.

ANSWERS

27.1   **C.** Uteroplacental insufficiency and early onset preeclampsia provide strong clinical suspicion for antiphospholipid syndrome. Therefore, maternal testing with lupus anticoagulant, anticardiolipin antibodies, and anti–beta-2 glycoprotein-I is an important part of this particular evaluation. Routine testing for diabetes, thyroid disease, and TORCH infections is generally not recommended.

27.2   **C.** There is evidence that a pregnancy interval less than 6 months is associated with an increased risk of stillbirth, but no increased risk after this duration.

Clinical Pearls

See US Preventive Services Task Force Study Quality levels of evidence in Case 1

➤ Fetal autopsy, placental evaluation, and karyotype are the most important tests in the evaluation of a stillbirth (Level II-2).

➤ Testing for lupus anticoagulant, anticardiolipin antibodies, and anti–beta-2 glycoprotein-I is recommended as treatment may improve outcome in subsequent pregnancy (Level II-2).

➤ "TORCH titers" (serology for toxoplasmosis, rubella, cytomegalovirus, and herpes simplex) are rarely helpful and routine testing is not recommended (Level III).

➤ Antenatal testing at 32 to 34 weeks is recommended in healthy women with a history of prior stillbirth (Level III).

CONTROVERSIES

- Routine testing for inherited thrombophilias is controversial and should be reserved for selected cases where clinical suspicion is strong.

REFERENCES

1. Management of stillbirth. ACOG Practice Bulletin No. 102. American College of Obstetricians and Gynecologists. *Obstet Gynecol.* 2009;113:748-761.

2. MacDorman MF, Kirmeyer S. Fetal and perinatal mortality, United States, 2005. *Natl Vital Stat Rep.* 2009;57:1-19 (Level II-3).

3. Chu SY, Kim SY, Lau C, et al. Maternal obesity and risk of stillbirth: a meta-analysis. *Am J Obstet Gynecol.* 2007;197:223-228.
   A meta-analysis of nine high-quality studies identifying an increased risk of stillbirth in overweight and obese women (meta-analysis).

4. Fretts RC, Schmittdiel J, McLean FH, Usher RH, Goldman MB. Increased maternal age and the risk of fetal death. *N Engl J Med.* 1995;333:483-489.
   Analysis of a large Canadian database over 30 years demonstrating the decline of stillbirth and the association of advanced maternal age (Level II-3).

5. Silver RM, Varner MW, Reddy U, et al. Work-up of stillbirth: a review of the evidence. *Am J Obstet Gynecol.* 2007;196:433-444.
   A review article examining the evidence for the workup of stillbirth from the five centers involved in the Stillbirth Collaborative Research Network (Level II-2).

6. Wapner RJ, Lewis D. Genetic and metabolic causes of stillbirth. *Semin Perinatol.* 2002;26:70-74 *(Level III).*

7. Rodger CS, Creasy MR, Fitchett M, Maliszewska CT, Pratt NR, Waters JJ. Solid tissue culture for cytogenetic analysis: a collaborative survey for the Association of Clinical Cytogeneticists. *J Clin Pathol.* 1996;49:638-641 *(Level II-2).*

8. Silver RM. Fetal Death. *Obstet Gynecol.* 2007;109:153-167.
   Clinical expert series reviewing fetal death in depth (Level III).
9. Cundy T, Gamble G, Townend K, Henley PG, MacPherson P, Roberts AB. Perinatal mortality in type 2 diabetes mellitus. *Diabet Med.* 2000;17:33-39.
   Large observational study conducted in New Zealand over 12 years documenting the perinatal mortality on pregnancies complicated by type 2 diabetes mellitus (Level II-2).
10. Goldenberg RL, Thompson C. The infectious origins of stillbirth. *Am J Obstet Gynecol.* 2003;189:861-873.
    Excellent review of the literature examining infectious causes related to stillbirth (Level III).
11. Rey E, Kahn SR, David M, Shrier I. Thrombophilic disorders and fetal loss: a meta-analysis. *Lancet.* 2003;361:901-908.
    A meta-analysis of 31 prospective and retrospective observational studies, which found that FVL and PTGM were associated with a two-to threefold increase in both early recurrent pregnancy loss and late, nonrecurrent fetal loss (meta-analysis).
12. Preston FE, Rosendaal FR, Walker ID, et al. Increased fetal loss in women with heritable thrombophilia. *Lancet.* 1996;361:913-916.
    A large multicenter prospective cohort evaluating inherited thrombophilias and fetal loss (Level II-2).
13. Dizon-Townson D, Miller C, Sibai B, et al. The relationship of the factor V Leiden mutation and pregnancy outcomes for the mother and fetus. *Obstet Gynecol.* 2005;106:517-524.
    Prospective observational multicenter study conducted by the NICHD Maternal-Fetal Medicine Units Network which evaluated almost 5000 women and found no differences in pregnancy outcomes in heterozygous factor V Leiden carriers and a low-risk of venous thromboembolism in pregnancy (Level II-2).
14. Fretts RC. Etiology and prevention of stillbirth. *Am J Obstet Gynecol.* 2005;193:1923-1935.
    Widely quoted review article on stillbirth (Level III).
15. Salihu HM, Aliyu MH, Rouse DJ, Kirby RS, Alexander GR. Potentially preventable excess mortality among higher-order multiples. *Obstet Gynecol.* 2003;102:679-684.
    A retrospective cohort study of multiple gestations and mortality delivered in the United States from 1995 to 1997 (Level II-2).
16. Dickinson JE. Misoprostol for second-trimester pregnancy termination in women with a prior cesarean delivery. *Obstet Gynecol.* 2005;105:352-356.
    A review of women with prior cesarean deliveries undergoing abortion at 14 to 28 weeks gestation for fetal anomaly using misoprostol with the most effective being 400 µg vaginally every 6 hours for a total of 48 hours (Level II-2).
17. Reddy UM. Prediction and prevention of recurrent stillbirth. *Obstet Gynecol.* 2007;110:1151-1164 *(Level III).*
18. Conde-Agudelo A, Rosas-Bermudez A, Kafury-Goeta AC. Birth spacing and risk of adverse perinatal outcomes: a meta-analysis. *JAMA.* 2006;295:1809-1823.
    A large meta-analysis of observational studies investigating the association between interpregnancy interval and untoward perinatal health events that are entwined with neonatal mortality (meta-analysis).
19. Antepartum fetal surveillance. ACOG Practice Bulletin No. 9. American College of Obstetricians and Gynecologists. 1999.

Case 28

A 34-year-old G2P1001 Caucasian woman at 22 weeks' gestation has noticed a painless lump in her right breast. She has no breast discharge and no family history of breast cancer. On examination, the patients has a 2.0 cm firm mobile mass of the right upper outer quadrant. There is no nipple retraction and no adenopathy. The left breast is unremarkable. The patient is referred to a breast center. The mass is noted to be solid on ultrasound examination, and the patient has a core needle biopsy of the mass revealing infiltrating intraductal carcinoma.

➤ What are the best options for therapy for this patient?

➤ What are the effects of chemotherapy on the pregnancy?

➤ What are the important considerations in managing her pregnancy?

ANSWERS TO CASE 28:
Breast Cancer in Pregnancy

Summary: A 34-year-old G2P1001 Caucasian female at 22 weeks' gestation has 2 cm right breast mass, which on biopsy reveals an infiltrating intraductal carcinoma. There are no skin changes or adenopathy.

> **Best options for therapy:** Because of the pregnancy and the size of the lesion, a breast conserving procedure would be difficult in this case since radiotherapy to the chest wall should not be used. Thus, mastectomy with axillary lymph node dissection is likely the best option.

> **Effects of chemotherapy on the pregnancy:** Chemotherapy appears to be safe in pregnancy in the second and third trimesters.

> **Important considerations in managing her pregnancy:** Excising the local lesion and lymph node sampling to properly stage the patient, followed by chemotherapy if nodes are positive for metastasis.

ANALYSIS

Objectives

1. Be able to describe the clinical presentations of breast cancer, cervical cancer, and leukemia in pregnancy.
2. Be able to describe the diagnostic approaches of breast cancer, cervical cancer, and leukemia in pregnancy.
3. Be able to discuss the complications of management of each of the cancers described in the first objective in pregnancy.
4. Describe the effect of pregnancy on the malignancies outlined in the first objective.

Considerations

The patient described this case has at least a stage II breast cancer and clearly needs therapy. At 22 weeks' gestation, there is no option of waiting until delivery, since this delay would almost certainly affect the patient's survival. Breast cancer therapy involves care of the local disease, dissection of the lymph nodes either by systematic dissection or sentinel node technique, and adjuvant therapy to prevent local recurrence. If this patient was not pregnant, then lumpectomy with sentinel node biopsy of the lymph nodes, and radiotherapy to the chest wall to help decrease recurrence to the chest would be standard therapy. Consideration should also be given to investigation of this patient for BRCA1 or BRCA2 mutations.

APPROACH TO
Malignancy in Pregnancy

Cervical cancer is the most frequent malignant neoplasm in pregnancy, followed by breast cancer and melanoma. The most common hematologic malignancy is Hodgkin lymphoma. The diagnosis of cancer in pregnancy can be delayed because of difficulties in distinguishing cancer-related symptoms from physiologic changes of pregnancy. Malignancy in pregnancy presents a significant dilemma in management as a result of conflict between maternal therapy and effects of treatment on fetal well-being. Due to the small number of cases and lack of large studies, there are no evidence-based guidelines to help with the management of pregnant patients with malignancies. The goal of cancer therapy in pregnant women is to provide the best cancer care for the patient while minimizing the potential harm to the fetus.[1]

Given the complex management involved in the care of a pregnant patient with cancer, a multidisciplinary team is essential to ensure that the mother, fetus, family, and all members of the health care team are well informed about the risks, benefits, and alternatives of the treatment choices and modalities. Management must be individualized to balance the ethical, moral, spiritual, and cultural issues that complicate such a diagnosis.

Breast Cancer

The definition of pregnancy-associated malignancy is breast cancer diagnosed during pregnancy or lactation up to 12 months postpartum. It is the second most common malignancy to complicate pregnancy.

Diagnosis of breast cancer in pregnancy is usually delayed up to 5 to 7 months due to physiologic changes. Because of diagnostic delays, pregnant women are at higher risk of presenting late in disease in comparison to non-pregnant women.[2] This is due to natural tenderness, engorgement, and increased nodularity of the breasts during pregnancy (see Table 28-1 for differential diagnosis). Stage for stage, however, the prognosis is the same as the nonpregnant woman.

A breast lump discovered during pregnancy should be adequately and urgently assessed, preferably by a specialist breast team. The sensitivity of mammography decreases during pregnancy due to the increase in size, vascularity, and glandular density of the breast tissue. The sensitivity of mammography ranges from 63% to 78%.[3] Adequate shielding is required during mammographic studies to decrease the radiation exposure to the fetus. Ultrasound has become the generally preferred imaging modality to evaluate a breast mass in pregnant women and may accurately differentiate between solid or cystic masses and is used as an adjunct to mammography.

Core biopsy under ultrasound guidance remains the gold standard in making the diagnosis of a breast mass.[1] When necessary, an open biopsy under local

Table 28–1 DIFFERENTIAL DIAGNOSIS OF BREAST MASS IN PREGNANCY OR LACTATING WOMEN

Breast cancer

Abscess

Lipoma

Lactating adenoma

Fibrocystic disease

Leukemia or lymphoma

Phyllodes tumor

Sarcoma

anesthesia is also appropriate. Clinically palpable lymph nodes should be evaluated by ultrasound-guided fine-needle aspiration (FNA) biopsy for pathology confirmation. Sentinel lymph node biopsy has not been fully evaluated in gestational breast cancer and is not recommended outside of clinical trials.[4]

Staging is according to the TMN system of the American Joint Committee on Cancer.[1] Chest x-ray for staging with abdominal shielding is considered safe during pregnancy. MRI of the thorax is preferred over CT imaging. Radiologic staging is indicated for the evaluation of metastasis to the lung, liver, or bone if the patient is symptomatic, has palpable lymph nodes, or has T3 or T4 lesions. An abdominal ultrasound can be performed to evaluate the liver. Bony metastasis may be evaluated by low-dose bone scans or MRI without contrast of the thoracic and lumbar spine.

Treatment of breast cancer in pregnancy is individualized according to the circumstances of each case: gestational age at diagnosis; surgical staging; surgical pathology of the tumor; hormonal receptor status; lymph node involvement; patient's choice regarding child bearing.[2] It is imperative that treatment is not delayed. Termination of pregnancy is usually not recommended but may be considered for an individual patient during treatment planning.[1] Continuation of pregnancy represents no threat to the fetus and the risk of transplacental metastasis is extremely rare.

Surgery is the definitive treatment for pregnancy-associated breast cancer.[1] Mastectomy with axillary dissection is traditionally considered the best choice for stage I, II, and some stage III breast cancers.[5] Axillary dissection is important for treatment and staging because nodal metastases are commonly found in pregnancy-associated breast cancer.

In pregnancy, modified radical mastectomy with lymph node dissection is performed in place of breast conserving surgery to decrease the need of chemotherapy or radiotherapy. Stages III and IV are inoperable and are treated by simple mastectomy as a palliative measure, followed by chemotherapy, hormone therapy, or radiotherapy.

Adjuvant chemotherapy is recommended in node-positive breast cancers or with tumors greater than 1 to 2 cm in diameter that are poorly differentiated. The most commonly used regimen in gestational breast cancer is doxorubicin with cyclophosphamide with or without 5-fluorouracil (FAC regimen).[1] Chemotherapy agents can cross the placenta and have known effects in the first trimester. Therefore, chemotherapy is usually deferred in the first trimester as long as the health of the mother is not compromised. Reports are lacking on adverse pregnancy outcomes after exposure to cyclophosphamide, doxorubicin, and 5-fluorouracil during the second and third trimester.[6] The use of tamoxifen in pregnancy has been contraindicated due to concerns over possible teratogenesis and its use for the treatment of hormone receptor-positive breast cancer is deferred until after delivery.[7]

In women less than 40 years, 30% will become amenorrheic and 90% of women over 40 years will cease menstruating following chemotherapy for breast cancer.[2] In those who continue to ovulate and desire pregnancy, the recommendation is to wait 2 years following treatment of breast cancer, as the risk of recurrence is highest within the first 2 years after diagnosis.[8] Nonhormonal methods should be used for contraception. Future pregnancy is safe unless the mother has an estrogen-receptor positive tumor and has not been in remission.

Women with pregnancy-associated breast cancer have the same survival stage for stage as nonpregnant women with breast cancer. They may do poorly, however, as an aggregate secondary to late diagnosis and aggressive disease.[8]

Cervical Cancer

Cervical cancer is the most common malignancy found in pregnancy. It most commonly presents as postcoital bleeding and a history of cervical dysplasia. Traditional signs and symptoms of early pregnancy overlap with the presenting complaints of invasive cervical cancer and can often be misinterpreted as threatened abortion.[2] Therefore, it should always be one of the differential diagnoses with vaginal spotting or discharge and postcoital bleeding.

Colposcopy plays an important diagnostic role. The increased vascularity of the cervix in pregnancy, however, can make the interpretation of colposcopic findings difficult. The likelihood of a high-grade lesion progressing to invasive disease during pregnancy is low and treatment is not warranted during pregnancy due to the risks. Biopsy should be avoided if no invasive disease is suspected. If invasive disease is suspected, colposcopic-directed biopsies should be taken. This is associated with risk of bleeding, infection, or preterm labor. Endocervical curettage is contraindicated. Bleeding should be controlled with routine hemostatic methods. In the event of an unsatisfactory colposcopy examination, a repeat colposcopy evaluation is recommended in 6 to 12 weeks as the eversion of the transformation zone occurs during pregnancy.[1]

Cervical conization during gestation is reserved only for suspicion of invasive cancer.[9] The safest time of doing a LEEP cone biopsy during pregnancy is during the middle second trimester, 14 to 20 weeks, or after fetal maturity has been documented. The procedure should be performed in the operating suite, with a knife, after the first trimester and after appropriate counseling about the risk of fetal loss and transfusion.

Invasive cervical cancer is clinically staged according to the International Federation of Gynecology and Obstetrics (FIGO). This involves clinical examination and chest x-ray with abdominal shielding. The use and timing of staging studies during pregnancy must be considered carefully because of the fetal exposure to ionizing radiation used with CT and fluoroscopy.

Pregnant women with cervical cancer are much more likely to have stage I disease and most have stage IB disease. Pregnancy does not affect the survival rate for cervical cancer.[1] Women with stage IA1 cervical cancer can be followed with periodic colposcopy and cytology and delivery when obstetrically indicated.

Management of invasive cervical cancer in pregnancy is dependent on the gestational age at diagnosis, stage of disease, mother's choice, and future childbearing desires. The choice of treatment modality for pregnant patients with cervical cancer is based on the same principles as those for nonpregnant patients. In general, vaginal delivery and reevaluation 6 weeks post-delivery is acceptable for those patients with stage microinvasive squamous cell carcinoma measuring 3 mm or less and without lymphovascular space involvement. With stage I disease (confined to the cervix), planned treatment delay, such as awaiting fetal lung maturity, is generally acceptable for those individuals whose pregnancies are greater than 20 weeks' gestation. Patients with early-stage disease can be treated surgically with radical hysterectomy and bilateral lymphadenectomy. Depending on the time of diagnosis, surgery may be done early in gestation with termination of the pregnancy or delaying therapy until delivery.

When the cervical cancer is beyond stage I disease, and prior to fetal viability, primary chemoradiation is offered to the patient. If advanced disease is detected after fetal viability, a classical cesarean is performed with fetal lung maturity; this reduces the chances of blood loss and cutting into the tumor. Radiation therapy is used to treat advanced disease that is not amenable to surgery. In the first trimester, radiation usually leads to spontaneous miscarriage at a cumulative dose of 30 to 50 Gy.

For stage IB1 and IB2 cervical cancer in young patients, there is increasing evidence that radical trachelectomy allows for future pregnancy. Some limited studies indicate success with this modality.

Leukemia

The leukemias are a heterogenous group of malignancies that arise from genetically altered, lymphoid or myeloid progenitor cells, located in the bone marrow.[10] This results in dysregulated growth and clonal expansion. Historically, the leukemias were classified into two basic groups: acute and chronic.

In pregnancy, most leukemias (90%) are classified as acute.[10] Acute leukemia may be separated into several subtypes, on the basis of their cell of origin and cytogenetic abnormalities. The most common acute leukemia during pregnancy includes acute myeloid leukemia (AML), acute promyelocytic leukemia (APL), and acute lymphoid leukemia (ALL).

The clinical manifestations of the acute leukemias are nonspecific and many of these symptoms are common in normal pregnancies, such as fatigue, weakness, dyspnea, and lack of energy. Patients may experience symptoms of epistaxis, easy bruisability, and recurrent infections. On physical examination, these patients often demonstrate pallor, petechiae, or ecchymosis.[10] Patients present with elevated white blood cell counts, neutropenia, anemia, thrombocytopenia, disseminated intravascular coagulation with associated bleeding or thrombosis, and, occasionally, lymphadenopathy. The diagnosis of acute leukemia in pregnancy requires a peripheral blood smear demonstrating a normocytic, normochromic anemia with a mild to severe thrombocytopenia, and blasts are almost always present. Bone marrow biopsy with flow cytometry may also be performed for the diagnosis of acute leukemia.

In a patient with acute leukemia, the primary goal of chemotherapy is the eradication of leukemic clone cells from the bone marrow and restoration of normal hematopoiesis.[10] Regardless of gestational age, the immediate induction of remission, as in the nonpregnant population, the immediate induction of remission remains the first objective in the management of the pregnant patient with acute leukemia. In a retrospective review of 37 women with acute leukemia during pregnancy, all cases were immediately started on chemotherapy, with therapeutic abortion recommended to the women presenting in the first trimester.[11] Multiagent chemotherapy consisted of anthracycline and cytarabine, cyclophosphamide, prednisone, and asparaginase.

Fetal risk was highest with chemotherapy exposure in the first trimester; however, combination chemotherapy must be considered for acute leukemia patients who are pregnant because of the likelihood of rapid disease progression and maternal complications without therapy. Potential risks from acute leukemia and its treatment during pregnancy include preterm delivery, low birth weight, disseminated intravascular coagulation, and maternal or fetal bleeding and infection because of thrombocytopenia and neutropenia. It does not seem that the course of leukemia is adversely affected by pregnancy.[12]

Comprehension Questions

28.1   A 37-year-old woman at 8 weeks' gestation is noted to have stage II
        breast cancer and she opts for radiotherapy. Which of the following
        statements is most accurate regarding this therapy?
        A. Radiation leads to an all or none effect at this stage of pregnancy.
        B. Typically miscarriage will not occur unless the radiation dose
           exceeds 30 Gy.
        C. This patient's prognosis is worse than a nonpregnant patient with
           a similar stage disease.
        D. Chemotherapy in this patient is deferred until 20 weeks' gestation.

28.2   What are the options for fertility-sparing procedure for stage IB cervi-
        cal cancer and management of future pregnancy?
        A. LEEP conization
        B. Radical trachelectomy
        C. Radical hysterectomy
        D. Local pelvic irradiation

28.3   Which of the following statements is most accurate regarding perform-
        ing colposcopy in the pregnant patient?
        A. Unsatisfactory examinations are less commonly seen in the preg-
           nant patient
        B. The hormonal changes of pregnancy make colposcopy in preg-
           nancy more challenging
        C. The colposcopist should limit the biopsy to the least visible area
        D. In general, visible lesions should be reevaluated with Pap smear or
           colposcopy about every 2 weeks.

ANSWERS

28.1   **B.** Usually miscarriage does not occur until the radiation dose exceeds
        30 Gy. Chemotherapy is usually avoided in the first trimester, but
        considered acceptable in the second and third trimesters.

DOSE (Gy)	EFFECT ON FETUS
< 0.1	No major effect
0.1-0.15	Increased risk
2.5	Malformation in most
> 30	Miscarriage

Because there is no dose of diagnostic radiation that is completely safe for the fetus, radiography should be avoided if possible at all times during pregnancy. At all stages of gestation, radiation-induced noncancer health effects are not detectable for fetal doses below 5 cGy. At a dose of 5 to 50 cGy between 8 and 15 weeks after conception, growth retardation and mental retardation can occur. After 25 weeks, prenatal radiation exposure with doses higher than 50 cGy leads to fetal death in a dose-dependent manner.[1] Therapeutic radiation for cervical cancer during pregnancy is lethal to a fetus.

28.2   **B.** Recent advances in surgical technique now allow patients with early invasive cervical cancer to maintain fertility. Radical trachelectomy with pelvic lymphadenectomy removes the tumor with adequate free margins, while retaining the uterine corpus for support of future pregnancies. This is possible for up to a small stage IB1 squamous cell tumor. The rate of first-trimester loss is the same as in the general population, but there is an increased rate of second-trimester loss. There is also an increased risk of preterm labor and the permanent cervical cerclage mandates cesarean delivery.[13]

Pelvic radiotherapy for cervical cancer leads to sterility as a result of the direct cytotoxic effect on the endometrium and ovarian injury.[1]

28.3   **B.** The challenge of performing an adequate colposcopic examination is related to pregnancy changes in the cervix: increased friability caused by related eversion of the columnar epithelium, cervical distortion from a low fetal presenting part, early effacement, and obstruction of visualization by the mucus plug.[14]

It is important that the health care provider performing the colposcopic examination be skilled in performing the test in pregnant women. An unsatisfactory colposcopy may be encountered in the early gestation, but a repeat colposcopy every 4 weeks or within 6 to 12 weeks may allow time for the migration of the transformation zone to the ectocervix, allowing a satisfactory examination.[15]

Clinical Pearls

See US Preventive Services Task Force Study Quality levels of evidence in Case 1

➤ Cervical cancer is the most common cancer in pregnancy (Level III).

➤ Pregnancy-associated breast cancer is defined as breast cancer diagnosed during pregnancy or lactation up to 12 months postpartum (Level III).

➤ Ultrasound-guided core biopsy is the gold standard for diagnosis of breast cancer in pregnancy (Level II-3).

➤ Benefit to mother is balanced against risks to pregnancy (Level III).

➤ Multidisciplinary input involving obstetrician, gynecology oncologist, medical oncologist, radiologist, perinatologist, neonatologist, and support staff is very important (Level III).

➤ Tumor markers play a very limited role during pregnancy (Level II-3).

➤ Chemotherapy can be safely used, if needed, after the first trimester (Level II-3).

➤ Melanoma and hematologic malignancies are the commonest tumors that may metastasize to the placenta. Sporadic cases with fetal metastases have also been observed (Level III).

REFERENCES

1. Cohn D, Ramaswamy B, Blum K. Malignancy and pregnancy. In: *Creasy and Resnik's Maternal-Fetal Medicine: Principles and Practice*. 6th ed. Philadelphia: Saunders, 2009.
2. Shah SA, Shafi MI. Cancer in pregnancy. Obstetrics, Gynaecology and Reproductive Medicine. 2008;18(10):279-284.
3. Ahn BY, Kim HH, Moon WK, et al. Pregnancy- and lactation-associated breast cancer: mammographic and sonographic findings. *J Ultrasound Med*. 2003;22:491-499.
4. Lyman GH, Giuliano AE, Somerfield MR, et al. American Society of Clinical Oncology guideline recommendations for sentinel lymph note biopsy in early-stage breast cancer. *J Clin Oncol*. 205;23:7703-7720.
5. Woo JC, Yu T, Hurd TC. Breast cancer in pregnancy: a literature review. *Arch Surg*. 2003;138:91-98.
6. Berry DL, Theriault RL, Holmes FA, et al. Management of breast cancer during pregnancy using a standardized protocol. *J Clin Oncol*. 1999;17:855-861.
7. Issacs RJ, Hunter W, Clark K. Tamoxifen as systemic treatment of advanced breast cancer during pregnancy—case report and literature review. *Gynecol Oncol*. 2001;80:405-408.
8. Leslie KK, Lange CA. Breast cancer and pregnancy. *Obstet and Gynec Clin N Am*. 2005;32:547-558.
9. Muller CY, Smith HO. Cervical neoplasia complicating pregnancy. *Obstet Gynecol Clin N Am*. 2005;32:533-546.
10. Hurley TJ, McKinell, JV, Irani MS. Hematologic malignancies in pregnancy. *Obstet Gynecol Clin N Am*. 2005;32:595-614.

11. Chelghoum Y, Vey N, Raffoux E, et al. Acute leukemia during pregnancy. *Cancer.* 2005;104:110-117.
12. Caligiuni MA, Mayer RJ. Pregnancy and leukemia. *Semin Oncol.* 1989;16:388-396.
13. Ramirez PT, Schmeler KM, Soliman PT, Frumovitz M. Fertility preservation in patients with early cervical cancer: radical trachelectomy. *Gynecol Oncol.* 2008;110(Suppl2):S25-S28.
14. Brown D, Berran P, Kaplan KJ, et al. Special situations: abnormal cervical cytology during pregnancy. *Clin Obstet Gynecol.* 2005;48:178-185.
15. Nguyen C, Montz FJ, Bristow RE. Management of stage I cervical cancer in pregnancy. *Obstet Gynecol Surv.* 2000;55:633-643.

Case 29

A 43-year-old G1 is currently at $7^3/_7$ weeks' gestation, conceived by IVF (donor eggs) with a resultant dichorionic/diamniotic twin gestation. She presents for prenatal care. She denies a history of medical problems although endorses a history of three operative laparoscopic procedures due to a long history of chronic pelvic pain secondary to endometriosis. She got married earlier this year and desired to conceive. She failed to conceive due to infertility and ultimately required IVF. She admits to a history of depression since the age of 20. She has sought counseling and has been on antidepressants intermittently throughout the years. Most recently she was on sertraline; however, she stopped taking it prior to pregnancy because she thought this was contributing to her infertility issues. She is very excited about her pregnancy and thinks that she is doing "okay" off medications. She is a dentist and reports being happily married. There is no history of suicide attempts, substance abuse, or domestic violence.

➤ How would you screen this patient for depression?

➤ What are some neonatal/maternal risks associated with *untreated* depression during pregnancy?

ANSWERS TO CASE 29:
Depression in Pregnancy

Summary: A 43-year-old G1 at $7^3/_7$ weeks with twin gestation conceived by IVF and history of depression presents for prenatal care.

➤ **Screening patient for depression:** Screening questionnaires, such as the Edinburgh postnatal depression scale (EPDS) or Patient Health Questionnaire (PHQ) and clarification of the patient's responses will help to determine whether she requires further assessment and/or treatment.

➤ **Reasons for some neonatal/maternal risks associated with untreated depression during pregnancy:** Neonatal irritability has been associated with untreated maternal depression. There is an increased risk of maternal stress/anxiety, poor weight gain, poor prenatal care, substance abuse, and postpartum depression/psychosis when depression goes untreated during pregnancy.

ANALYSIS

Objectives

1. Understand how to screen pregnant patients for depression.
2. Review pharmacologic options and their effect on pregnancy.
3. Understand which patients are candidates for treatment during pregnancy.

Considerations

This is a 43-year-old woman who presents with symptoms of depression. It is not uncommon that a patient provides a history of depression at her first prenatal care visit. Reproductive age women are at risk of developing a depressive disorder and the **perinatal period** (defined as pregnancy and up to 1 y postpartum) represents a time of increased vulnerability. The incidence of depressive disorders during pregnancy is in the order of 10% to 16% of women.[1] Major depression as defined by the diagnostic and statistical manual-IV occurs in 3% to 5%, while the remainders of cases are minor depression[2] (Level III). This may actually be an underestimation since the diagnosis is not always an easy one to make because symptoms of depression may overlap with those of pregnancy.

The strongest risk factor for perinatal depression is a history of depression. Additional risk factors include a history of **postpartum depression (onset of symptoms within 4 wk),** low-income status, ethnic minority, domestic violence, financial hardship, poor social support, high-risk pregnancy, and family history of depression. Despite increasing knowledge of risk factors, it is difficult to identify which women will actually develop perinatal depression. That said, screening for depression during pregnancy is an important part of prenatal care and all women should be screened.

Depression screening is recommended "at least once during each trimester" per the American College of Obstetricians and Gynecologists.[3] Postpartum depression screening is also recommended and this most commonly occurs in conjunction with the 6 week visit. However, it should be noted that the most vulnerable period after delivery is 10 to 19 days followed by 3 months, with most cases occurring by 5 months. A widely quoted rule of thumb for postpartum depression screening is "2 weeks, 6 weeks, 6 months"[2] (Level III). Although it is challenging to coordinate multiple postpartum screening visits, it should be considered for high-risk women. It is also important to distinguish postpartum depression from *postpartum blues*. The latter occurs in 80% of women. Symptoms are mild and self-limiting, typically resolving by 2 to 3 weeks postpartum.

Self-report screening is routinely used in clinical practice during the perinatal period. It is important to note that these questionnaires are not diagnostic but rather are used to determine which patient requires further assessment and treatment. The **Edinburgh postnatal depression scale** is a 10-item questionnaire and perhaps the most widely used tool for depression screening during the perinatal period. A score of *15 or more* in the antenatal period and *13 or more* in the postnatal period is considered a validated cutoff score for probable major depression.[4] (Level III). The detection rates are better for severe depression with specificity of approximately 78% to 96%. The nine-item **patient health questionnaire** is also a validated screening instrument and has been studied in the obstetric-gynecologic setting[5] (Level II-2). This questionnaire takes 3 minutes to complete and permits planning and monitoring of treatment.

It is not unreasonable for this patient to be observed off of medication if she is currently euthymic and does not have other risk factors for relapse. If she becomes symptomatic, the patient can be restarted on pharmacotherapy and referred for adjunct psychotherapy (individual, couples, or group) as well. Based on a recent cohort study, she can be informed that her risk of relapse may be as high as 68% by having discontinued medication as compared to a lower risk of 25% if she remains on medication during pregnancy[6] (Level II-2). The risks of untreated depression as well as the risk of prenatal exposure to antidepressants should be reviewed with the patient.

Untreated depression during pregnancy has been associated with stress, poor prenatal care, substance abuse, and postpartum depression/psychosis, all of which can impact fetal/neonatal outcome. Based on the available evidence, infants born to mothers with a depressive disorder have increased risk of irritability making them more difficult to console. They are also less attentive and have fewer facial expressions[7] (Level III). Increased cortisol levels, as seen in those with depression, may precipitate preterm birth (PTB). At present, the data looking at the association between *untreated* depression during pregnancy and adverse pregnancy outcomes such as miscarriages, PTB, or small-for-gestational-age infants (SGA) are inconsistent. Some studies report an association while others do not, thus a definitive conclusion is difficult to make based on the available data[8,9] (Level III).

Healthy lifestyles should be supported and treatment of any addictions (ie, tobacco, alcohol) should be offered in order to optimize maternal/fetal outcome. It is also important to review the patient's medication list given that side effects from antihypertensive medications (ie, beta blockers), diuretics, corticosteroids, and sedatives can mimic depression. This patient should be provided with education material such as perinatal/postpartum depression booklets and resource contact numbers/and or web sites.

APPROACH TO
Depression in Pregnancy

CLINICAL APPROACH

A large majority of women who fulfill criteria for depressive disorder may experience symptoms during pregnancy. Those who are considered at high risk for relapse during pregnancy and therefore would benefit from continued or initiation of treatment during pregnancy include those with a history of severe or recurrent major depression, psychosis, history of suicide, coexisting panic or bipolar disorders, and history of relapse after discontinuation of antidepressants. The decision on whether to treat or discontinue pharmacotherapy during pregnancy can be made based on severity of symptoms, risk factors, and individual preference. Collaboration between the obstetrician and psychiatrist is important when considering this decision. It goes without saying that a patient with suicidal or psychotic features should be seen immediately by a psychiatrist who can optimize treatment. Those with coexisting bipolar disorders should also be managed by a psychiatrist as initiation of antidepressant monotherapy may trigger mania and psychosis[8,9] (Level III).

Those who are on antidepressant medication during pregnancy and are asymptomatic (preferably > 6 mo) can be offered a trial off medication with a slow taper provided they do not have any of the above risk factors for relapse and are willing to be off medication. If the patient is motivated to have a trial off medication, it is important to monitor her closely for signs/symptoms of relapse. Again it is important to review with the patient that her risk of relapse is higher after discontinuing medication during pregnancy and that this risk must be weighed against the potential risks of antidepressant medication use during pregnancy. It is always reasonable to refer a patient for psychotherapy especially when a trial off medication is considered. If a patient chooses to continue on medication during pregnancy or is not a candidate for discontinuing medication, then she should remain on the same medication at the lowest effective dose.

Those who have symptoms of major depression but are not receiving any treatment can be offered initiation of antidepressant therapy and adjunct psychotherapy. Sometimes a patient may choose psychotherapy before starting pharmacotherapy. This is a reasonable option as long as the patient is not debilitated and is without risk factors such as a prior failed trial of psychotherapy alone or recurrent, severe relapses. If a patient requires pharmacotherapy, the drug safety profile should be factored into the particular antidepressant that is selected. It is also reasonable to select an antidepressant that the patient has responded well to in the past. Selective serotonin reuptake inhibitors (SSRIs) remain the first-line choice for treatment. Counseling regarding the risks and benefits of antidepressant use during pregnancy should be undertaken and weighed against the risks of untreated depression. Electroconvulsive therapy is also a safe and effective alternative to treatment in those with severe depression unresponsive to pharmacotherapy.

There are two recent publications by representatives from the American Psychiatry Association and the American College of Obstetricians and Gynecologists who convened a working group to critically evaluate the existing literature on the risks of depression and antidepressants during pregnancy[8,9] (Level III). Some studies have reported an increased risk of miscarriage in the first trimester in those exposed to various antidepressants; however, it is difficult to establish this association when confounding variables such as substance abuse and maternal age were not well controlled in these studies.[10] Conflicting evidence exists with regard to the use of antidepressants and SGA infants. Selective serotonin reuptake inhibitors (SSRIs) have been associated with an increased risk of SGA infants, albeit very small, compared to unexposed group after controlling for confounding variables[11] (Level II-2). Although some studies suggest that the use of SSRIs during pregnancy may be associated with an increased risk of PTB[12] (Level II-2), data are not consistent across all studies.

With regard to structural malformations, the current data on SSRI exposure during pregnancy do not provide consistent information to support major or specific teratogenic risks[8,9] (Level III). Although linked databases have found that pregnancies exposed to paroxetine during the first trimester have an increased risk of cardiac malformations[13] (Level II-2), other large cohort studies have not supported this association[14] (Level II-2). A higher incidence of congenital heart defects has been seen with the use of SSRI in combination with benzodiazepine as compared to SSRI alone[15] (Level II-2) and therefore monotherapy in the treatment of depression is recommended. The majority of tricyclic antidepressants (TCAs) have not been associated with structural defects. Other antidepressants are not as well studied; however, no specific malformation has been associated with the use of bupropion or venlafaxine.

Infants born to mothers who used TCAs during pregnancy have an increased risk of neonatal behavioral symptoms such as jitteriness, irritability, and convulsions[16] (Level II-2). Approximately one-third of women using SSRIs in late pregnancy had infants with transient **"poor neonatal adaptation"** with symptoms in the immediate newborn period consisting of hypoglycemia, irritability, temperature instability, seizures, tachypnea, and/or weak absent cry. The absolute risk of **persistent pulmonary hypertension (PPH)** among newborns has also been shown to be increased in mothers who used SSRIs late in pregnancy (3-6 per 1000 infants compared to 0.5-2 per 1000 infants baseline)[8,9] (Level III). The data on the use of antidepressants (sertraline, fluoxetine, paroxetine, fluvoxamine, citalopram) during lactation show that exposure through breast milk is considerably lower than transplacental exposure during pregnancy. Sertraline is considered the safest for lactation and therefore the first choice when considering which antidepressant to start during pregnancy and in the postpartum period[2] (Level III). TCAs have been well studied and similarly considered safe for use during lactation although one report of respiratory depression was reported with the use of doxepin.[1] Other antidepressants are less well studied and therefore patients need to be counseled appropriately.

In summary, depression in reproductive age women is common. Awareness of this illness is important given that pregnancy and the postpartum period are times when a woman is at high risk for developing depression or having a relapse. Collaboration of care between the obstetrician and the mental health provider will ensure optimal maternal health care. The decision to initiate or discontinue treatment needs to be individualized based on the patient's symptoms and psychiatric history. The risks and benefits of untreated depression need to be weighed against the potential fetal/neonatal risks of antidepressant use during pregnancy.

Postpartum Depression

Postpartum depression, which usually occurs within the first 3 to 4 months after delivery, affects 10% to 15% of women. The clinical symptoms and diagnostic criteria are identical to depression that can occur any other time in a woman's life. Women in the postpartum period are most vulnerable to develop psychiatric illness. Women who have suffered one major episode of postpartum depression have about 25% recurrence risk. Those at highest risk are those with a personal history of depression, previous episode of postpartum depression, or depression during pregnancy. In addition to a history of depression, recent stressful life events, lack of social support, unintended pregnancy, and uninsured status are also risk factors.

Usually, postpartum depression develops slowly over the first 3 to 4 months after delivery although the disorder presents more abruptly. Postpartum blues are more mild and do not meet the same diagnostic criteria as postpartum depression. Screening for, diagnosing, and treating depression are critical to proper intervention. Women with current depression or a history of major depression are at particular risk, and should be monitored carefully.

Unfortunately, too many women tragically fall "through the cracks" such that they themselves or their children become victims to the depression. Pregnancy and the postpartum period represent an incredibly important time to assess for mood disturbance.

There are multiple depression screening tools available for use. These tools usually can be completed in less than 10 minutes. Most have a specificity ranging from 77% to 100%. Thus, it can be argued that sensitivity should be the determining factor to maximize the number of depressed patients identified. Many of these screening tools have been validated with specific ethnic populations. Examples of highly sensitive screening tools include the Edinburgh postnatal depression scale.

Comprehension Questions

29.1   A 28-year-old G1P0 at 18 weeks' gestation reports a history of sertraline use for the treatment of depression. What is the best management for this patient?

    A. Recommend to discontinue medication.

    B. Recommend fetal echocardiogram.

    C. Recommend anatomy scan at 18 to 20 weeks gestation and continue treatment.

    D. Recommend termination of the pregnancy.

29.2   A 30-year-old G2P1 woman at 32 weeks' gestation is noted to have a history of postpartum depression. She required SSRI antidepressant therapy after the last delivery. She asks about the possibility of postpartum depression after this current pregnancy. Which of the following statements is most accurate?

    A. Each pregnancy is independent and the prior postpartum depression should have no impact on this pregnancy.

    B. The criteria for postpartum depression is identical to that of nonpregnant patients.

    C. The Edinburgh depression scale is more valid for nonpregnant than pregnant individuals.

    D. Postpartum depression affects approximately 1% to 3% of postpartum women.

ANSWERS

29.1   **C.** This patient should be encouraged to continue on treatment as
        the risks of untreated depression are greater than the risks of treat-
        ment during pregnancy. Data on SSRI exposure during pregnancy do
        not provide consistent information to support major or specific ter-
        atogenic risks and therefore routine anatomy scan is a reasonable
        start for the evaluation of this patient. If there is a cardiac abnormal-
        ity on ultrasound then she can be referred for fetal echocardiogram.

29.2   **B.** The criteria for postpartum depression are identical to that of
        depression outside of pregnancy. A history of depression is a risk fac-
        tor for postpartum depression. The Edinburgh depression scale was
        developed to identify postpartum depression. Postpartum depression
        affects approximately 10 to 15 of women after delivery.

Clinical Pearls

See US Preventive Services Task Force Study Quality levels of evidence in Case 1

➤ Perinatal depression is common and is associated with increased risk of
  maternal and neonatal adverse outcomes (Level III).

➤ Pharmacotherapy should be continued during pregnancy in those who
  are at high risk of relapse (Level III).

➤ SSRIs are the drug class of choice when treating depression during
  pregnancy or postpartum (Level III).

➤ SSRIs are associated with a small increased risk of SGA infants, poor neonatal
  adaptation, and persistent pulmonary hypertension in the newborn (Level II-2).

➤ Current data on SSRI exposure (in aggregate) during pregnancy do not
  provide consistent information to support major or specific teratogenic risks
  (Level II-2).

CONTROVERSIES

• Association of antidepressants and increased risk of miscarriages and PTB.
• First-trimester use of paroxetine and increased risk of cardiac malformations.

REFERENCES

1. Use of psychiatric medications during pregnancy and lactation. ACOG Practice
   Bulletin No. 102. American College of Obstetricians and Gynecologists. *Obstet
   Gynecol.* 2008;111(4):1001-1020.
2. Dossett EC. Perinatal depression. *Obstet Gynecol Clin N Am.* 2008;35:419-434
   (Level III).
3. American College of Obstetricians and Gynecologists. ACOG Committee
   Opinion No. 343. *Obstet Gynecol.* 2006;108:469-477.

4. Matthey S, Henshaw C, Elliot S, Barnett B. Variability in use of cut-off scores and formats on the Edinburgh postnatal depression scale—implications for clinical and research practice. *Arch Womens Ment Health*. 2006;9:309-315 (Level III).

5. Spitzer RL, Williams JBW, Kroenke K, Hornyak R, McMurray J. Validity and utility of the PRIME-MD patient health questionnaire in assessment of 3000 obstetric-gynecologic patients: the PRIME-MD patient health questionnaire obstetric-gynecologic study. *Am J Obstet*. 2000;183(3):759-769 (Level II-2).

6. Cohen LS, Altshuler LL, Harlow BL, et al. Relapse of major depression during pregnancy in women who maintain or discontinue antidepressant treatment [published erratum appears in JAMA 2006;296:170]. *JAMA*. 2006;295:499-507. *A prospective cohort of 201 pregnant women with a history of depression who were recently or currently on antidepressant medication. Of those who remained on treatment during pregnancy, 26% relapsed compared to 68% who discontinued treatment (Level II-2).*

7. Field T, Diego M, Hernandez-Reif M. Prenatal depression effects of the fetus and newborn: a review. *Infant Behav Dev*. 2006;29:445-455 (Level III).

8. Yonkers KA, Wisner KL, Steward DE, et al. The management of depression during pregnancy: a report from the American Psychiatric Association and the American College of Obstetricians and Gynecologists. *Obstet Gynecol*. 2009;114(3):703-713. *Representatives from the American Psychiatry Association and the American College of Obstetricians and Gynecologists convened a working group to critically evaluate the existing literature on the risks of depression and antidepressants during pregnancy (Level III).*

9. Yonkers KA, Wisner KL, Steward DE, et al. The management of depression during pregnancy: a report from the American Psychiatric Association and the American College of Obstetricians and Gynecologists. *Gen Hosp Psychiatry*. 2009;31(5):403-413. *See reference number 8 (Level III).*

10. Hemels M, Einarson A, Koren G, Lanctot K, Einarson T. Antidepressant use during pregnancy and the rates of spontaneous abortions: a meta-analysis. *Ann Pharmacother*. 2005;39:803-809.

11. Oberlander T, Warburton W, Misri S, Aghajanian J, Hertzman C. Neonatal outcomes after prenatal exposure to selective serotonin reuptake inhibitor antidepressants and maternal depression using population-based linked health data. *Arch Gen Psychitary*. 2006;63:898-906 (Level II-2).

12. Chambers CD, Johnson KA, Dick LM, Felix RJ. Birth outcomes in pregnant women taking fluoxetine. *N Eng J Med*. 1996;335:1010-1015 (Level II-2).

13. Kallen BA, Otterbald Olaussan P. Maternal use of selective serotonin reuptake inhibitors in early pregnancy and infant congenital malformations. *Birth Defects Res A Clin Mol Teratol*. 2007;79:301-308 (Level II-2).

14. Louik C, Lin A, Werler M, Hernandez-Diaz S, Mitchell A. First trimester use of selective serotonin-reuptake inhibitors and the risk of birth defects. *N Eng J Med*. 2007;356:2675-2683 (Level II-2).

15. Oberlander TF. Major congenital malformations following prenatal exposure to serotonin reuptake inhibitors and benzodiazepines using population-based health data. *Birth Defects Res B Dev Reprod Toxicol*. 2008;83:68-76 (Level II-2).

16. Kallen B. Neonate characteristics after maternal use of antidepressants in late pregnancy. *Arch Pediatr Adolesc Med*. 2004;158:312-316 (Level II-2).

Case 30

A 23-year-old Caucasian woman, G1P0, at 33 weeks' gestation is undergoing induction of labor for severe preeclampsia. She has a functioning epidural catheter in place and has been pushing for 20 minutes. The fetal heart rate (FHR) tracing has been normal (category I) throughout the labor but you are called to the bedside for a prolonged deceleration to 60 beats per minute (bpm) lasting 3 minutes. You perform a sterile vaginal examination that rules out a prolapsed umbilical cord, and confirms complete dilation of the cervix with the fetal head at +2 station. Now at 7 minutes the FHR remains in the 60s.

➤ What is the most likely diagnosis?

➤ What is your next step?

➤ What complications are associated with your method of management?

ANSWER TO CASE 30:

Operative Vaginal (Forceps) Delivery for Fetal Indication

Summary: A nulliparous woman with severe preeclampsia at 33 weeks' gestation is being induced with oxytocin. She has reached the second stage of labor and now manifests a fetal indication for expeditious delivery.

> **Most likely diagnosis:** Prolonged deceleration of the FHR in the second stage of labor.

> **Next step:** Forceps-assisted delivery.

> **Complications:** Maternal complications include hemorrhage from genital tract lacerations and possible damage to the anal sphincter with future risk of fetal incontinence. Newborn complications include birth trauma and hypoxia.

ANALYSIS

Objectives

1. Select a method of management appropriate to the clinical circumstances of this case.
2. Identify the prerequisites for operative vaginal delivery.
3. Be aware of possible complications that may arise.

Considerations

The etiology of the FHR deceleration in this case is uncertain. The differential diagnosis includes abruption of the placenta (made more likely by the woman having severe preeclampsia), an umbilical cord complication (occult compression, tight nuchal cord, true knot in the cord), or often unexplained, even in retrospect. Management depends heavily on the training and experience of the accoucheur, but the best option in this setting is forceps delivery.

APPROACH TO

Operative Vaginal Delivery for Fetal Indication

DEFINITIONS

ENGAGEMENT: The biparietal diameter of the fetal head has passed through the pelvic inlet (inferred clinically when the leading bony edge is at or below zero station).

PROLONGED DECELERATION: A visually apparent decrease in FHR from baseline that is ≥ 15 bpm, lasting ≥ 2 minutes, but < 10 minutes.

LOW FORCEPS DELIVERY: A forceps delivery performed when the leading point of the fetal skull is at station ≥ +2 cm and not on the pelvic floor. Subsets include rotation ≤ 45 degrees (usually straightforward) or > 45 degrees (can be more difficult).

CLINICAL APPROACH

The first task confronting the caregiver is to select a method of management. When the woman is first seen at 3 minutes, conservative measures like turning off the oxytocin, repositioning, and administering oxygen should be tried. However, when the heart rate is still down at 7 minutes, active intervention is warranted. Prematurity is a relative contraindication to vacuum extraction. Midwives and most family physicians are not trained in the use of forceps. Depending on the facility, it may take time to set up for an emergency cesarean delivery and it cannot be known with certainty when or if the FHR will improve. Thus, if the operator has adequate training and experience, forceps delivery is the best option.

Prior to applying the forceps, a quick check should be made to ensure that the prerequisites for forceps delivery (Table 30–1) are satisfied.[1] The operator must accurately diagnose the position of the fetal head and apply the forceps accordingly. The application should be checked to ensure that the sagittal

Table 30–1 PREREQUISITES FOR OPERATIVE VAGINAL DELIVERY
Ruptured membranes
Complete cervical dilation
Engagement of fetal head
Known position of fetal head
Experienced operator
Adequate fetopelvic relationship
Informed consent—risks, benefits, alternatives
Adequate anesthesia
Empty bladder/rectum
Appropriate instrument
Satisfactory maternal position

suture bisects the plane of the shanks, that the posterior fontanel is one fin-gerbreadth above the plane of the shanks and that, if a fenestrated blade is used, the operator's finger cannot be inserted into the posterior aspect of the fenestra (Figures 30–1 and 30–2). Next, any necessary rotation of the head should be accomplished. After rechecking the application, traction can be applied manually using a Pajot-Saxtorph maneuver or a Bill axis traction han-dle. Given that this case involves a 33-week fetus, descent of the head should be observed on the first traction attempt. Some operators prefer to remove the forceps prior to delivering the head. An episiotomy may or may not be per-formed according to the judgment of the operator.

For those with training and experience the preceding may seem almost trivial. However, many contemporary training programs do not adequately prepare trainees to confidently and competently perform these procedures. If, instead of the case described, there was a term fetus with a deep transverse

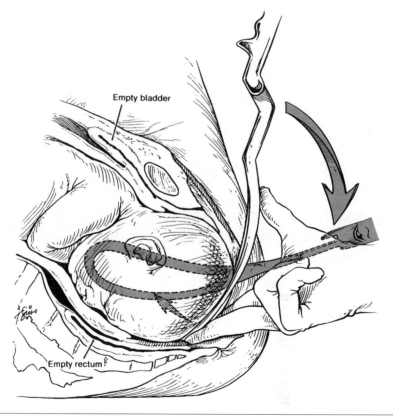

Figure 30–1. Sagittal view of the first blade application. The fetus is presenting as vertex and with occiput anterior. The application of the left blade Simpson forceps is shown. (*Reproduced, with permission, from Cunningham FG, Leveno KJ, Bloom SL, et al. Williams Obstetrics. 23rd ed. New York, NY: McGraw-Hill; 2010.*)

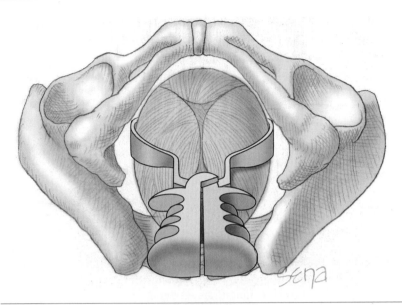

Figure 30-2. After the right blade is inserted, and forceps are symmetrically placed and articulated. *(Reproduced, with permission, from Cunningham FG, Leveno KJ, Bloom SL, et al. Williams Obstetrics. 23rd ed. New York, NY: McGraw-Hill; 2010.)*

arrest following a prolonged second stage of labor, the requirement for skill, judgment, and careful assessment of fetopelvic relationships is much more stringent and difficult to achieve. With a forceps delivery rate in the United States of only 1%,[2] compared to a cesarean delivery rate of 32%, relatively few individuals acquire and maintain these technical skills.

Once a woman begins the second stage of labor, all types of deliveries have risks. Therefore, it is appropriate to consider the risks and benefits of each possible method of delivery: forceps, vacuum extraction, cesarean, or awaiting spontaneous delivery. For one specific complication of the newborn, intracranial hemorrhage, the risks for forceps, vacuum, and cesarean in the second stage of labor were found to be comparable.[3]

Maternal risks of operative vaginal delivery include hemorrhage from genital tract lacerations and anal sphincter injury with a future risk of fecal incontinence. These injuries are attributable not only to the instrument itself, but also to the use of the instrument. A case in point would be a laceration of the external anal sphincter caused by prolonged downward traction on the fetal head with forceps. The operator must be cognizant of the fact that the axis of traction must change continuously as the fetal head descends in the pelvis. The same principle applies to vacuum extraction.

Neonatal morbidity associated with operative vaginal delivery can be reduced by employing good judgment and proper technique. Fractures of clavicle and skull, the latter uncommonly, facial nerve and brachial plexus palsies, and the previously cited intracranial hemorrhage all have been associated with instrumental delivery. Subgaleal hemorrhage occurs more often with vacuum extraction than with forceps.[4]

Faced with a decision between operative vaginal delivery and cesarean delivery, the operator should be reminded that there is more at stake than the current case. If a first delivery is by cesarean, the next is highly likely to be by cesarean as well.[5] The incidence of placenta previa, placenta accreta, uterine rupture, and various maternal complications all increase with each successive cesarean. In contrast, if the first delivery is vaginal, the next one is also likely to be vaginal.[6]

Lastly, even though the case presented would not be appropriate for vacuum extraction (VE), it is evident that VE is on the rise in the United States. When VE is selected for an appropriate case, the operator is advised to pay particular attention to cup position, which should be symmetric and centered approximately 3 cm anterior (toward the fetal face) to the posterior fontanel. VE should not be used for gestations less than 34 weeks. The incidence of shoulder dystocia may be greater with VE than with forceps. As with forceps, good judgment and good technique are essential.

For many reasons, operative vaginal delivery is on the decline in the United States and several other parts of the world. It is being replaced by cesarean delivery despite the lack of evidence that shows an advantage of cesareans to either mothers or babies. Unless physicians receive adequate training in either forceps delivery, vacuum extraction, or both, operative vaginal delivery will no longer be a viable alternate to abdominal delivery.

Comprehension Questions

30.1 What is the range in minutes of prolonged deceleration?
 A. 1 to 3
 B. 2 to 5
 C. 2 to 10
 D. 10 to 15

30.2 In the case scenario, which of the following missing pieces of information is most important before proceeding with forceps delivery?
 A. Whether there was meconium in the amniotic fluid.
 B. The estimated fetal weight.
 C. The bispinous diameter of the maternal pelvis.
 D. The position of the fetal head.

30.3   When the biparietal diameter of the fetal head has passed through the pelvic inlet, at what station is the leading bony edge usually palpated?
A. −2
B. 0
C. +2
D. +5

30.4   Which of the following statements regarding episiotomy is most accurate when forceps are used?
A. It should be performed routinely.
B. It is seldom indicated.
C. It should be left up to the judgment of the operator.
D. Mediolateral is preferred over midline.

ANSWERS

30.1   **C. 2 to 10 minutes:** This answer is found in "Definitions" section of the chapter.

30.2   **D. An accurate diagnosis of position is most important, although attention should be paid to the other choices also.** This answer is found in the second paragraph of "Clinical Approach" and also in Table 30–1.

30.3   **B.** Zero station. Answer is found in "Definitions" section.

30.4   **C.** Answer is found in the second paragraph of "Clinical Approach."

Clinical Pearls

See US Preventive Services Task Force Study Quality levels of evidence in Case 1

➤ Lacerations of the external anal sphincter at forceps delivery are technique-dependent, not simply an inherent risk of the instrument (Level III).
➤ Forceps delivery has some specific indications where VE is not possible, for example, the premature infant (Level III).
➤ Training in forceps techniques is a very important element of all obstetric residency programs (Level III).
➤ All forceps applications should be checked by the most experienced person in the room **prior** to initiating traction (Level III).

REFERENCES

1. Dennen EH. *Forceps Deliveries*. Philadelphia, PA: F.A. Davis Company; 1955.
2. Martin JA, Hamilton BE, Sutton PD et al. Births: Final data for 2005. National Vital Statistics Reports. Hyattsville, MD: NCHS; 2007:56.
3. Towner D, Castro MA, Eby-Wilkens E, Gilbert WM. Effect of mode on delivery in nulliparous women on neonatal intracranial injury. *NEJM.* 1999;341(23):1709-1714.
4. Clinical management guidelines for obstetrician-gynecologists. Operative vaginal delivery. ACOG Practice Bulletin No. 17. Washington, DC: American College of Obstetricians and Gynecologists; June 2000.
5. Yeomans ER. Operative vaginal delivery. *Clinical Obstetrics—The Fetus and Mother.* 3rd ed. Malden, MA: Blackwell Publishing; 2007:1077-1084.
6. Patel RR, Murphy DJ. Forceps delivery in modern obstetric practice. *BMJ.* 2004;1302-1305.

Case 31

A 28-year-old African American woman, G2P0101, with sickle cell anemia presented at 21 weeks of gestation with back and hip pain, typical symptoms of her acute painful episodes. She was admitted to the hospital for management. Laboratory studies revealed a hematocrit of 18%, reticulocyte count 27%, total bilirubin 8.2 mg/dL, and direct bilirubin 2.8 mg/dL.

On hospital day 2 the patient developed left-sided chest pain, tachypnea, and progressively worsening hypoxemia. Her oral temperature was 38.8°C and her respiratory rate was 24 per minute. Chest x-ray showed a left lower lobe infiltrate. Repeat hematocrit was 16%.

➤ What is the most likely diagnosis?

➤ What is your next step?

➤ What are potential complications of this patient's disorder?

ANSWERS TO CASE 31:
Sickle Cell Disease

Summary: This is a 28-year-old African American female, G2P0101, with sickle cell anemia admitted at 21 weeks of gestation with symptoms of an acute vaso-occlusive episode. She developed worsening hypoxemia and her chest x-ray showed a left lower lobe infiltrate.

➤ **Most likely diagnosis:** Acute chest syndrome.

➤ **Next steps:** Transfer to ICU or OB critical care unit, supplemental oxygen and respiratory support, transfusion, antibiotics.

➤ **Potential complications:** Early mortality, restrictive and obstructive lung disease, interstitial fibrosis, pulmonary hypertension, fetal hypoxemia.

ANALYSIS

Objectives

1. Understand the utility and necessity of hemoglobin electrophoresis in the diagnosis of the various sickle hemoglobinopathies.
2. Be able to diagnose and manage the acute chest syndrome.
3. Learn how to provide optimal prenatal care to women with sickle cell anemia.

Considerations

The acute chest syndrome is the second most common cause of hospitalization and the leading cause of admission to an intensive care unit and of premature death among patients with sickle cell disease (SCD). It is generally defined as development of a new pulmonary infiltrate involving at least one complete lung segment, not due to atelectasis, in a patient with SCD.[1] Chest pain, fever, tachypnea, wheezing, and cough are usually present in addition to the imaging findings. The syndrome typically develops 24 to 72 hours after the onset of a vaso-occlusive episode, and is often preceded by a drop in hemoglobin level and/or platelet count. Three major causes have been proposed: pulmonary infection, fat embolism, and pulmonary infarction due to intravascular sickling and occlusion.[1] A recent case report describes a woman in the third trimester of pregnancy who developed acute chest syndrome precipitated by a lower respiratory infection.[2] Surprisingly, this was her first ever manifestation of her underlying sickle cell disease.

Treatment is primarily supportive. Supplemental oxygen and, if needed, mechanical ventilation to maintain a PaO_2 of at least 70 mm Hg are essential to prevent further sickling and avoid fetal hypoxemia. Inhaled bronchodilators should be given if there is evidence of bronchospasm. Antibiotic coverage for community-acquired organisms should be administered. Simple or exchange transfusion to increase the hematocrit and reduce the hemoglobin S level often leads to clinical improvement. Opioid analgesics and intravenous hydration should be administered with caution because they may lead to respiratory depression and pulmonary edema.

APPROACH TO

Sickle Cell Disease With Acute Vaso-Occlusive Episode and Acute Chest Syndrome

DEFINITIONS

SICKLE CELL DISEASE (SCD): A group of inherited structural hemoglobinopathies caused by a change in the normal amino acid content of hemoglobin.

ACUTE PAINFUL EPISODE: An episode of acute pain caused by vaso-occlusion in a patient with SCD, previously called sickle cell crisis.

ACUTE CHEST SYNDROME: Development of a new pulmonary infiltrate involving at least one complete lung segment, not due to atelectasis, in a patient with SCD, often accompanied by chest pain, fever, tachypnea, wheezing, and cough.

CLINICAL APPROACH

Etiology

Sickle cell disease refers to a group of inherited structural hemoglobinopathies caused by a change in the normal amino acid content of hemoglobin. Normal adult hemoglobin A is a tetramer composed of two α chains and two β chains. The substitution of valine or lysine for glutamic acid at the sixth position in the β chain produces the two most common structurally abnormal hemoglobins, S and C, respectively. Thalassemia refers to decreased synthesis of normal hemoglobin. Thalassemia syndromes are named by the type of chain that is inadequately produced; for example, in β thalassemia the beta-globin chain is underproduced.

The most common sickle cell diseases, sickle cell anemia (hemoglobin SS disease), hemoglobin SC disease, and hemoglobin S-β thalassemia, are all characterized by chronic hemolytic anemia and vaso-occlusive phenomena. Hemoglobin S polymerizes when oxygen saturation is low, causing erythrocytes to become rigid and distorted in shape, which then leads to structural damage to the cell membrane.[3] These changes and other functional red cell alterations lead to impaired blood flow in small vessels, vaso-occlusion, and hemolysis.

Clinical Presentation

The chronic hemolysis of SCD produces a mild to moderate anemia with high-normal or elevated mean corpuscular volume (MCV), reticulocytosis, unconjugated hyperbilirubinemia, elevated LDH, and low serum haptoglobin. Peripheral blood smear usually shows normochromic erythrocytes. Sickled red cells, polychromasia, and Howell-Jolly bodies reflecting hyposplenia may be seen. The characteristic clinical picture in patients with SCD is acute and chronic multisystem organ failure due to repeated episodes of vaso-occlusion. The most common acute event is the acute painful episode, formerly called sickle cell crisis. Patients present with acute pain, most frequently in the back, extremities, joints, and abdomen. Fever and worsening anemia may also be present. Standard laboratory tests cannot distinguish an acute vaso-occlusive episode from the baseline condition. Other causes of pain, fever, and worsening anemia must be excluded. Acute chest syndrome is the second most common acute event, the clinical presentation of which has been discussed previously. Patients with SCD are at increased risk for infection due to splenic dysfunction, especially from encapsulated organisms such as *Streptococcus pneumoniae* and *Haemophilus influenzae*. Vaccines against both of these infectious agents are recommended.[4] Urinary tract infections are common, particularly in pregnant patients.

Pregnant patients are at increased risk for maternal complications[5] because of increased metabolic demands, hypercoagulable state, and venous stasis, and for fetal complications related to compromised placental blood flow. Maternal and fetal complications of SCD are listed in Table 31–1.

Diagnosis

SCD is inherited in a straightforward autosomal recessive pattern. Cellulose acetate gel hemoglobin electrophoresis is the definitive test to identify carriers and those affected with SCD. Individuals of African, African American, Mediterranean, Middle eastern, and Asian Indian descent should be offered this testing because of increased carrier frequencies in these populations. Solubility tests such as Sickledex are not appropriate for screening[6] because they will fail to identify carriers of β thalassemia and abnormal hemoglobins other than hemoglobin S. Prenatal diagnosis is available for couples at risk for fetal hemoglobinopathy by analysis of fetal DNA from chorionic villi or amniotic fluid.

Table 31–1 MATERNAL AND FETAL COMPLICATIONS OF SICKLE CELL DISEASE IN PREGNANCY

MATERNAL	FETAL
Acute chest syndrome	Intrauterine growth restriction
Infection	Prematurity
Thrombosis/thromboembolism	Perinatal death
Preeclampsia/eclampsia	
PROM/preterm labor	
Placental abruption	
Death	

PROM = premature rupture of membranes.

Treatment

All patients with SCD should be seen regularly for health care maintenance. For pregnant women, meticulous prenatal care with attention to known complications of SCD may improve outcome. A team approach is optimal, including obstetrics/maternal-fetal medicine, hematology, pain management, and social services. Baseline physical findings and laboratory values should be established. Patients should be immunized against S pneumoniae, H influenzae type B, hepatitis B virus, and influenza. Folic acid requirements are increased due to intense hematopoiesis; a dose of 4 mg/d is recommended.[6] Iron stores are increased in most women with SCD due to chronic hemolysis and/or blood transfusions; however, iron deficiency may be present in up to 20%. Accordingly, iron supplementation should be reserved for patients with low plasma iron or serum ferritin. Frequent screening for and treatment of bacteriuria are essential to prevent pyelonephritis, which may precipitate a vaso-occlusive episode.

Pregnant women with SCD are at increased risk for fetal growth restriction, preterm labor, and perinatal mortality. Serial sonograms to monitor fetal growth are recommended. Antepartum testing should be initiated if complications develop; the benefit of routine fetal surveillance in patients with SCD has not been established. The signs and symptoms of preterm labor should be reviewed with the patient at each prenatal visit.

The value of prophylactic blood transfusion in pregnancy is debated. Transfusion has been shown to reduce the incidence of acute painful episodes, but a randomized trial showed no improvement in perinatal outcome.[7] Risks include hemolytic transfusion reactions, alloimmunization, and hepatitis.

In most centers management is individualized, with transfusion reserved for patients with prior poor obstetrical outcome or frequent vaso-occlusive episodes.

Acute painful episodes may have no identifiable cause or may be precipitated by infection, dehydration, stress, or weather conditions. Episodes usually last for 2 to 7 days. The mainstays of treatment are exclusion of causes other than vaso-occlusion, hydration, and aggressive opiate pain relief. Supplemental oxygen may reduce sickling in small vessels. Nonsteroidal anti-inflammatory drugs, hydroxyurea, and 5-azacytidine, which are commonly used in nonpregnant patients, may have adverse fetal effects and should be avoided. Fetal assessment may demonstrate a nonreactive non-stress test, which will often become reactive with resolution of the painful episode.

Spontaneous labor at term and vaginal delivery are preferred. The patient should have adequate pain relief, oxygenation, and hydration. Epidural analgesia is recommended. Compatible blood should be available and consideration given to preoperative transfusion for severely anemic patients when cesarean section is contemplated. A cord blood sample collected at delivery is useful to screen for hemoglobinopathy in the newborn. Breast-feeding is not contraindicated unless the patient is taking medications that would make it inadvisable. Combined oral contraceptives do not affect the course of SCD, but some recommend against their use because of the potential for thrombosis related to the estrogen component. Intrauterine devices should not be used routinely because of increased risk of infection. Progesterone-only pills, contraceptive implants, and intramuscular medroxyprogesterone may be the best contraceptive options for women with SCD because **progesterone has been shown to decrease the incidence of painful episodes.**[4]

Comprehension Questions

31.1   In the sickle mutation of the beta-globin gene, what amnio acid is substituted for glutamic acid?
A. Glycine
B. Valine
C. Lysine
D. Arginine

31.2   Which species of Streptococcus is an encapsulated organism?
A. S pyogenes
B. S agalactiae
C. S pneumoniae
D. S fecalis

31.3 Which of the following methods of contraception is the best option for women with sickle cell disease?
   A. Estrogen-containing oral contraceptives
   B. Intrauterine device
   C. Nuva ring (etonogestrel/ethinyl estradiol vaginal ring)
   D. Implanon (etonogestrel) implant

ANSWERS

31.1 **B.** Valine is substituted for glutamic acid in the sixth position of the beta-globin chain.

31.2 **C.** S *pneumoniae*, also known as the pneumococcus, is an encapsulated organism that affects asplenic patients preferentially. Individuals with homozygous SS sickle cell anemia most often suffer auto-infarction of the spleen at an early age.

31.3 **D.** Preferred contraceptives for women with sickle cell disease are progesterone-only methods: IM medroxyprogesterone, the progesterone-only mini-pill, and implants such as Implanon.

Clinical Pearls

See US Preventive Services Task Force Study Quality levels of evidence in Case 1

➤ Hemoglobin electrophoresis is the recommended test to identify carriers of abnormal hemoglobin and those affected with SCD. Solubility tests such as Sickledex are not appropriate for screening (Level II-3).

➤ Pregnant patients with SCD are at increased risk for maternal and fetal complications including infection, thrombosis, preeclampsia, abruption, preterm labor, fetal growth restriction, and perinatal mortality (Level II-2).

➤ The most common acute events in patients with SCD are painful episodes and acute chest syndrome. The mainstays of treatment of an acute painful episode are oxygen administration, hydration, aggressive opiate pain relief, and exclusion of causes other than vaso-occlusion (Level II-2).

➤ Pregnant patients with SCD should receive folic acid supplementation of 4 mg/d. Iron supplementation should be reserved for those with evidence of iron deficiency (Level III).

➤ Progesterone-only contraceptive pills, implants, and intramuscular medroxyprogesterone may be the best contraceptive options for women with SCD (Level II-3).

REFERENCES

1. Gladwin MT, Vichinsky E. Pulmonary complications of sickle cell disease. *N Engl J Med.* 2008;359(21):2254-2265.
2. Campbell K, Ali U, Bahtiyar M. Acute chest syndrome during pregnancy as initial presentation of sickle cell disease: A case report. Am J Perinatol 2008;25:547-550.
3. Stuart MJ, Nagel RL. Sickle-cell disease. *Lancet.* 2004;364:1343-60.
4. Dauphin-McKenzie N, Gilles JM, Jacques E, Harrington T. Sickle cell anemia in the female patient. *Obstet Gynecol Surv.* 2006;61(5):343-352.
5. Villers MS, Jamison MG, De Castro LM, James AH. Morbidity associated with sickle cell disease in pregnancy. *Am J Obstet Gynecol.* 2008;199(2):125.e1-125.e5.
6. ACOG Practice Bulletin No. 78. Hemoglobinopathies in pregnancy. *Obstet Gynecol.* 2007;109(1):229-237.
7. Koshy M, Burd L, Wallace D, Moawad A, Baron J. Prophylactic red-cell transfusions in pregnant patients with sickle cell disease: a randomized cooperative study. *N Engl J Med.* 1988;319(22):1447-1452.

Case 32

A 20-year-old G1P0 at 32 weeks' gestation presents for her first prenatal visit. One year ago, she was hospitalized overnight for symptomatic anemia. At that time she had heavy menses which lasted longer than usual for her just prior to her hospitalization. She also states that she bruises easily. She denies any family history of bleeding disorders or any other significant medical history.

Her antepartum course has been complicated by some spotting in the first trimester. She is feeling fetal movement, and denies leaking of fluid, vaginal bleeding, or contractions. She also states that she has not experienced any headaches, nausea or vomiting, or problems with her eyesight. Her blood pressure in clinic is 120/60 mm Hg with a heart rate of 80 beats per minute, and a negative urine protein. Her abdomen is soft and nontender, with a fundal height of 32 cm. On her extremities, there are several bruises at various stages. Ultrasound shows normal fetal anatomy and is consistent with her last menstrual period. Routine prenatal labs drawn at 32 weeks were normal except for a platelet count of 40,000/mm^3.

➤ What is the most likely diagnosis?

➤ What is the next step?

➤ What are potential complications of the patient's disorder?

ANSWERS TO CASE 32:

Idiopathic Thrombocytopenic Purpura

Summary: This is a 20-year-old G1P0 at 32 weeks' gestation with a past history of menorrhagia, symptomatic anemia requiring transfusion, and easy bruising. She denies any family history of bleeding disorders.

➤ **Most likely diagnosis:** Idiopathic thrombocytopenic purpura (ITP).

➤ **Next step:** Evaluate the patient for bleeding disorders.

➤ **Potential complications:** Hemorrhage, neonatal thrombocytopenia.

ANALYSIS

Objectives

1. Review the differential diagnosis of thrombocytopenia.
2. Outline the evaluation and management of ITP in pregnancy.
3. Describe the indications for and efficacy of treatment modalities for ITP in pregnancy.
4. Discuss delivery mode and neonatal complications associated with ITP in pregnancy.

Considerations

This is a 20-year-old G1P0 with a past history of symptomatic anemia who now presents with thrombocytopenia at 32 weeks. Causes of thrombocytopenia that should be considered in this patient include preeclampsia and HELLP syndrome, gestational thrombocytopenia, and ITP. Less common causes include systemic lupus erythematosus, antiphospholipid antibody syndrome, HIV-associated thrombocytopenia, thrombotic thrombocytopenic purpura (TTP), and medication use.[1] In this patient who is normotensive with negative urine protein, the likelihood of preeclampsia or HELLP syndrome is low. Gestational thrombocytopenia is relatively unlikely since this is usually asymptomatic and platelet count rarely drops below 70,000/mm³. Lupus and TTP can be ruled out by lack of associated symptoms or signs. Antiphospholipid antibodies (lupus anticoagulant, anticardiolipin IgG and IgM, and beta glycoprotein) and HIV can be ruled out by laboratory evaluation. ITP is the most likely diagnosis in this patient since platelet count is less than 50,000/mm³; there are no symptoms or signs of systemic disease and no evidence of HIV, antiphospholipid antibodies, or medication use.

APPROACH TO
Idiopathic Thrombocytopenic Purpura

DEFINITIONS

THROMBOCYTOPENIA: This is defined by some authorities as a platelet count of less than $150 \times 10^9/L$ (150,000/mm^3) and by others as a platelet count of less than $100 \times 10^9/L$ (100,000/mm^3). It is one of the most common hematologic complications of pregnancy.

GESTATIONAL THROMBOCYTOPENIA: This entity can be difficult to distinguish from ITP, and it occurs much more commonly than ITP (7/100 compared to 1/1000). GTP usually has a platelet count above $70 \times 10^9/L$, produces no symptoms, is confined to pregnancy, remits after pregnancy, and is very rarely associated with fetal or neonatal thrombocytopenia.[1]

PLATELET GLYCOPROTEINS: These act as antigens on the platelet surface. A large number of platelet glycoproteins have been identified, among which are IIb/IIIa, Ib/IX, Ia/II, IV, and V. In ITP, autoantibodies bind to these glycoprotein antigens resulting in rapid clearance from the circulation, predominately in the liver and spleen. An increase in megakaryocytes in the bone marrow cannot compensate for the destruction of platelets and the peripheral platelet count drops, sometimes to very low levels.[2]

CLINICAL APPROACH

Thrombocytopenia, defined as a platelet count of less than $150 \times 10^9/L$ (150,000/mm^3), is one of the most common hematologic complications of pregnancy. Idiopathic thrombocytopenic purpura accounts for only a small percentage of thrombocytopenia occurring in pregnancy; however, it does carry substantial risks for both the mother and fetus. Therefore, it is necessary that obstetricians be aware of the diagnosis of this disease and its treatment.

Pathologically, ITP is an autoimmune disorder in which IgG antibodies are formed to platelet antigens. Up to 50% to 60% of patients with the disorder have antibodies to platelet glycoproteins IIb/IIIa. Both direct and indirect tests are available for measuring the antiplatelet antibodies. For the direct test, the patient's platelets are combined with anti-IgG ^{125}I and the resulting level of radioactivity is measured. For the indirect test, the patient's plasma is combined with normal platelets. A wash is then applied, and the radioactivity measured as with the direct test. These antiplatelet antibody assays have a specificity above 90%; however, IgG antibody levels are not elevated in all patients with ITP. In up to 30% of patients, there are normal levels of platelet-associated IgG but elevated levels of platelet-associated C3. The utility of antiplatelet antibody testing is uncertain.[4] Therefore, ITP remains primarily a clinical diagnosis of exclusion and confirmatory laboratory studies are not required.

The established criteria for diagnosis of ITP originally described by Cines et al[3] include the following:

- Normal blood count indices apart from thrombocytopenia
- Bone marrow biopsy which shows increased size and number of megakaryocytes
- Peripheral blood smear showing an increased percentage of large platelets
- Normal coagulation panel
- No other obvious causes of thrombocytopenia (ie, preeclampsia, TTP)

Bone marrow biopsy is usually not required to make the diagnosis. Once a diagnosis of ITP has been made, the pregnant patient is generally treated according to the guidelines for nonpregnant adults. These guidelines are based on the patient's current platelet count and symptomatology (presence of petechiae or easy bruising), and include stepwise introduction of corticosteroids, immunosuppressive therapy, and splenectomy. The current recommendations from the American Society of Hematology[4] are shown in Table 32–1.

If platelet count is less than $50,000/mm^3$, prednisone is usually recommended at a starting dose of 1 to 2 mg/kg. Intravenous immunoglobulin (IVIg) should be considered as first-line treatment in patients with platelet counts less than $10,000/mm^3$ or in those with platelet counts between 10,000 and $30,000/mm^3$ accompanied by significant bleeding. It would be appropriate second-line therapy for those with similar platelet counts who have not shown improvement following 2 to 4 weeks of prednisone treatment. Splenectomy should be reserved for those patients in the second trimester

Table 32–1 THROMBOCYTOPENIA: CLINICAL MANIFESTATIONS AND TREATMENT

PLATELET COUNT(MM³)	SYMPTOMS	RECOMMENDATIONS
> 50,000	None or mild purpura	No treatment
30,000-50,000	Asymptomatic	May consider prednisone
	Minor purpura	Prednisone
	Mucous membrane or vaginal bleeding	Prednisone; may consider hospitalization, IVIg
	Severe, life-threatening bleeding	Hospitalization, prednisone, IVIg
< 30,000	With or without symptoms	Prednisone +/− IVIg

IVIg = Intravenous immunoglobulin

who have failed glucocorticoid and IVIg therapy, are bleeding, and have platelet counts of less than 10,000/mm^3. One key difference between the treatment of ITP in pregnant and nonpregnant adults is that the alternative immunosuppressive agents such as cyclophosphamide, vincristine, vinblastine, danazol, and azathioprine are usually avoided during pregnancy.

The goal of therapy in patients with ITP in pregnancy is to induce remission and support the platelet count until delivery can occur. Neither corticosteroids nor IVIg provide cures for a patient with ITP. Studies of the efficacy of corticosteroids have found a transient response in 75% of patients, but in only 14% to 33% of cases was the response sustained.

While the antiplatelet antibodies responsible for ITP are of the IgG class and can cross the placenta, there is little correlation between maternal and neonatal platelet count. If maternal platelet count is less than 50,000/mm^3, the fetus has a 6% to 10% risk of thrombocytopenia at birth, and only a 1% to 5% risk of severe thrombocytopenia.[5] The overall risk of intraventricular hemorrhage (IVH) is less than 1%. Due to this relatively low risk of IVH, cordocentesis and fetal scalp sampling to assess fetal platelet count prior to deciding on route of delivery are no longer recommended. The presence and level of platelet-associated IgG are also not predictive of neonatal platelet count. Finally, there is substantial evidence that shows that vaginal delivery of women with ITP does not increase neonatal morbidity. Thus, cesarean section should be reserved for obstetrical indications.[6]

Comprehension Questions

32.1   A 25-year-old patient at 24 weeks' gestation presents to your office with a known history of ITP and a platelet count of 30,000/mm^3. She denies bleeding. The only notable physical examination finding is the presence of mild purpura on her lower extremities. Which of the following is the most appropriate treatment for this patient?

A. No treatment
B. Prednisone
C. IVIg
D. Splenectomy

32.2   A 32-year-old woman with known ITP at 34 weeks' gestation presents to your office for consultation regarding a plan for labor and delivery. What should you recommend?

A. Percutaneous umbilical blood sampling weekly.
B. Elective cesarean delivery at 37 weeks.
C. Awaits spontaneous labor.
D. Induce labor at 37 weeks.

32.3 Which of the following is helpful for the diagnosis of ITP?
  A. Antiplatelet antibodies
  B. Normal complete blood count except for thrombocytopenia
  C. Presence of small platelets on peripheral smear
  D. A coagulation panel suggestive of DIC

ANSWERS

32.1 **B.** In a patient with a platelet count of 30,000 who is either asymptomatic or has only mild purpura, prednisone is the most appropriate initial therapy. IVIg might be considered in this patient if she does not respond to the prednisone, or if her clinical circumstances worsen. This patient is not an appropriate candidate for splenectomy.

32.2 **C.** Multiple studies have failed to show reduction in intracranial hemorrhage among infants of mothers who underwent elective cesarean section. Induction of labor increases the risk of cesarean. The best choice is to await spontaneous labor, reserving cesarean for obstetric indications.

32.3 **B.** While the presence of antiplatelet antibodies is supportive, there is a subset of ITP patients in whom the antiplatelet antibody level will not be elevated. In ITP, the peripheral smear shows enlarged platelets. The coagulation panel is normal in patients with ITP.

Clinical Pearls

See US Preventive Services Task Force Study Quality levels of evidence in Case 1

➤ Patients with ITP have isolated thrombocytopenia, enlarged platelets on peripheral smear, and no other cause of thrombocytopenia (Level II-3).
➤ Patients with ITP may or may not have elevated antiplatelet antibody levels; the diagnosis is clinical (Level III).
➤ Treatment of ITP is generally not indicated with platelet count above 50,000 (Level III).
➤ If indicated, treatment should consist of prednisone and/or IVIg depending on platelet count and symptoms (Level III).
➤ Neither maternal platelet count nor antiplatelet antibody levels are reliable predictors of neonatal thrombocytopenia (Level II-3).
➤ Cesarean section is not beneficial in reducing neonatal intracranial hemorrhage (Level II-3).

REFERENCES

1. ACOG Practice Bulletin No. 6. Thrombocytopenia in Pregnancy, September 1999.
2. Sukenik-Halevy R, Ellis MH, Fejgin MD. Management of immune thrombocytopenic purpura in pregnancy. *Obstet Gynecol Survey*. 2008;63:182-188.
3. Cines DB, Blanchett VS. Immune thrombocytopenic purpura. *N Eng J Med*. 2002;346:995.
4. George JN, Woolf SH, Raskob GE, et al. Idiopathic thrombocytopenic purpura: a practice guideline developed by explicit methods for the American Society of Hematology. *Blood*. 1996;88:3-40.
5. Kelton JG. Idiopathic thrombocytopenia purpura complicating pregnancy. *Blood Rev*. 2002;16:43-46.
6. Gernsheimer T, McCrae KR. Immune thrombocytopenic purpura in pregnancy. *Curr Opin Hematol*. 2007;14:574-580.

Case 33

A 26-year-old female, G3P2002 at 25 weeks' gestation, presents to the labor and delivery suite with a complaint of 5 days of coughing and flu-like symptoms and shortness of breath. She states that one of her children has had similar symptoms. She has had fever and chills but no nausea or vomiting. Her medical history is significant for seasonal allergies. On initial evaluation she is found to have a respiratory rate of 42 breaths/min, temperature 101°F, blood pressure 136/82 mm Hg, pulse 122 bpm. A pulse oximeter is applied and her saturation (SpO_2) is 90%. Her physical examination shows a weight of 230 lb, a height of 64 in, a nontender gravid uterus of appropriate size, coarse breath sounds bilaterally with few expiratory wheezes, and diminished sounds at both lung bases. She has no jugular venous distention, and her heart is regular in rhythm, without murmurs, rubs, or gallop. Electronic fetal monitoring reveals irregular low-amplitude contractions and fetal heart rate of 177 beats per minute with minimal variability. Arterial blood gas values are pH: 7.26, CO_2: 52 mmHg, PaO_2: 65 mmHg, HCO_3: 21 mEq/L. Her hematocrit is 34%, with a WBC of 14,000/mm^3 and a slight bandemia. Her platelet count is 160,000/mm^3. A shielded chest x-ray is obtained and reveals a pattern of diffuse patchy infiltrates in all lung fields and consolidation in the right lower lobe. It is interpreted as possible early acute respiratory distress syndrome (ARDS) or pneumonia.

➤ What are possible initial diagnoses?

➤ What should be your initial steps?

➤ What are potential complications from her disorder?

ANSWERS TO CASE 33:
Ventilator Management

Summary: A 26-year-old woman who is at 25 weeks' gestation has respiratory insufficiency, and arterial blood gas findings of hypoxemia and hypercarbia.

➤ **Initial diagnoses:** Viral upper respiratory infection, pneumonia secondary to URI, bronchospastic process like asthma, acute lung injury/early ARDS.

➤ **Initial steps:** IV access and cautious hydration, oxygenation, obtain arterial blood gases and chest x-ray, ICU/anesthesiologist consultation.

➤ **Potential complications:** Respiratory failure, fetal compromise from prolonged hypoxemia, sepsis, potential multiple organ failure.

ANALYSIS

Objectives

1. Recognize the differential diagnoses for respiratory failure.
2. Be familiar with the respiratory changes in pregnancy that will impact mechanical ventilation.
3. Learn about the use of ventilator support and potential lung injury and hemodynamic compromise.
4. Recognize complications from ventilatory support (barotrauma, oxygen toxicity).

Considerations

The physiologic changes of pregnancy predispose a pregnant woman to develop severe respiratory compromise from what can appear at times to be a non-severe insult. Oxygen consumption rises by nearly 20% in pregnancy, therefore, there are many changes in respiratory function to ensure that this increased demand for O_2 is met. Maternal minute ventilation is increased by 50% in pregnancy. As there is essentially no increase in respiratory rate in pregnancy, this increase in minute ventilation results from the almost 40% increase in tidal volume. Concomitant with this is a decrease in the functional residual capacity. These changes induce a respiratory alkalosis that is compensated for by an increase in bicarbonate excretion by the kidneys. The maternal end result is a state of compensated respiratory alkalosis with an almost normal pH (7.4-7.44) and a decrease in the $PaCO_2$ to 30 to 31 mm Hg, and a serum bicarbonate level of 18 to 22 mEq/L. The overall effect is to optimize fetal O_2 exchange and eliminate fetal CO_2. However, these changes also mean that the pregnant woman is more likely to experience rapid declines in oxygenation and be less able to buffer an acidosis, thus making her susceptible to significant compromise by smaller insults. Due to a decrease in plasma colloid osmotic pressure, the pregnant patient is also at increased risk for developing pulmonary edema.

APPROACH TO
Ventilator Management

DEFINITIONS

ACUTE RESPIRATORY DISTRESS SYNDROME (ARDS): Formerly "adult" instead of "acute", its origin dates back to the 1960s. To diagnose it, there should be no evidence of heart failure. Diffuse infiltrates on chest x-ray are caused by noncardiogenic pulmonary edema and the result is severe hypoxemia that does not usually respond to supplemental oxygen. A key component of the definition of ARDS is a PaO_2 to FIO_2 ratio of less than 200.

BAROTRAUMA: A term which encompasses complications like pneumothorax and pneumomediastinum. It can accompany the high ventilatory pressures sometimes needed to achieve adequate oxygenation. Any of several pressures—high PEEP, high peak inspiratory pressure or plateau pressure—associated with positive pressure mechanical ventilation may cause barotrauma.

CLINICAL APPROACH

This 26-year-old gravida presents with symptoms and signs of respiratory failure. Respiratory failure in the pregnant woman can result from conditions that may or may not be related to pregnancy such as infection, trauma, drug overdose, cardiogenic pulmonary edema, hypertension, hemorrhage, asthma, aspiration, and pulmonary emboli. Pregnancy-specific conditions such as preeclampsia, HELLP syndrome, pulmonary edema due to tocolytic agents, chorioamnionitis, and amniotic fluid embolism should also be considered in the differential diagnoses. The initial goals for the patient in respiratory failure are stabilization and a thorough investigation for an underlying cause. Immediate respiratory support is often necessary. Options for therapy range from conservative management with face-mask oxygenation, bronchodilators, and diuresis to mechanical ventilatory support. A thorough history and physical examination, combined with laboratory findings such as hematocrit, white blood cell count, arterial blood gases, and electrolytes as well as selected imaging studies (shielded chest x-rays, CT scanning, ultrasound, or echocardiograms) should help to determine the etiology and guide therapy. ARDS typically yields diffuse interstitial infiltrates on the chest x-ray (Figure 33–1). In the pregnant woman at or beyond the stage of viability (24 wk), fetal status

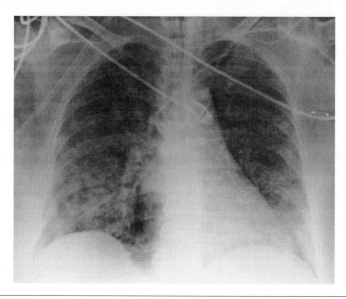

Figure 33–1. A chest radiograph showing the exudative phase of ARDS with diffuse interstitial and alveolar infiltrates. *(Reproduced, with permission, from Fauci AS et al (eds).* Harrison's Principles of Internal Medicine. *17th ed. New York, NY: McGraw-Hill; 2008:1681.)*

will also need to be considered in the initial assessment and a plan outlining timing and route of delivery may be necessary. Fetuses remote from term may best be served by remaining in utero during maternal therapy. Those with a high likelihood of survival may be better managed by delivery when an opportunity arises. In any case, the safety of the mother must be placed first. In the mother with respiratory failure, measures to ensure maternal safety will also be the best initial steps for the fetus.

Steps to relieve hypoxemia, preserve airway, and improve ventilation must be among the first actions. A patient who presents with hyperventilation in the face of a rising CO_2 and diminished PO_2 has impending respiratory failure and should be considered a candidate for mechanical ventilation. Several factors have to be weighed simultaneously. The overall goal is to restore oxygenation, maintain a near-normal pH if possible, and eliminate excess CO_2. Choices in optimum ventilatory rate, tidal volume, oxygen percentage, and the possible addition of positive end expiratory pressure (PEEP) must be weighed against the potential for barotrauma and worsening hemodynamic performance secondary to increased intrathoracic pressure and lower intravascular volume. Similarly, in choosing the mode of ventilation (pressure vs volume-driven modes), lung compliance and the possibility of inducing bronchospasm must be considered. Table 33–1 presents choices in ventilation with their benefits and drawbacks.

Table 33–1 VENTILATION METHODS AND MODES

VENTILATION METHODS

	BENEFITS	DRAWBACKS	COMMENTS
Pressure-targeted ventilation	Improved control over airway pressure and increased ability to work synchronously with patient respiratory efforts.	Decreased control over volume in the face of decreased compliance or resistance.	Preferred choice if overdistension/barotrauma key concern (barotrauma still possible with this modality).
Volume assist-control ventilation (VACV)	Improved control over minute ventilation and CO_2 elimination.	Decreased control over airway and alveolar pressure.	May be preferred choice if CO_2 clearance is key concern.

VENTILATOR MODES (TRADITIONAL)

	DESCRIPTION	BENEFITS	RISKS/DRAWBACKS
Controlled mechanical ventilation (CMV)	Ventilator does all respiratory work at present volume and rate with no patient effort.		
Assist-control ventilation (ACV)	Patient triggers breath but ventilator provides set tidal volume breath. If spontaneous rates fall below set value, ventilator initiated breath delivered.	Work of breathing minimized.	Patients with tachypnea may develop respiratory alkalosis. Attempts to exhale against ventilator-driven inspiration can cause significant barotraumas.
Intermittent mandatory ventilation (IMV)	Combination of fully spontaneous breaths at patient-driven rate and tidal volume and additional ventilator breaths at preset rate and tidal volume.	Decreased risk of alkalosis, decreased risk of increased intrathoracic pressures, less requirement for patient sedation or paralysis.	Increased work of breathing and patient fatigue.
Synchronized intermittent mandatory ventilation (SIMV)	Patient-activated demand valve that allows mechanical breath in concert with patient's respiratory effort.	Greater patient comfort. Lower airway pressures.	Increased work of breathing and patient fatigue.

(Continued)

Table 33–1 VENTILATION METHODS AND MODES (CONT.)

VENTILATOR MODES (NEW)
Developed to address management challenges associated with ARDS

	DESCRIPTION	BENEFITS	RISKS/DRAWBACKS
Inverse ratio ventilation (IRV)	Instead of a one-third inspiration and two-thirds expiration in each cycle this ratio is inversed to achieve better oxygenation through higher mean alveolar pressure and volume with lower peak airway pressures (due to expanded inspiration time).	Good for recruitment of atelectatic areas in patients with worsening lung compliance. Reduced peak airway pressure.	Patient will require heavy sedation or paralysis. Hyperinflation may occur with air-trapping leading to trauma or hemodynamic compromise secondary to increased intrathoracic pressure.
Pressure support ventilation (PSV)	Ventilator provides preset level of pressure to patient-initiated inspiration. Passive exhalation.	Reduced breathing workload. Good weaning strategy.	No set rate so may have variable minute ventilation which may be suboptimal if patient has inconsistent respiratory drive.
Proportional assist ventilation	Ventilator provides inspiration assistance to patient-initiated inspiration that is proportional to patient effort.	Reduced working load. More consistent minute ventilation.	Not well studied.

ADDITIONAL VENTILATION STRATEGIES			
	DESCRIPTION	BENEFITS	RISKS/DRAWBACKS
High-frequency ventilation	Administration of small tidal volumes at high frequency.	Minimizes airway pressure.	May have impaired CO_2 removal.
Positive end expiratory pressure (PEEP)	Threshold resistor in exhalation that impedes flow if expiratory pressure is low.	Increases functional residual capacity and may reinflate collapsed alveoli.	May result in cardiovascular alterations and thus requires hemodynamic monitoring.

Data from Van Hook JW. Acute respiratory distress syndrome in pregnancy. *Semin Perinatol.* 1997;21(4):320-327; and Whitty JE. Airway management in critical illness. In: Dildy GA, Belfort MA, Saade GR, et al. (eds). *Critical Care Obstetrics.* 4th ed. London: Wiley-Blackwell Publishing; 2003.

Ventilator and Hemodynamic Management

Initial settings for mechanical ventilation should attempt to establish the optimal minute ventilatory rate to improve oxygenation with the lowest risk for barotrauma. For example, with volume-driven modes such as assist control, volume control, or synchronized intermittent mandatory ventilation (SIMV), a tidal volume of approximately 5 to 8 cc/kg, with a rate of 12 breaths per minute would deliver a reasonable 6 to 7 L per minute respiratory volume to a 100 kg woman. Whether or not to maintain this volume should be determined by its impact on peak and mean airway pressures and the risk of lung trauma. If a volume mode appears to generate unacceptably high airway pressures, a pressure-regulated mode may be preferable. In that case, pressures should be established that result in volumes adequate to achieve oxygenation and CO_2 elimination. Initially a fractionally inspired oxygen (FIO_2) of 100% should be chosen.[1] It is a generally acceptable practice to attempt weaning of FIO_2 to a level below 50% as soon as it can be done while maintaining oxygen saturation levels above 94%. Weaning must be gradual, due to the fact that when a critical PaO_2 to PAO_2 ratio is reached, small changes in FIO_2 can produce large drops in oxygenation. In order to improve oxygen delivery, and achieve a lowering of the FIO_2, addition of positive end expiratory pressure (PEEP) can be considered. This, however, may induce two factors that can have a negative impact on lung dynamics and systemic oxygen delivery. First, the addition of PEEP will often increase peak airway pressures and increase the risk of barotrauma. It is therefore considered prudent to try to maintain peak and mean airway pressures below 35 cm H_2O. Second, with a patient who has poor intravascular filling either from prolonged work of breathing and insensible fluid losses, or hemodynamic shifts from third spacing, the addition of PEEP may lead to cardiovascular compromise and a decrease in cardiac output, venous return, and delivery of oxygen to the fetus. Maintaining euvolemia is also an integral part of management. Because of the need for close monitoring of hemodynamic status, an arterial line should be placed, and serious consideration should be given to early placement of a pulmonary arterial catheter for monitoring cardiac output and preload values (CVP, PAWP).

ARDS

A reasonable assumption for the patient presented in the preceding discussion is that her compromise is due to a persistent upper respiratory infection, with a possible underlying opportunistic bacterial pneumonia. Her history and physical examination, as well as laboratory and imaging results, are strongly suggestive of acute respiratory distress syndrome. The presentation and current status of this patient makes her a candidate for mechanical ventilation with possible hemodynamic support. Sedation and/or paralysis of the patient may be necessary if long-term mechanical ventilation is required.

Table 33–2 DEFINITION OF ACUTE LUNG INJURY AND ACUTE
RESPIRATORY DISTRESS SYNDROME

Acute lung injury
- Acute onset
- $Pao_2/FiO2 \leq 300$ mm Hg (regardless of PEEP)
- Bilateral infiltrates on chest x-ray
- Pulmonary artery occlusion pressure of ≤ 18 mm Hg

ARDS
All of the above except:
- $Pao_2/FiO2 \leq 200$ mm Hg (regardless of PEEP)

Data from Bernard GR, Artigas A, Brigham KL, et al. Report of the American-European Consensus conference on acute respiratory distress syndrome: definitions, mechanisms, relevant outcomes, and clinical trial coordination. Consensus Committee. *J Crit Car.* 1994;9(1):72-81.

As defined by the American-European Consensus Committee (Table 33–2), acute respiratory distress syndrome (ARDS) is the most severe form of acute lung injury (ALI).[2] This injury is a result of an inflammatory process that produces diffuse alveolar damage in both lungs which, in turn, leads to flooding of the alveoli and compromises pulmonary gas exchange and leads to decreased lung compliance and increased pulmonary arterial pressure. As in the case described in the preceding discussion, patients with ARDS will typically present with signs and symptoms of both the underlying/precipitating disease and of the ARDS—which can include chest pain, cough, tachypnea, dyspnea, tachycardia, and hypoxemia. A key feature of ARDS is the development of a large shunt. Patients with this disorder, therefore, will have poor or minimal response to supplemental oxygen therapy. Mechanical ventilation will, therefore, almost always be required in the management of a patient with ARDS. Regardless of treatment modality, **ARDS in pregnancy is associated with a high fetal and maternal mortality.** Maternal mortality is reported to be between 14% and 44%.[3-6] The most common cause of maternal death in pregnant patients with ARDS is multiple organ dysfunction syndrome (MODS).

The main goal of management in the presence of ARDS is to provide respiratory support while the underlying condition is treated and/or resolved and the acute lung injury healed. Concurrent goals are to minimize barotrauma, provide adequate nutritional support, and prevent complications such as nosocomial infections and deep vein thrombosis (DVT).[7] There is not a clearly preferred method of mechanical ventilation in ARDS, but there are some basic principles to bear in mind when choosing a mode of ventilatory support in ARDS. The goal is to "recruit" undamaged alveoli. It is a fine balance to obtain desirable gas exchange using these undamaged alveoli without causing additional damage. High tidal volume ventilation can damage unaffected alveoli, so ventilation strategy should aim to limit overdistension of these unaffected alveoli, therefore, lower tidal volume may be needed. Peak plateau airway pressure of less than 35 cm H_2O is preferable.[7] The respiratory rate will need to be increased in order to compensate for decreases in tidal volume. Airway pressure release ventilation (APRV) or high-frequency oscillatory ventilation (HFOV) may be needed in patients with persistent respiratory failure in the face of low-tidal ventilation.

One strategy that is employed to reduce the risk of tidal volume-related barotrauma in ARDS is that of "permissive hypercapnia" in which the tidal volume is lower than that conventionally used and the arterial PCO_2 is allowed to rise above normal. A theoretical negative effect of this strategy is difficulty removing carbon dioxide from the fetal compartment, and therefore it should be used with caution during pregnancy. An important goal in caring for pregnant women with respiratory failure is to optimize fetal outcomes. Delivery is often necessary, and while some studies have suggested that delivery improves the respiratory status of the critically ill gravida, these studies are limited. There is currently not enough data to clearly guide decisions regarding timing and route of delivery.[3,8] When immediate delivery is not necessary or not possible due to maternal status, attempt at a vaginal delivery appears to be a reasonable option as it is associated with smaller fluid shifts and avoids other risks of surgery—all are desirable goals in this population. In one case series that included 43 pregnant women on ventilator support, 86% of the women delivered during their admission (mean EGA [estimated gestational age] was 31.6 wk).[3] Of these, 65% underwent cesarean delivery primarily for obstetric complications. Maternal mortality in this study was 14% and perinatal mortality was 11%. The leading cause of perinatal mortality was complications of prematurity.

Summary

Respiratory failure in the pregnant patient presents significant challenges. Early recognition of respiratory failure and prompt initiation of respiratory support are essential. Identification and treatment of underlying causes of respiratory failure/ARDS is also critical. Throughout management of these patients, the physiologic changes of pregnancy that affect respiratory function must be continuously considered. A plan for delivery based on ensuring maternal safety is also important. A coordinated response and management by a team that includes an obstetrician and an intensivist (either obstetric or medical) as well as anesthesiologists, a neonatologist, and skilled nursing care will help to optimize outcomes for these critically ill mothers and their fetuses. When ventilation will be prolonged, supportive care to include DVT prophylaxis with heparin and/or sequential compression devices, adequate nutrition, and medical management to reduce gastrointestinal stress should also be provided.

Comprehension Questions

33.1 A pregnant patient at 32 weeks EGA presents with respiratory failure; her fetal heart rate tracing reveals a baseline of 160 beats per minute, minimal variability, and late decelerations. Which of the following is the best approach regarding delivery?

A. Deliver the patient as soon as possible as this will maximize the chance of fetal survival and will help improve maternal status.

B. Stabilize and intubate the patient and deliver for obstetric indications.

C. Stabilize and intubate the patient and then proceed with a cesarean section.

D. Proceed to delivery only if there is maternal cardiac arrest.

33.2 Which of the following statements regarding ARDS in the obstetric patient is true?

A. Fetal/perinatal mortality is high when there is ARDS in pregnancy, but maternal mortality is low.

B. Most cases of ARDS respond to management with supplemental oxygen.

C. Pregnant women with ARDS will almost always require mechanical ventilation.

D. Sepsis is the leading cause of death among pregnant women with ARDS.

33.3 It is preferable in the management of ARDS to maintain peak and mean airway pressures below which level?

A. 30 cm H_2O
B. 35 cm H_2O
C. 40 cm H_2O
D. 45 cm H_2O

ANSWERS

33.1 **B.** By stabilizing and intubating the patient, oxygenation will be improved, and the fetal heart rate pattern is likely to normalize.

33.2 **C.** ARDS in pregnant woman often requires mechanical ventilation.

33.3 **B.** It is optimal to maintain peak and mean airway pressures below 35 cm H_2O to minimize the risk of barotrauma.

Clinical Pearls

See US Preventive Services Task Force Study Quality levels of evidence in Case 1

➤ Respiratory adaptations of pregnancy that promote increased oxygen availability and facilitate CO_2 elimination also make pregnant women particularly susceptible to respiratory failure (Level III).

➤ Early recognition of respiratory failure, and endotracheal and mechanical ventilation intubation to restore oxygenation and adequate CO_2 elimination is crucial in order to optimize maternal and fetal outcomes (Level III).

➤ Avoiding both barotrauma and oxygen toxicity is important in ventilator management. This may involve permissive hypercapnia to limit both peak and plateau inspiratory pressures (Level II-3).

➤ Positive end expiratory pressure (PEEP) is often necessary to obtain adequate oxygenation in ARDS. PEEP, however, increases the risk of cardiovascular compromise and, therefore, hemodynamic monitoring is indicated (Level II-3).

➤ With respiratory failure, fetal status will be optimized when maternal status is optimized (especially in the initial period of stabilization). When determining when and how to deliver the obstetric patient with ARDS, maternal safety must drive decision-making. In almost all cases, emergent cesarean section of the gravida on mechanical ventilation should be undertaken for obstetric and maternal indications (worsening preeclampsia, HELLP, maternal cardiac arrest) and not for fetal indications (Level III).

REFERENCES

1. Parrillo JE. Adult respiratory distress syndrome. In: *Current Therapy in Critical Care Medicine*. St Louis, MO: Mosby; 1997.
2. Bernard GR, Artigas A, Brigham KL, et al. Report of the American-European Consensus conference on acute respiratory distress syndrome: definitions, mechanisms, relevant outcomes, and clinical trial coordination. Consensus Committee. *J Crit Car.* 1994;9(1):72-81.
3. Jenkins TM, Troiano NH, Graves CR, Baird SM, Boehm FH. Mechanical ventilation in an obstetric population: characteristics and delivery rates. *Am J Obstet Gynecol.* 2003;188:549-552.
4. Mabie WC, Barton JR, Sibai BM. Adult respiratory distress syndrome in pregnancy. *Am J Obstet Gynecol.* 1992;167:950-957.
5. Chen CY, Chaen CP, Wang KG, Kuo SC, Su TH. Factors implicated in the outcome of pregnancies complicated by acute respiratory failure. *J Reprod Med.* 2003;48:641-648.
6. Cole DE, Taylor TL, McCullough DM, Shoff CT, Derdak S. Acute respiratory distress syndrome in pregnancy. *Crit Care Med.* 2005;33:269S-278S.
7. Van Hook JW. Acute respiratory distress syndrome in pregnancy. *Semin Perinatol.* 1997;21(4):320-327.
8. Tomlison MW, Caruthers TJ, Whitty JE, Gonik B. Does delivery improve maternal condition in the respiratory-compromised gravida? *Obstet Gynecol.* 1998;91:108-111.

Case 34

An 18-year-old G1P0 woman at 22 weeks' gestation was admitted to the hospital with a 2-day history of fever, chills, and flank pain. Examination revealed a temperature of 103°F and marked costovertebral angle tenderness on the right. Urinalysis showed 4+ bacteria and many WBCs. Urine and blood cultures were obtained intravenous and ceftriaxone was begun for presumptive pyelonephritis. Lactated Ringer solution was ordered intravenously at 125 cc/h. The next morning, the patient was found to have a blood pressure of 70/30 mm Hg, a temperature of 96°F, pulse of 140 bpm, and respirations of 36 breaths per minute. Her urine output over the previous 12 hours was 200 cc.

➤ What complication of pyelonephritis has she developed?

➤ What is the pathophysiology of this condition?

➤ How should this condition be managed?

ANSWER TO CASE 34:
Septic Shock

Summary: An 18-year-old G1P0 at 22 weeks was admitted to the hospital, diagnosed with pyelonephritis and begun on a suitable intravenous antibiotic. In less than 24 hours, she developed septic shock.

➤ **Complication of pyelonephritis developed:** Septic shock. Shortly after initiating IV antibiotic therapy for pyelonephritis is a time of increased risk for the development of septic shock.

➤ **Pathophysiology of this condition:** Most cases of pyelonephritis in pregnancy are due to infection by gram-negative aerobic bacteria, *Escherichia coli* being the most frequent causative agent. Antibiotic therapy causes lysis of bacteria, and this in turn leads to release of endotoxin. Endotoxin triggers a host inflammatory response culminating in hypotension, decreased tissue perfusion, and septic shock.

➤ **Management of this condition:** The short answer to this question is that septic shock must be managed aggressively. The plan of management consists of early goal-directed therapy characterized by fluid resuscitation, broad spectrum antibiotics, and, if needed, vasopressors to maintain mean arterial pressure above 65 mm Hg. Details are provided in the section Clinical Approach.

ANALYSIS

Objectives

1. Identify the most common obstetric antecedents of septic shock.
2. Review the characteristics of the bacteria that are most commonly etiologic in septic shock in pregnancy.
3. Outline the evolving management of septic shock in pregnancy and the immediate postpartum period.

Considerations

The woman in the case scenario presented with classic signs and symptoms of pyelonephritis. Most cases of pyelonephritis in pregnancy are caused by infection with gram-negative aerobic bacteria, but an increasing number are due to group B *Streptococcus*. In this series of 440 pregnant women hospitalized with acute pyelonephritis, more than half of whom were in their second trimester (as in our case), there were no cases of septic shock specifically mentioned.[1] However, 7% of the women developed pulmonary insufficiency, presumably related to release of endotoxin. In contrast, when the question is reversed, that is, not how many cases of septic shock occurred in pregnant women diagnosed with pyelonephritis, but instead how many cases of pyelonephritis were found in a series of pregnant women with septic shock, pyelonephritis was the leading cause of septic shock in one report[2], accounting for 6 of 18 cases. It is not definitely known whether early diagnosis and aggressive treatment of pyelonephritis in pregnancy would interdict its progression to septic shock, but it makes sense that it would.

APPROACH TO
Septic Shock

DEFINITIONS

ENDOTOXIN: A bacterial toxin not freely released into the surrounding tissue or fluid. It is a lipopolysaccharide component of the cell wall of especially gram-*negative* aerobic bacteria. Its release occurs only upon injury or damage to the bacterial cell wall, which, as in the case described, occasionally occurs after the initiation of treatment.

EXOTOXIN: Also a bacterial toxin, but produced by gram-*positive* bacteria and readily liberated into tissue or fluid. Exotoxins are very potent and rapidly active even when secreted in very small amounts. In the recent obstetric literature exotoxins have accounted for an increasing percentage of cases of sepsis syndrome, septic shock representing the most extreme manifestation of the sepsis syndrome.

SYSTEMIC INFLAMMATORY RESPONSE SYNDROME (SIRS): A response of the host, in our setting generated by infection (but in other settings capable of being caused by noninfectious entities like trauma or burns). It is manifested by two or more of the following criteria: hyperthermia (> 38°C) or hypothermia (< 36°C), tachycardia (HR > 90 bpm), tachypnea (> 20 breaths per minute) or hypocarbia ($PaCO_2$ < 32 mm Hg), abnormal white blood cell count (> 12,000 or < 4000), bandemia (> 10% bands). Importantly, SIRS criteria have not been developed specifically for pregnancy. Also, the definition of SIRS excludes hypotension. Once hypotension develops and persists despite adequate fluid resuscitation, the condition has progressed to septic shock.

CLINICAL APPROACH

This section of the chapter is organized around the three objectives previously stated. According to one expert, septic shock, which accounts for 215,000 deaths per year in the United States, is one of the most challenging problems in all of critical care medicine.[3] Fortunately for obstetricians, it is relatively rare in pregnancy, occurring with a frequency of 1 per 8000 deliveries.[4] Accordingly, there are relatively few reports on septic shock complicating either pregnancy or the puerperium and no trials of therapy conducted exclusively in pregnant women. The most common obstetric antecedents of septic shock are: pyelonephritis, septic abortion, chorioamnionitis, endometritis, and necrotizing fasciitis. Prior to the Supreme Court ruling on Roe v. Wade, septic abortion was the most common of these and it still predominates in countries where abortion is illegal. At the present time in the United States, pyelonephritis is the leading cause of septic shock in pregnant women.

Although many different bacteria are capable of inciting septic shock, only relatively few are important causes of obstetric infection. The predominant gram-negative causes of septic shock can be remembered by the acronym EEKPP—*Escherichia, Enterobacter, Klebsiella, Proteus,* and *Pseudomonas.* Endotoxin released by these agents incites an intense inflammatory response in the host, which then leads to vasodilation, hypotension, inadequate tissue perfusion, lactic acidosis, and, if not reversed, death. Monomicrobial infection is most often seen with pyelonephritis, whereas most other obstetric infections are polymicrobial, and therefore require broad-spectrum antimicrobial therapy, often with multiple agents.

More recently, there has been an upsurge of infections caused by gram-positive organisms including Staphylococci (especially methicillin-resistant subtypes that are either hospital-acquired or community-acquired), group A Streptococci, and *Clostridium sordellii.* These bacteria elaborate powerful exotoxins that can cause widespread tissue destruction.[5-7] The obstetric literature pertaining to these gram-positive infections consists mainly of case reports or very small series. Andrews et al[5] described a woman who developed toxic shock due to methicillin-resistant *Staphylococcus aureus* (MRSA) 4 weeks after a cesarean delivery. The staphylococcus was not identified until hospital day 9, when culture of a left-breast aspirate identified the organism. A toxin assay after discharge from the hospital confirmed the presence of enterotoxin B, one of the three toxins (the other two are enterotoxin C and toxic shock syndrome toxin 1) known to be associated with staphylococcal toxic shock; half of all cases are nonmenstrual.

Obstetric cases have been reported after vaginal and cesarean deliveries, postpartum wound infections, and mastitis. A heart-wrenching case of necrotizing fasciitis after cesarean delivery was reported by deMoya and colleagues.[6] In this case the infecting organism was group A *Streptococcus,* reported to be more lethal than *Staphylococcus.* Group A *Streptococcus* elaborates several exotoxins, for example, exotoxin A, along with other proteins that act as superantigens, triggering massive release of cytokines. The unfortunate patient survived, but with loss of her entire abdominal wall, uterus, tubes, ovaries, gallbladder, right colon, and all four extremities. Lastly, Cohen and colleagues[7] reported four cases of toxic shock following either medical or spontaneous abortion associated with infection by *Clostridium* species, two with perfringens and two with sordellii. *Clostridium sordellii* secretes a potent exotoxin identified as cytotoxin L (L for lethal). All four patients had a rapidly progressive illness with necrotizing endomyometritis and three of the four died.

It is apparent, then, that bacteria and/or their component toxins can produce a sepsis syndrome that, unchecked, will develop into septic shock. The cornerstone of management is early diagnosis, but often that is not easy. A program of early goal-directed therapy[8] has been shown to reduce mortality from septic shock. However, not all patients with septic shock require the same treatment interventions. The woman in our case scenario, for example, requires aggressive fluid resuscitation and transfer to an intensive care unit. Per hour 1 to 2 L (not the 125 cc/h she was receiving) would be appropriate. The total volume needed should be determined by monitoring central venous pressure. An arterial catheter should be placed to monitor blood pressure and obtain timely pH and blood gas measurements. If adequate fluid resuscitation has not elevated the mean arterial pressure above 65 mm Hg, then vasopressors would be indicated. Adequate oxygenation should be maintained, with endotracheal intubation and mechanical ventilation, if necessary. The ceftriaxone she was receiving likely does not need to be changed, but some authorities[1] prefer ampicillin and gentamicin for the treatment of pyelonephritis in pregnancy. Surgical intervention is seldom necessary for septic shock secondary to pyelonephritis, but prolonged hypotension and ischemia can lead to gangrene of the extremities and amputation in severe cases. When septic shock results from necrotizing fasciitis, extensive debridement of necrotic tissue is an essential component of management. Antibiotic therapy should include vancomycin for methicillin-resistant *Staphylococcus* and clindamycin for *Streptococcus*; there is evidence that clindamycin may directly inhibit synthesis of group A streptococcal toxins.

The sequelae of septic shock depend on the duration and severity of the insult. Conditions that are associated with septic shock like acute renal failure, acute respiratory distress syndrome (ARDS), DIC, and abnormal liver function are best managed in an intensive care unit. From the literature, the more organ systems that are involved, the worse the prognosis.

The high mortality associated with septic shock has engendered an impressive number of randomized clinical trials of adjunctive therapies of agents including high-and low-dose corticosteroids, ibuprofen, vasopressin, insulin, activated protein C, and others. The results of such trials are conflicting, inconclusive, or negative in most instances.

Finally, three of the five obstetric antecedents (chorioamnionitis, endometritis, and septic abortion) of septic shock involve infection of the uterus. Necrosis of the uterus, tubes, and ovaries can also complicate necrotizing fasciitis.[6] Therefore, laparotomy with hysterectomy and possible adnexectomy are crucial interventions that an obstetrician-gynecologist may need to undertake to save the life of his or her patient.

Comprehension Questions

34.1 In obstetrics which of the following diagnoses is the leading cause of septic shock?
A. Necrotizing fasciitis
B. Pyelonephritis
C. Chorioamnionitis
D. Endometritis

34.2 Which of the following bacteria elaborates cytotoxin L?
A. Group A *Streptococcus*
B. *Escherichia Coli*
C. MRSA
D. *Clostridium sordellii*

34.3 Which of the following criteria for systemic inflammatory response syndrome (SIRS) is most likely to be affected by altered physiology in pregnancy?
A. Temperature of 39°C
B. Pulse > 90 bpm
C. P_{CO_2} < 32 mmHg
D. WBC > 12,000/mm³

ANSWERS

34.1 **B.** As mentioned in the chapter, there are very few series of septic shock in pregnancy. The answer to this question can be found on page 676 of reference 4.

34.2 **D.** Cytotoxin L has been found in cases of *Clostridium sordellii* infection related to abortion (for extended discussion, see reference 7).

34.3 **C.** Progesterone increases during pregnancy stimulates the respiratory center and minute volume increases. P_{CO_2} is inversely related to minute volume and is therefore reset to a mean of 30 mm Hg. This is the best answer, but choice B has merit as well, since heart rate increases physiologically during pregnancy.

Clinical Pearls

See US Preventive Services Task Force Study Quality levels of evidence in Case 1

➤ Pyelonephritis is one of the most common serious medical complications of pregnancy. Only a few cases result in serious sequelae like ARDS or septic shock—stay alert! (Level III)

➤ Systemic vascular resistance normally decreases in pregnancy, but nowhere near the level seen in septic shock ($\leq$ 400 dyne/sec/cm^{-5}). Such profound vasodilation necessitates aggressive fluid resuscitation and possibly exogenous vasopressors (Level II-3).

➤ Necrotizing fasciitis complicates 1 to 2 per 1000 cesarean deliveries and the cesarean rate is steadily rising. Risk factors include diabetes, obesity, and hypertension—all commonly encountered in pregnant women. Early diagnosis and extensive debridement may prevent septic shock (Level III).

REFERENCES

1. Hill JB, Sheffield JS, McIntire DD, Wendel GD Jr. Acute pyelonephritis in pregnancy. *Obstet Gynecol.* 2005;105:18-23.
2. Mabie WC, Barton JR, Sibai B. Septic shock in pregnancy. *Obstet Gynecol.* 1997;90:553-561.
3. Parillo JE. Septic shock—vasopressin, norepinephrine, and urgency. *N Engl J Med.* 2008;358:954-956.
4. Martin SR, Foley MR. Intensive care in obstetrics: an evidence-based review. *Am J Obstet Gynecol.* 2006;195:673-689.
5. Andrews JI, Shamshirsaz AA, Diekema DJ. Nonmenstrual toxic shock syndrome due to methicillin-resistant staphylococcus aureus. *Obstet Gynecol.* 2008;112:933-938.
6. deMoya MA, del Carmen MG, Allain RM, Hirschberg RE, Sephard JO, Kradin RL. Case 33-2009: A 35-year-old woman with fever, abdominal pain, and hypotension after cesarean section. *N Engl J Med.* 2009;361:1689-1697.
7. Cohen AL, Bhatnagar J, Reagan S, et al. Toxic shock associated with Clostridium sordellii and Clostridium perfringens after medical and spontaneous abortion. *Obstet Gynecol.* 2007;110:1027-1033.
8. Rivers E, Nguyen B, Havstad S, et al. Early goal-directed therapy in the treatment of severe sepsis and septic shock. *N Engl J Med.* 2001;345:1368-1377.
9. Russel JA. Management of sepsis. *N Engl J Med.* 2006;355:1699-1713.
10. Sheffield JS. Sepsis and septic shock in pregnancy. *Crit Care Clin.* 2004;20:651-660.

Case 35

An 18-year-old primigravida at term is admitted to labor and delivery with regular uterine contractions and a history of rupture of the fetal membranes 2 hours prior to admission. She has a positive vaginal culture for group B β-hemolytic *Streptococcus* (GBS) noted at 36 weeks gestation and denies allergies to medications. On examination, she is afebrile, blood pressure is 110/70 mm Hg, pulse is 88 beats per minute, and she is having regular contractions every 3 to 4 minutes. Examination reveals a term size uterus with vertex presentation, fetal heart tones are detected at 140 beats per minute, and cervix is dilated to 6 cm. Amniotic fluid pooling is noted in the vagina at the time of the examination.

An IV is started, and penicillin G, 5 million units is administered intravenously for GBS prophylaxis. As the infusion of penicillin is begun, the patient complains of itching on her arms and head, and hives are noted by her nurse. Within 30 seconds, the patient becomes restless and complains of shortness of breath and dizziness. Her lungs are clear to auscultation and a diffuse urticarial rash is noted. Her pulse is noted to be 160 beats per minute and her blood pressure is noted to be 90/60 mm Hg. The fetal heart rate slows to a rate of 70 beats per minute.

➤ What is the most likely diagnosis?

➤ What is your next step?

➤ What are potential complications of the patient's disorder?

ANSWERS TO CASE 35:
Anaphylactic Reaction to Penicillin

Summary: This is a healthy 18-year-old primigravida at term gestation in labor with the acute onset of urticaria, tachycardia, and hypotension upon administration of penicillin.

> **Most likely diagnosis:** Anaphylaxis to penicillin.

> **Next step:** Discontinue penicillin infusion, begin supportive measures, and administer epinephrine.

> **Potential complications:** Maternal death, fetal anoxic injury, and death.

ANALYSIS

Objectives

1. Describe the pathophysiology of anaphylaxis.
2. Describe the clinical presentation of acute allergic reactions and anaphylaxis.
3. Describe the treatment of anaphylaxis.

Considerations

This healthy 18-year-old woman experienced the acute onset of urticaria, tachycardia, and hypotension upon intrapartum administration of penicillin. While other obstetric emergencies may cause hypotension and tachycardia (such as amniotic fluid embolism, massive pulmonary embolism, or uterine rupture), the combination of rapid appearance of cutaneous manifestations and hemodynamic compromise immediately after penicillin infusion makes anaphylaxis highly likely.

Anaphylaxis is a serious allergic reaction that is rapid in onset and may cause death. It is caused by the interaction of a specific antigen with IgE. The subsequent release of inflammatory mediators results in the **acute onset of symptoms,** usually within minutes of antigen exposure, including wheezing, urticaria, angioedema, flushing, itching, diarrhea and abdominal pain, hypotension, rhinorrhea, and bronchorrhea. The inciting agent may be a food, drug, latex, or insect sting. In up to 50% of cases the culprit allergen is never identified. Antibiotics are arguably the most common cause of drug-induced anaphylaxis, and **β-lactams account for roughly 20% of all drug-related episodes.** Anaphylaxis occurs in approximately 1 in 5000 to 10,000 courses of penicillin therapy.

Immediate intervention is similar to that in the nonpregnant patient and consists of discontinuation of penicillin infusion and provision of **supportive care**. An adequate airway and intravenous access are secured, **aggressive fluid resuscitation** begun, and the mother positioned in left lateral decubitus with Trendelenburg in an effort to **maximize venous return**. **Epinephrine should then be administered (0.2-0.5 mg of a 1:1000 solution intramuscularly every 5 min as needed).** Second-line therapy includes **diphenhydramine, ranitidine, and glucocorticoids**.

In pregnancy, vasoconstriction associated with maternal anaphylaxis may precipitate fetal bradycardia. The first priority is to stabilize the mother; once this is accomplished it is likely that the fetal heart rate will recover, and labor may be allowed to continue. Emergent cesarean delivery has been described, with varying maternal and neonatal outcomes. Successful supportive management with delayed delivery has also been reported. The optimal delivery plan will involve an assessment of the entire clinical picture once all measures have been undertaken to stabilize the mother.

APPROACH TO
Anaphylactic Reaction to Penicillin

Diagnosis

In 2006, the National Institute of Allergy and Infectious Disease/Food Allergy and Anaphylaxis Network symposium set forth clinical criteria for diagnosing anaphylaxis. Anaphylaxis is highly likely when **any one of the following three criteria** is fulfilled:

1. Acute onset of an illness (minutes to several hours) with involvement of the skin, mucosal tissue, or both, and at least one of the following:
   a. Respiratory compromise
   b. Hypotension or associated evidence of end-organ dysfunction
2. Two or more of the following that occur rapidly after exposure to a likely allergen:
   a. Involvement of the skin-mucosal tissue
   b. Respiratory compromise
   c. Hypotension or associated evidence of end-organ dysfunction
   d. Persistent gastrointestinal symptoms
3. Hypotension after exposure to a known allergen (for adults, systolic BP < 90 mm Hg or > 30% decrease from that person's baseline).

Pathophysiology

Anaphylactic reactions are mediated through antigen-induced IgE mast cell and basophil degranulation. Release of histamine and other inflammatory mediators causes spasm of the bronchial, gastrointestinal, and coronary artery smooth muscle, vasodilation, increased vascular permeability, and tachycardia. Wheezing, nausea, vomiting, diarrhea, myocardial ischemia, flushing, hypotension, urticaria, and angioedema may result. Intravascular fluid can be transferred to the extravascular space at a rapid rate (50% within 10 min), so aggressive volume resuscitation is imperative. The loss of intravascular volume invokes compensatory responses, which seem to have variable effects; in some patients, peripheral resistance is elevated to an exaggerated degree, and in others it falls inappropriately despite catecholamine release. From a therapeutic standpoint, it is important to remember that patients in later stages of anaphylactic shock may not respond to pressors if they are already maximally vasoconstricted. Intravenous fluid resuscitation and volume expansion is the treatment of choice in such cases.

Anaphylaxis in pregnancy has been described following laminaria insertion, exercise, induction of general anesthesia, and exposure to latex, antibiotics, iron, ranitidine, local anesthesia, insect stings, and snake antivenom. Strictly speaking, only IgE-dependent events can be termed anaphylaxis. Such a reaction to penicillin occurs when the β-lactam ring is opened and bound to protein in the penicilloyl configuration, forming an antigenic hapten called the major determinant, or when protein binds a minor product of penicillin metabolism (penicilloate or penilloate).

Immediate Management

When faced with a patient with an anaphylactic reaction to penicillin, the obstetrician's first concern is maternal stabilization. The drug infusion should be stopped immediately, and help sought to secure an adequate airway. As described earlier, rapid fluid shifts may deplete intravascular volumes such that massive infusions of crystalloid (up to 7 L) may be necessary. Accordingly, a large (1-2 L) bolus of normal saline should be administered as quickly as possible, and multiple wide-bore intravenous access sites obtained. The gravida should be placed in the left lateral decubitus position with Trendelenburg as tolerated to promote venous return and maximize cardiac output. Oxygen may be administered by face mask or endotracheal tube as necessary, and monitors applied to assess pulse oximetry and maternal and fetal heart rates continuously.

Aqueous epinephrine 1:1000 dilution (1 mg/mL) 0.2 to 0.5 mL intramuscularly or subcutaneously is given every 5 minutes as necessary to control symptoms and increase blood pressure. Available data suggest that the intramuscular route results in faster absorption. The preferred site is the anterior lateral thigh. In patients who do not respond, it may be given intravenously. It may be dosed intermittently (0.1-0.3 mL of 1:1000 concentration diluted in 10 mL of normal saline and given over several minutes), or as a continuous infusion. For a continuous infusion, 1 mg of a 1:1000 solution may be mixed in 250 mL of normal saline and infused at a rate of 1 μg/min to a maximum of 10 μg/min. This technique has been used in pregnancy with success.

Continuous cardiac monitoring is essential in this situation due to the risk for cardiac arrhythmia. Some controversy exists regarding the effect of epinephrine on the pregnant uterus.

Adjunctive measures include histamine receptor antagonists, inhaled β-agonists, and glucocorticoids. The combination of an H_1 and H_2 antagonist is superior to either one alone, but note that these are considered second-line therapy for anaphylaxis and should never be used in isolation. Diphenhydramine 25 to 50 mg and ranitidine 50 mg may be given parenterally. If bronchospasm unresponsive to epinephrine occurs, inhaled β-agonist (nebulized albuterol 2.5-5 mg in 3 mL saline) should be considered. Glucocorticoids are not usually acutely helpful, but in theory may prevent recurrent or prolonged anaphylaxis and should be used in patients with asthma or severe or prolonged anaphylaxis (methylprednisolone 1-2 mg/kg or its equivalent IV every 6 h).

Individuals taking beta-blockers may be refractory to treatment if their response to epinephrine is blunted. Though unproven, glucagon may be helpful in such patients by independently activating adenylate cyclase to alleviate hypotension and bronchospasm. It is given in a dosage of 1 to 5 mg IV over 5 minutes, then infused (5-15 g/min titrated to clinical response). Vasopressors may be necessary to maintain blood pressure if epinephrine and fluid resuscitation fail. In the event of cardiac arrest, high-dose intravenous epinephrine is used (1-3 mg [1:10,000 dilution] administered over 3 min, 3-5 mg administered over 3 min, and then a 4-10 mg/min infusion).

Fetal Considerations

Maternal vasodilation and hypoxia will predictably lead to fetal bradycardia and eventually hypoxemia and death. Efforts should primarily be focused on stabilization of the mother, since successful maternal resuscitation will make in utero resuscitation more likely. Adverse neonatal outcomes including anoxic injury and death have been described following both emergent cesarean delivery and delayed delivery. If maternal cardiac arrest occurs, management should include continued efforts at maternal cardiopulmonary resuscitation, followed by delivery of the viable fetus within an appropriate amount of time.

Prevention of Anaphylaxis to Penicillin

It is clear that penicillin should not be given to individuals with a documented history of anaphylaxis to penicillin. Because anaphylaxis can occur in patients with no prior reaction or no prior exposure to penicillin, history alone cannot prevent all serious allergic reactions. However, since penicillin allergy is often overdiagnosed and situations arise in pregnancy where penicillins are the most appropriate or the only treatment option, it is incumbent upon the clinician to take a detailed history of the nature of past reactions to penicillin. This history should include the patient's age at the time of the reaction and whether the patient actually recalls the reaction or was told of it by a reliable informant, the duration from penicillin exposure to onset of symptoms, the nature of the reaction, route of and reason for penicillin administration, concurrent medications, and reactions to penicillin-like medications (see diagnostic criteria for anaphylaxis earlier). **It is rare for life-threatening reactions to penicillin to present more than 1 hour following exposure.**

Because of its narrow spectrum of antimicrobial activity and effectiveness against GBS, penicillin is the drug of choice for intrapartum prophylaxis. The Centers for Disease Control and Prevention guidelines for prophylaxis against GBS were revised in 2002 in the face of increasing resistance to clindamycin and erythromycin. Adherence to these guidelines now requires knowledge of the nature of a past reaction to penicillin. Penicillin and cefazolin are withheld from patients with history of immediate hypersensitivity to penicillin and those in whom anaphylaxis would be more difficult to treat (ie, asthmatics or individuals on beta-blockers). In patients who have a history of penicillin allergy but do not meet these conditions, cefazolin is given.

Skin Testing

Approximately 10% of the US population reports allergy to penicillin. It is estimated that 80% to 90% of these patients are not truly allergic. A detailed history suggesting penicillin allergy approximately doubles the likelihood that an individual will have positive skin testing to penicillin; its absence reduces this likelihood by roughly half. Skin testing is highly accurate for identification of penicillin allergy; at least 98% of individuals with a negative skin test result can tolerate penicillin without sequelae.

Skin testing is appropriate for those patients with a history of immediate hypersensitivity reaction who require penicillin therapy. It has been performed safely during pregnancy. If an initial skin-prick test with the major determinant penicilloyl polylysine (PPL) and either penicillin G or a mixture of minor determinants is negative after 15 minutes, then intracutaneous testing is performed. A positive result is an increase in the wheal diameter of at least 3 mm compared to negative control. Negative skin testing only implies the absence of an IgE-mediated reaction and does not predict IgE-independent allergy. Patients with a history of serious but non-IgE-related allergy (Stevens-Johnson syndrome, toxic epidermal necrolysis, hemolytic anemia, hepatitis, or interstitial nephritis) are not appropriate candidates for skin testing and should continue to avoid penicillins.

The major limitation of skin testing is that PPL has not been manufactured in the United States since 2004, and it is unclear whether or when production will resume. An alternative radioallergosorbent test (RAST) correlates only with the major determinant. A combination approach involving RAST with minor determinant skin testing may be accurate but has not been tested.

Therefore, those individuals with a history suggesting immediate hypersensitivity to penicillin who require its use (notably pregnant women with syphilis) should undergo desensitization if skin testing reagents are not available.

Desensitization

In patients with IgE-mediated penicillin allergy who require penicillin therapy, immune tolerance can be produced by administering successively increasing doses of penicillin. This process takes approximately 4 hours and should be performed in a setting where close observation and immediate intensive care are available, because adverse reactions occur in approximately 30% of patients. Tolerance lasts only for as long as the drug is given; the risk of an immediate hypersensitivity reaction returns after 24 hours and repeat desensitization is necessary. Both oral and intravenous desensitization protocols have been used in pregnancy with good results. It is important that the patient understands she is still allergic to penicillin after undergoing desensitization.

Comprehension Questions

35.1   Which of the following histories is highly suggestive of anaphylaxis?
   A. Maculopapular rash beginning 5 days after PCN exposure
   B. Nausea and vomiting without rash, respiratory symptoms, or hypotension
   C. Urticaria and wheezing beginning 30 minutes after penicillin infusion
   D. Fever and epidermal necrosis with skin sloughing requiring intensive care

35.2   All of the following are appropriate initial steps in the management of severe anaphylaxis EXCEPT:
   A. Intravenous fluid bolus
   B. Oxygen by face mask
   C. Epinephrine 0.2 mL of 1:1000 aqueous solution IM
   D. Diphenhydramine 25 mg po

35.3   A 30-year-old G1P0 at 36 weeks' gestation arrives by ambulance, having become unresponsive 40 minutes after a bee sting. She is tachycardic, hypotensive, and stridorous. She had IV lines placed in the ambulance and is receiving fluids. The fetal heart rate is 70 beats per minute. Which of the following is the best initial step?
   A. Perform an emergent cesarean delivery.
   B. Give methylprednisolone 100 mg IV.
   C. Position her in left lateral decubitus with Trendelenburg.
   D. Begin an epinephrine drip.

35.4   A 17-year-old G1P0 is diagnosed with primary syphilis at 26 weeks'
        gestation. Her mother reports she developed hives and wheezing
        shortly after taking penicillin as a child. Which of the following is the
        most appropriate next step?
        A. Benzathine penicillin G 2.4 million units IM single dose
        B. Doxycycline 100 mg po bid for 14 days
        C. Azithromycin 2 g po single dose
        D. Desensitization to penicillin and treatment with penicillin

ANSWERS

35.1   **C.** Idiopathic maculopapular eruptions occur in 1% to 4% of patients
        receiving penicillin but have many other causes, and cutaneous man-
        ifestations of anaphylaxis typically arise within minutes to hours of
        exposure. Gastrointestinal symptoms must be accompanied by cuta-
        neous, respiratory, or hemodynamic signs in order to constitute an
        anaphylactic reaction. Fever with skin sloughing suggests a severe
        IgE-independent allergic reaction such as Stevens-Johnson syn-
        drome or toxic epidermal necrolysis.

35.2   **D.** Although histamine receptor antagonists may be helpful in coun-
        teracting the effects of mast cell degranulation, they are considered
        a second-line therapy and should not be given in isolation. The com-
        bination of an H_1 and an H_2 blocker is superior to either one alone.
        In severe cases they should be given parenterally.

35.3   **C.** While this patient may require emergent delivery, the fetal heart
        rate may respond to efforts at maternal resuscitation, and the poten-
        tial harm from emergency anesthesia and blood loss with surgery will
        only add further insult to her condition. Steroids may be helpful in
        preventing prolonged or biphasic anaphylaxis but are not useful in
        the acute management. Maternal stabilization with positioning to
        maximize venous return will make in utero resuscitation more likely.
        Epinephrine drip has been used successfully in pregnancy with ana-
        phylaxis, but intramuscular injection should be tried first.

35.4   **D.** This patient has a history suggestive of anaphylaxis to penicillin.
        Ideally, she should undergo skin testing to determine whether she
        can tolerate penicillin; however, since skin testing reagents are
        unavailable, she should undergo desensitization and treatment with
        penicillin. Doxycycline is not used in pregnancy because offspring
        exposed to tetracyclines in utero may have permanently discolored
        teeth. Treatment failure and resistance to azithromycin has been
        reported, so this is not an appropriate choice.

Clinical Pearls

See US Preventive Services Task Force Study Quality levels of evidence in Case 1

➤ The following measures constitute an appropriate response to anaphylaxis to penicillin in pregnancy:
  ➤ Discontinue penicillin infusion.
  ➤ Assess airway, breathing, circulation, and position gravida to maximize venous return (Level III).
  ➤ Give intravenous fluid bolus (1-2 L normal saline) (Level III).
  ➤ Administer epinephrine (Level II-2) or ephedrine (Level III).
  ➤ Consider histamine receptor antagonists, inhaled β_2-agonists, and glucocorticoids (Level III).
  ➤ Assess response to maternal resuscitative efforts and consider delivery.
➤ Epinephrine should be given intramuscularly in the anterior lateral thigh (Level II-2).
➤ The vast majority (80%-90%) of patients who report penicillin allergy have negative skin testing, and 98% of these patients can tolerate penicillin without serious adverse effects (Level II-2).
➤ Penicillin skin testing may be performed safely in pregnancy (Level III).
➤ Since skin testing reagents are currently unavailable, desensitization is necessary if a pregnant penicillin-allergic woman requires penicillin therapy (Level III).

CONTROVERSIES

Epinephrine versus Ephedrine

Concern has been raised regarding the potential for the alpha-adrenergic stimulation associated with epinephrine to cause uterine vessel constriction, contributing to uteroplacental insufficiency and fetal hypoxia. Some authors argue that ephedrine should be the first-line therapy for anaphylaxis in pregnancy; since it is a less potent α-agonist, it may spare uterine blood flow by increasing cardiac output through β_1-agonist activity. Given its popularity for treating post-anesthesia hypotension, ephedrine is readily available and familiar in the obstetric suite. For these reasons it may be appropriate to try ephedrine as initial therapy in the pregnant woman experiencing anaphylaxis. However, since epinephrine is the mainstay of treatment in severe anaphylaxis, epinephrine should be used if ephedrine does not bring about a favorable response quickly.

Steroids

The use of corticosteroids in anaphylaxis is extrapolated from their utility in treating other allergic disorders, but has not been tested in placebo-controlled trials. Biphasic anaphylactic reactions have been described, and experts postulate that steroids might prevent a prolonged or biphasic reaction. Like most aspects of anaphylaxis therapy, data demonstrating the effectiveness of steroids are lacking.

Overdiagnosis of Penicillin Allergy

It is commonplace for clinicians to accept a diagnosis of penicillin allergy without taking a history regarding the details of the reaction, thereby unnecessarily withholding penicillin from patients without a true allergy. Through careful history-taking, patients in whom anaphylaxis is highly likely may be identified. Those without such a history could probably receive penicillin safely. However, the current lack of availability of skin testing reagents makes this issue difficult to approach and may contribute to the overdiagnosis of penicillin allergy, since there is no logical next step except to choose an alternative antibiotic. In those cases for which penicillin is the only acceptable treatment, it is likely that many subjects reporting a history of penicillin allergy will undergo unnecessary, costly, and time-consuming desensitization procedures.

Cephalosporins

Although the cross-reactivity rate for penicillin and cephalosporins has been reported as 10%, the true figure is unknown. In a review of studies documenting penicillin allergy with skin testing, only 4% of skin-test positive subjects experienced cephalosporin reactions. Again, the lack of availability of skin testing means that those with a history of penicillin allergy will need to receive an alternate antibiotic, a graded challenge to cephalosporin, or desensitization.

REFERENCES

1. Chisholm CA, Katz VL, McDonald TL, Bowes WA Jr. Penicillin desensitization in the treatment of syphilis during pregnancy. *Am J Perinatol.* 1997;14(9):553-554.
2. Entman SS, Moise KJ. Anaphylaxis in pregnancy. *South Med J.* 1984;77(3):402.
   This case report describes a pregnant woman who experienced anaphylaxis after receiving snake antivenin at 28 weeks. She was given multiple doses of epinephrine and other therapies. Six weeks later she delivered; the infant had evidence of intracranial hemorrhage and died at 4 days of age. The argument is made that epinephrine compromised uteroplacental perfusion, and that ephedrine is a better choice.

3. Gei AF, Pacheco LD, Vanhook JW, Hankins GDV. The use of a continuous infusion of epinephrine for anaphylactic shock during labor. *Obstet Gynecol.* 2003;102(6):1332-1335.
   Case report of anaphylaxis to intrapartum ampicillin, treated with epinephrine in intermittent doses followed by a continuous infusion. Pharmacology of epinephrine and ephedrine are reviewed.
4. Gruchalla RS, Pirmohamed M. Antibiotic allergy. *N Engl J Med.* 2006;354:601-609.
5. Lieberman PL. Anaphylaxis and anaphylactoid reactions. In: Adkinson NF Jr, Yunginger J, Busse W, Bochner B, Holgate S, Simons F, eds. *Middleton's Allergy: Principles and Practice.* Philadelphia, PA: Mosby; 2003:1497-1518.
6. Lieberman P, Kemp S, Oppenheimer J, Lang D, Bernstein I, Nicklas R. The diagnosis and management of anaphylaxis: an updated practice parameter. *J Allergy Clin Immunol.* 2005;115(Suppl):483S-523S.
   An extensive, evidence-based review of anaphylaxis management with accessible algorithms.
7. Salkind AR, Cuddy PG, Foxworth JW. Is this patient allergic to penicillin? An evidence-based analysis of the likelihood of penicillin allergy. *JAMA.* 2001;285(19):2498-2505.
   A good review of history-taking tips, as well as the utility and limitations of history and skin testing.
8. Sampson HA, Munoz-Furlong A, Campbell RL, et al. Second symposium on the definition and management of anaphylaxis: Summary report—Second National Institute of Allergy and Infectious Disease/Food Allergy and Anaphylaxis Network symposium. *J Allergy Clin Immunol.* 2006 Feb;117(2):391-397.
   Latest guidelines for diagnosis of anaphylaxis, critique of the evidence behind current management, and suggested avenues for further research.
9. Wendel GD Jr, Stark BJ, Jamison RB, Molina RD, Sullivan TJ. Penicillin allergy and desensitization in serious infections during pregnancy. *N Engl J Med.* 1985;312(19):1229-1232.

Case 36

A 23-year-old African American G3P2002 at $22^0/_7$ weeks by LMP consistent with a first-trimester ultrasound presents as a new patient because she has recently moved to the area. Her medical history is significant for asthma since the age of 7. Her asthma has always been well controlled rarely requiring the use of her albuterol inhaler. One month before conception, however, she had "several" mild exacerbation relieved easily with the use of her inhaler. Last month she had four asthma exacerbations which required a visit to the emergency room for nebulizer treatment. It was recommended that she start a "new inhaler" but she did not fill the prescription prior to relocating.

She is currently using her albuterol inhaler daily for symptoms and has exacerbations 2 to 3 times per week. She also reports chest tightness, wheezing, and waking up 1 to 2 times per week at night. In addition, she has congestion with yellow nasal discharge and sinus tenderness for 1 month not relieved with over-the-counter decongestants. She denies allergies, fever, or sick contacts. She denies prior intubations, use of steroids, and has never measured a baseline peak flow. Her obstetrical history is significant for two prior vaginal deliveries without asthma complications. With her last delivery she had postpartum hemorrhage requiring blood transfusion due to a "floppy" immediately after delivery. She is otherwise healthy and denies other medical problems. Prenatal labs are unremarkable.

Her BP is 100/78 mm Hg, weight 135 lb, height 5 ft 1 in, urine dips negative for protein, glucose, ketones. Her examination is significant for sinus tenderness bilaterally, erythematous nasal mucosa bilaterally, purulent nasal discharge, no nodes palpable, throat and tympanic membranes are clear bilaterally. Bilateral expiratory wheezing throughout all lung fields is noted. Fetal hear tones are detected.

➤ What is your next step?

➤ How would you classify this patient's asthma?

➤ What are the potential maternal complications associated with asthma in pregnancy?

➤ What are the potential fetal complications?

ANSWERS TO CASE 36:

Asthma in Pregnancy

Summary: This is a 23-year-old woman G3P2002 at $22^0/_7$ weeks gestation with a history of asthma that has worsened during this pregnancy.

➤ **Next step:** Evaluate patient with peak expiratory flow rate (PEFR).

➤ **Classify this patient's asthma:** This patient has moderate persistent asthma because she has daily symptoms with exacerbations > 2 times/wk and nocturnal symptoms > 1 time/wk. Patients with moderate persistent asthma also have pulmonary function test 60% to 80% of predicted and may experience some interference with normal activities.

➤ **Potential maternal complications associated with asthma in pregnancy:** Patients with moderate or severe asthma may have increased number of exacerbations, hospitalizations, and unscheduled visits. The risk of cesarean delivery may also be increased in these women. Women with severe asthma may have an increased risk of preeclampsia and gestational diabetes mellitus (GDM). Women with mild or well-controlled asthma tend do well in pregnancy with outcomes similar to nonasthmatics. Although rare, potential life-threatening complications of *untreated* severe asthma include pneumothorax, pneumomediastinum, acute cor pulmonale, and respiratory arrest.

➤ **Potential fetal complications:** Preterm birth (< 37 wk) and small-for-gestational-age infants (SGA) may complicate pregnancies in those with severe asthma or those who require the use of oral corticosteroids.

ANALYSIS

Objectives

1. Review current asthma classification guidelines.
2. Understand implications of asthma on maternal/perinatal outcome.
3. Review management of asthmatics in outpatient and inpatient setting.

Considerations

This patient's asthma has progressively worsened during this pregnancy. New environmental triggers and an upper respiratory infection have contributed to her recent asthma exacerbations. With suboptimal treatment, this patient is unlikely to improve and both maternal and perinatal morbidity may be increased.

Asthma is one of the most common medical conditions complicating pregnancy, with an incidence of 4% to 9%[1] (Level III). The clinical course of asthma in pregnancy is relatively unpredictable; however, there is evidence to suggest that worsening of asthma may be related to baseline asthma severity. Approximately one-third of pregnant asthmatics experience worsening of symptoms while one-third improve and one-third remain the same. Exacerbations are more common in the second and third trimester and are less frequent in the last 4 weeks of pregnancy. Asthma typically follows a similar clinical course with successive pregnancies. As such, this patient would be expected to do relatively well given that her symptoms were well controlled prior to this pregnancy and in previous pregnancies. This patient has not received appropriate treatment and her asthma severity has deteriorated. This case underscores the importance that *all* asthmatics, even those with mild or well-controlled disease, need to be monitored for symptoms and treated accordingly during pregnancy.

Asthma symptoms correlate poorly with objective measures of pulmonary function.[2] Therefore, the next step in the evaluation of this patient is to perform an objective measure of airway obstruction. The single best measure is the **forced expiratory volume (FEV$_1$),** which is the volume of gas exhaled in 1 second by a forced exhalation after a full inspiration. This value, however, can only be obtained by spirometry, thus limiting its clinical use. The **peak expiratory flow rate (PEFR)** correlates well with FEV$_1$ and can be measured with inexpensive, disposable portable peak flow meters. Both the FEV$_1$ and PEFR remain unchanged throughout pregnancy and may be used as measures of asthma control and severity.

A patient who presents to the outpatient setting with worsening symptoms but is without evidence of a severe exacerbation may be treated and followed closely as an outpatient. This patient has **moderate persistent asthma** according to the current classification system by the 2004 National Asthma Education and Prevention Program Working Group on Asthma and Pregnancy (NAEPP)[3] (Level III). In addition to the clinical history, a PEFR of 60% to 80% of personal best or predicted will support this diagnosis. One of the recommended treatments for moderate persistent asthma is a low-dose inhaled corticosteroid (ICS), such as budesonide plus a long-acting β$_2$-agonist (salmeterol). This patient also has a chronic sinus infection which is evident by the purulent nasal discharge and sinus tenderness. A broad-spectrum antibiotic would be effective in treating her sinus infection. Sinusitis, rhinitis, and gastroesophageal reflux are all conditions that may exacerbate asthma and their treatment is an integral part of asthma management.

This patient should be counseled to recognize the signs and symptoms of early asthma exacerbations such as coughing, chest tightness, dyspnea, wheezing, or a 20% decrease in PEFR so that therapy can be initiated promptly. She should also be educated on how to control her environmental triggers such as cold air, dust, strong fumes, exercise, inhaled irritants, emotional stress, food additives (sulfites), drugs (aspirin and beta-blockers) and smoke. Measures that can be taken include removing carpets, changing filters in the home heating and cooling systems, avoiding smokers, moving pets outside, avoiding the home for 1 hour after vacuuming or dusting, encasing mattresses and pillows in airtight covers, washing bed linens weekly in 130°F water, lowering home humidity to no more than 50%, closing windows, and using air conditioning[4,5] (Level III).

Finally, it is also important to discuss the effect of asthma on pregnancy. Recent data from large prospective studies indicate that classification of asthma severity and appropriate treatment may result in favorable pregnancy outcome. These studies have shown that excellent maternal and fetal outcomes can be achieved in women with mild or well-controlled asthma. Those with severe and poorly controlled asthma may have an increased risk of preeclampsia, GDM, and preterm birth < 37 weeks. Cesarean delivery may also be increased in women with moderate or severe asthma. In a large prospective study in pregnant subjects, the exacerbation and hospitalization rates for mild asthmatics were 12.6% and 2.3%, respectively. In moderate asthma, the exacerbations and hospitalization rates were 25.7% and 6.8%, respectively while in those with severe, these rates were 51.9% and 26.9%, respectively[6] (Level II-2).

It is very reasonable to be cautiously optimistic about this patient's pregnancy outcome. Nonetheless, she should be followed closely until her asthma is back to her baseline. She should be instructed to follow-up in several days but to notify her physician if symptoms are not improving or are worsening. If her asthma control is difficult to achieve with the previously recommended interventions, then a multidisciplinary team approach, including maternal-fetal medicine and pulmonary specialists, is recommended.

APPROACH TO
Asthma in Pregnancy

Optimal management of asthma during pregnancy includes severity classification, subjective and objective monitoring of asthma control, avoiding or controlling asthma triggers, educating patients, and individualizing pharmacologic therapy to maintain normal pulmonary function. The ultimate goal of the management of asthma is to prevent hypoxic episodes in the mother which in turn ensures adequate oxygenation of the fetus.

The 2004 NAEPP established a classification scheme of asthma according to clinical symptoms and objective tests of pulmonary function[3] (Level III). Asthma is graded according to the patient's most severe symptoms while on or off controller medication and therapy is tailored accordingly (Table 36–1). It is important to remember that approximately 30% of those initially thought to be mild asthmatics may be reclassified as moderate or severe during pregnancy. Each prenatal visit should therefore include an evaluation of asthma

Table 36–1 2004 NATIONAL ASTHMA EDUCATION & PREVENTION PROGRAM CLASSIFICATION AND TREATMENT

	MILD INTERMITTENT	MILD PERSISTENT	MODERATE PERSISTENT	SEVERE PERSISTENT
Symptoms	≤ 2 times a week	> 2 times a week but < 1 time a day	Daily	Continual
	Asymptomatic between exacerbations		Exacerbations occur ≥ 2 times a week	Frequent exacerbations
Nocturnal awakening	≤ 2 times a month	> 2 times a month	> 1 time a week	Frequent
Pulmonary function tests	Normal PEFR between exacerbations FEV_1 or PEF ≥ 80% of predicted PEF variability < 20 %	FEV_1 or PEF ≥ 80% of predicted PEF variability 20%-30%	FEV_1 or PEF 60%-80% of predicted PEF variability > 30%	FEV_1 or PEF ≤ 60% of predicted PEF variability > 30%
Interference with daily activities	None	Mild	Some interference with normal activities but rare severe exacerbation	Limitations of physical activity
Rescue therapy	Inhaled short-acting β_2-agonist as needed	Inhaled short-acting β_2-agonist as needed	Inhaled short-acting β_2-agonist as needed	Inhaled short-acting β_2- agonist as needed
Preferred treatment	No daily medication	Low-dose ICS	Low-dose ICS and long-acting β_2-agonist or Medium-dose ICS or Medium-dose ICS and long-acting β_2-agonist	High-dose ICS and long-acting β_2-agonist and if needed, oral corticosteroids maintenance or taper

(Continued)

Table 36–1 2004 NATIONAL ASTHMA EDUCATION & PREVENTION PROGRAM CLASSIFICATION AND TREATMENT (CONT.)

	MILD INTERMITTENT	MILD PERSISTENT	MODERATE PERSISTENT	SEVERE PERSISTENT
Alternative treatment		Cromolyn, leukotriene modifiers, or theophylline (listed alpha)	Low-dose ICS and theophylline or leukotriene modifiers If needed, medium-dose ICS and theophylline or leukotriene modifiers	High-dose ICS and theophylline

severity and symptom frequency, nocturnal symptoms, medications, emergency visits, and hospital admissions for exacerbations. The 2004 NAEPP guidelines recommend spirometry at initial assessment and PEFR for routine monitoring at subsequent follow-up visit. Patients should be instructed to record PEFR immediately upon rising in the morning and again 12 hours later. They should establish their *personal best* PEFR during a period when their asthma is under good control. This value can then be used to recognize worsening of symptoms and subsequent response to treatment.

It is important to also ascertain a detailed asthma history. Patients with potentially fatal asthma include those with a history of prior intubation for asthma; two or more hospitalizations for asthma in the past year; three or more emergency care visits for asthma in the past year; hospitalization or an emergency care visit for asthma within the past month; current use of systemic corticosteroids or recent withdrawal from systemic corticosteroids; past history of syncope or hypoxic seizure due to asthma; prior admission for asthma to a hospital-based intensive care unit; and serious psychiatric disease or psychosocial problems. Patients with one or more of these risk factors are particularly concerning and any changes in their symptoms should prompt immediate medical attention in the outpatient or inpatient setting as appropriate.

It is also imperative to establish accurate determination of gestational age with a first-trimester ultrasound so that comparison may be made later for fetal growth. Routine obstetric monitoring for the pregnant asthmatic should include Doppler assessment of fetal heart tones and daily kick counts. Once fetal viability is achieved, the need for fetal surveillance may be based on asthma severity. Ultrasound for fetal growth and antenatal surveillance with either nonstress test (NST) or biophysical profile (BPP) testing may be considered in those with moderate or severe asthma, fetal growth restriction, asthma exacerbation, or decreased fetal movement.

Treatment

Since asthma is a disease of chronic airway inflammation and acute episodes of bronchospasm, treatment is directed at reducing this inflammation and reversing bronchospasm. The aim of therapy is to use the minimum medication needed to maintain control with the least risk of adverse effects. The 2004 NAEPP guidelines recommend a **"step" therapy** approach to pharmacologic treatment of asthma during pregnancy. With this approach, the number and frequency of medications are increased as necessary to establish control (step up) and reduced when possible to maintain control (step down). It is safer for women to be treated with asthma medications than to have asthma symptoms and exacerbations during pregnancy.

Asthma medications may be divided into two arms: rescue therapy and long-term control therapy. **All pregnant asthmatics should have an inhaled short-acting β_2-agonist for rescue treatment of acute symptoms.** β_2-Agonists relax the smooth muscle of the bronchioles and are used for relieving acute symptoms as well as preventing exacerbations from exposure to a trigger. Their onset of action is less than 5 minutes with duration of only 4 to 6 hours, and repetitive administration produces incremental bronchodilation. Albuterol is preferred over other short-acting β_2-agonists due to extensive safety-related information during pregnancy (category C). However, there is no evidence of fetal adverse effects with the use of other short-acting inhaled β_2-agonists. Inhaled **albuterol** can be delivered via a metered dose inhaler (MDI) or by nebulizer (2.5 mg or 0.5 mL of a 0.5% solution diluted in 2.5 mL normal saline).

Long-term control medications are used for prevention of asthma exacerbations. **Long-acting inhaled β_2-agonists** are used for moderate or severe persistent asthma. Salmeterol and formoterol have limited data in pregnancy, however, their pharmacologic and toxicologic profiles are considered to be similar to albuterol with the expected safety profile. **Inhaled corticosteroids (ICS)** are the first-line controller therapy for persistent asthma in pregnancy. Budesonide has been well studied in pregnancy (category B) and has not been shown to be teratogenic or associated with adverse perinatal outcome. Although budesonide is the ICS of choice, there are no data to indicate safety concerns with other ICS and maintaining a previously established treatment regimen may be more beneficial. Low, medium, and high doses of ICS can be used according to asthma severity (Table 36–2). Oral corticosteroids can be used as both maintenance and rescue therapy. Oral corticosteroids may increase the risk of cleft lip/palate if used in the first trimester. Whether they increases the risk of preeclampsia, preterm birth, and low-birth-weight infants remains uncertain as the available data make it difficult to separate the effects of oral corticosteroids from the effects of severe or uncontrolled asthma on pregnancy.

Table 36–2 EXAMPLES OF INHALED CORTICOSTEROIDS AND DOSES					
Drug	Budesonide DPI 200 µg/ inhalation	Beclomethasone CFC 42 or 84 µg/ inhalation	Beclomethaso HFA 40 or 80 µg/ inhalation	Fluticasone MDI 44, 110, or 220 µg/ inhalation	Flunisolide 250 µg/ inhalation
Low dose	200-600 µg	168-504 µg	80-240 µg	88-264 µg	500-1000 µg
Medium dose	600-1200 µg	504-840 µg	240-480 µg	264-660 µg	1000-2000 µg
High dose	> 1200 µg	> 840 µg	> 480 µg	> 660 µg	> 2000 µg

DPI = dry powder inhaler
MDI = metered-dose inhaler

Alternative drugs may be used as add-on controller therapy when using the step-therapy approach (Table 36–1). For example, cromolyn sodium (category B) is a mast cell stabilizer that can be used for the management of mild persistent asthma as an alternative to low-dose ICS. Leukotriene modifiers such as montelukast and zafirlukast (both category B) may be used as alternative add-on therapy; however, there is limited data of use in pregnancy. Theophylline (category C) is another alternative add-on controller therapy for persistent asthma. The disadvantage of this drug is that it has a very narrow therapeutic index and requires serum monitoring. Although animal data have raised concerns of fetal growth abnormalities with theophylline use, human data have not confirmed this or any additional maternal or fetal risks.

Acute Asthma Exacerbation

Treatment of an acute exacerbation during pregnancy is similar to that of nonpregnant asthmatics. Patients should be taught how to recognize the signs and symptoms of early exacerbations so that they may begin treatment at home promptly. **Initial treatment consists of a short-acting inhaled β_2-agonist** (albuterol) of 2 to 4 puffs by MDI at 20 minute intervals for up to three treatments, or single nebulizer treatment for up to 1 hour. A good response is characterized by PEFR greater than 80% of personal best and resolution of symptoms sustained for 4 hours. Patients may be continued on β_2-agonists every 3 to 4 hours for 24 to 48 hours. Inhaled corticosteroids should be initiated or if already taking ICS, the dose should be doubled. Follow-up appointment with their physician should be made as soon as possible. Inadequate response to initial therapy (PEFR < 80%) or decreased fetal activity warrants immediate medical attention.

Table 36–3 CRITERIA FOR INTUBATION OF A PREGNANT ASTHMATIC

- Maternal $Pao_2 \leq 60$ mm Hg
- Maternal $Paco_2 \leq 45$ mm Hg
- Evidence of maternal exhaustion
- Worsening acidosis (pH < 7.35)
- Altered maternal consciousness

Prevention of hypoxia is the ultimate goal for the pregnant woman who presents to the hospital during an acute asthma attack. Initial assessment should include a brief history and physical examination to assess the severity of asthma and possible trigger factors such as a respiratory infection. Patients with imminent respiratory arrest include those who are drowsy or confused, have paradoxical thoracoabdominal movement, absence of wheeze, bradycardia, and absence of pulsus paradoxus. Intubation and mechanical ventilation with 100% oxygen should be performed in these circumstances and the patient should be admitted to the intensive care unit. A $Paco_2$ greater than 35 mm Hg, with a pH less than 7.35 in the presence of a falling Pao_2 is a sign of impending respiratory failure in a pregnant asthmatic. Intubation is warranted when the $Paco_2$ is 45 mm Hg or more and rising (Table 36–3).

If intubation is not immediately warranted, measurement of PEFR or FEV_1 and arterial blood gas is important to determine the severity of asthma. **Initial treatment should include supplemental oxygen to maintain a PaO_2 greater than 60 mm Hg or an oxygen saturation of at least 95% with the patient on continuous pulse oximetry.** Because the fetus operates on the steep portion of the oxygen dissociation curve, decreases in maternal PaO_2, especially below 60 mm Hg, can result in profoundly decreased fetal PaO_2 and fetal hypoxia. Maternal oxygen saturation must remain greater than 95% to ensure adequate fetal oxygenation.

Intravenous access is essential for both administration of medicines and adequate hydration. Albuterol should be delivered by nebulizer every 20 minutes for a total of three doses. If the patient is moving air poorly, rendering the nebulizer ineffective, terbutaline 0.25 mg can be administered subcutaneously every 15 minutes for three doses. If the PEFR is < 40% of personal best, high-dose inhaled albuterol plus ipratropium by nebulizer or MDI should be used every 20 minutes or continuously for 1 hour.

Systemic steroids should be administered to those not responding immediately to bronchodilators and for those already taking regular oral corticosteroids. Intravenous methylprednisolone, 40 to 80 mg, is usually given every 6 to 8 hours. This may be substituted with prednisone orally (60 mg initially, then 60-120 mg daily tapered over several days). If the patient is too breathless to maintain oral intake, parenteral administration is preferred. Regardless of the route of administration, their onset of action is several hours so a β_2-agonist must be given as well. Response to treatment is considered good if PEFR or FEV_1 is 70% or more of baseline, patient is asymptomatic, and fetal status is reassuring. Patients who fail to respond to treatment within 4 hours warrant admission to the hospital for further monitoring and management.

Preterm labor may complicate an acute asthma exacerbation; however uterine contractions will usually abate with successful treatment of the exacerbation. If tocolytics are necessary, magnesium sulfate or calcium channel blockers can be administered. Indomethacin may induce bronchospasm in aspirin-sensitive asthmatics and should therefore be avoided.

Antepartum and Intrapartum Management

There are no standard guidelines for timing of delivery but it is generally accepted that delivery be undertaken at term, or when maternal health can be improved by delivery; however, it is important to avoid delivery of a patient during an acute exacerbation.

When the pregnant asthmatic presents for delivery, continuous monitoring of both mother and fetus is important. PEFR should be measured upon admission and again every 12 hours. Regularly scheduled medications should be continued throughout labor. **Stress-dose steroids should be administered to women who have taken systemic steroids in the preceding 4 weeks to avoid adrenal suppression.** This can be accomplished with 100 mg hydrocortisone intravenously every 8 hours until 24 hours postpartum. Labor induction can be safely accomplished with oxytocin or cervical ripening methods such as prostaglandin E_1 or E_2. The **analgesic** chosen during labor should be a **non-histamine-releasing narcotic,** such as fentanyl, as opposed to meperidine or morphine. Lumbar epidural or combined spinal epidural are appropriate options for pain management during labor. **If uterine atony results in postpartum hemorrhage, oxytocin and prostaglandin E_1 or E_2 are the uterotonics of choice. Prostaglandin $F_{2\alpha}$ and methylergonovine should be avoided as they both can cause bronchospasm.** The use of oral or ICS, β_2-agonists, antihistamines, and cromolyn is not contraindicated for breast-feeding women.

Comprehension Questions

36.1   A 19-year-old G1P0 at 9 weeks' gestation presents for prenatal care. She has mild persistent asthma well controlled on a low-dose inhaled corticosteroid, beclomethasone. What controller treatment plan would you recommend?

A. Start low-dose budesonide and discontinue current ICS.

B. Continue the same ICS.

C. Discontinue the ICS.

36.2   A 28-year-old woman at 20 weeks' gestation with asthma for 10 years
        comes into the OB triage area for exacerbation of her asthma. After
        two nebulized treatments, she is still dyspneic. Her arterial blood gas
        is as follows: pH 7.37, Po_2 85 mm Hg, Pco_2 35 mg Hg, and HCO_3
        18 mEq/L. Which of the following is the best description of her
        blood gas findings?
        A. Mild hypoxemia and normal ventilation
        B. Severe hypoxemia and normal ventilation
        C. Mild hypoxemia and significant hypercarbia
        D. Severe hypoxemia and metabolic acidosis
        E. Mild hypoxemia and metabolic acidosis

ANSWERS

36.1   **B.** Although budesonide is the preferred ICS for the treatment of
        mild persistent asthma due to favorable safety information of use in
        pregnancy, there are no concerns with other ICS. That being said, if
        a patient is well controlled on a previously established treatment reg-
        imen, it is reasonable to continue the same controller medication
        during pregnancy as well.

36.2   **C.** The Po_2 is slightly low, but more alarming is the Pco_2 which is
        elevated. The normal Pco_2 in pregnancy is 28 mm Hg. In an asth-
        matic exacerbation, typically the Pco_2 is decreased due to increased
        respiratory rate; when the Pco_2 is elevated, it illustrates CO_2 reten-
        tion and forbodes impending respiratory failure and possible need for
        intubation if the trend continues.

Clinical Pearls

See US Preventive Services Task Force Study Quality levels of evidence in Case 1

➤ It is safer for pregnant women with asthma to be treated with asthma medications than it is for them to have asthma symptoms and exacerbations (Level III).

➤ The ultimate goal of asthma therapy in pregnancy is maintaining adequate oxygenation of the fetus by preventing hypoxic episodes in the mother (Level III).

➤ Inhaled corticosteroids are first-line controller therapy for persistent asthma during pregnancy (Level II-3).

➤ Inhaled albuterol is recommended rescue therapy for pregnant women with asthma (Level III).

➤ Ultrasound assessment of fetal growth and antenatal fetal testing should be considered for women who have moderate or severe asthma during pregnancy (Level III).

➤ Mild and well-controlled asthma can be associated with excellent maternal and perinatal pregnancy outcomes (Level II-3).

➤ Severe and poorly controlled asthma may be associated with perinatal complications and maternal morbidity and mortality (Level II-2).

REFERENCES

1. Kwon HL, Belanger K, Bracken MB. Asthma prevalence among pregnant and childbearing-aged women in the United States: estimates from national health surveys. *Ann Epidemiol.* 2003;13:317-324 (Level III).

2. Stahl E. Correlation between objective measures of airway calibre and clinical symptoms in asthma: a systematic review of clinical studies. *Respir Med.* 2000 Aug;94(8):735-741.

3. National Heart, Lung and Blood Institute, National Asthma Education and Prevention Program. Working group report on managing asthma during pregnancy: recommendations for pharmacologic treatment-update 2004. NIH Publication No. 05-5236, March 2005.
    Since the 1993 recommendations, modification to the general asthma treatment guidelines, release of new asthma medications, revisions to the severity classification of asthma, and publication of new gestational safety data were sufficient to warrant an evidence-based update of these recommendations (Level III).

4. National Asthma Education Program: Report of the Working Group on Asthma and Pregnancy: Executive Summary: management of asthma during pregnancy. National Heart, Lung and Blood Institute. NIH publication 93-3279, March 1993.
    In 1993, the National Asthma Education and Prevention Program (NAEPP) published the Report of the Working Group on Asthma and Pregnancy, which comprehensively reviewed the data to date and presented recommendations for the management of asthma during pregnancy (Level III).

5. Gardner MO, Doyle NM. Asthma in pregnancy. *Obstet Gynecol Clin North Am.* 2004;31(2):385-413.

6. Dombrowski MP, Schatz M, Wise R, et al. Asthma during pregnancy. National Institute of Child Health and Human Development Maternal-Fetal Medicine Units Network and the National Heart, Lung, and Blood Institute. *Obstet Gynecol.* 2004;103:5-12.

    Multicenter, prospective, observational cohort study conducted over 4 years at 16 university hospital centers that looked at neonatal and maternal outcomes based on asthma severity during pregnancy. The study showed that when asthma is classified and therapy is tailored according to its severity, excellent maternal and infant outcomes can be achieved (Level II-2).

Case 37

A 27-year-old African American woman G1P0 is seen for prenatal care at 36 weeks' gestation. She has a history of lupus with her most recent flare occurring over 6 months prior to conception. An antiphospholipid (aPL) syndrome workup is negative. Her renal evaluation prior to pregnancy revealed a serum creatinine of 0.8 mg/dL and 24-hour urine collection at 8 weeks gestation contained 120 mg of protein. At that time, her blood pressure was 110/70 mm Hg and liver function tests and platelet counts were normal. Today, she describes a persistent headache for the past 12 hours and you note her blood pressure is 145/95 mm Hg. Her weight has increased 3 lb since her last visit 1 week ago, and her urine dipstick protein is 3+. Her fundal height is 36 cm, and she notes normal fetal movement. Admission lab in the hospital reveals a platelet count of 225,000/μL, normal liver function tests, serum creatinine of 0.8 mg/dL, and normal complement levels. Her antinuclear antibody (ANA) test is positive.

➤ What is the most likely diagnosis?

➤ What is your next step?

➤ What are potential complications of the patient's disorder?

ANSWERS TO CASE 37:
Preeclampsia in a Patient with SLE

Summary: This is a 27-year-old G1P0 patient at 36 weeks' gestation with underlying systemic lupus erythematosus (SLE) who has developed hypertension, proteinuria, and excessive weight gain with neurologic symptoms. Her labs indicate normal LFTs, platelets, and complement levels. Fundal height indicates a normally grown fetus.

➤ **Most likely diagnosis:** Preeclampsia.

➤ **Next step:** Evaluate the patient for lupus flare and if workup negative, schedule for delivery.

➤ **Potential complications:** Placental dysfunction, abruptio placenta, worsening preeclampsia, HELLP syndrome, or eclampsia.

ANALYSIS

Objectives

1. Describe the preconception and antenatal evaluation of a patient with SLE.
2. Understand the importance of evaluating the patient with SLE for concomitant aPL syndrome.
3. List the laboratory evaluation that helps to distinguish preeclampsia from a lupus flare.
4. Discuss the evaluation and treatment of aPL syndrome during pregnancy.

Considerations

This patient has a clinical presentation that could either be preeclampsia or an exacerbation of her lupus. SLE can present with proteinuria, seizures, and hypertension. Since the treatment is dramatically different: magnesium sulfate and delivery for preeclampsia, and corticosteroids and expectant management in SLE, distinguishing the two diseases is critical. One reliable method of distinguishing the two processes is by assessing the serum complement levels. In SLE, the serum complement levels will be dramatically lower due to the immune complex processes, whereas in preeclampsia, the serum complement levels will be normal.

APPROACH TO
Preeclampsia in a Patient With SLE

The term **lupus** (Latin for wolf) is attributed to the 13th century physician Rogerius who used it to describe erosive facial lesions that were reminiscent of a wolf's bite. In 1997 the American College of Rheumatology revised their 1982 criteria for the classification of systemic lupus erythematosus (SLE) to include 11 components (Table 37–1). For the diagnosis of lupus, the ACR recommends that a patient have at least 4 of the 11 criteria present in any order and over any time period. Patients who clinically have symptoms of lupus but who do not fulfill this 4/11 criteria are considered to have a "lupus-like" syndrome and may, in some cases, be treated as if they have the full syndrome.

The female to male ratio of lupus is between 8:1 and 13:1 with a prevalence between 4 and 250:100,000 persons. In the United States, the highest incidence is in Asians in Hawaii, African Americans, and Native Americans. The risk of an African American female developing SLE is 1:250 compared to 1:700 if the woman is Caucasian.

The etiology is unknown but is felt to have genetic, hormonal, immunologic, and environmental factors.

There are a number of classical clinical features, each with its own frequency (Table 37–2). Arthralgias/myalgias, fatigue, arthritis, hematologic changes, fever, alopecia, weight loss, and photosensitivity are seen most frequently in patients with SLE. There are also a number of lupus-inducing drugs, many of which are used during pregnancy. These are listed in Table 37–3. The prognosis for 5-year survival of 50% in the 1950s has improved markedly to over 90% for a 10-year survival in 1994. The prognosis is worse with CNS involvement, hypertension, azotemia, and an early age at onset, and the major cause of death remains infection.

Studies prior to 1985 suggested that pregnancy caused SLE exacerbations, but more recent publications find little or no increase in SLE flares during gestation. Older studies which indicated a worsening of the disease postpartum have been refuted by newer reports as well. Flares do occur during any trimester, and remission of SLE immediately before or at the time of conception probably do decrease the chances of an exacerbation during pregnancy and postpartum. Women with active lupus nephritis at the time of conception have a risk of flare during pregnancy that exceeds 50%. In a recent study of patients with lupus nephritis who became pregnant, 59% had no change in renal function, 30% had transient renal impairment, and 7% had permanent renal insufficiency after pregnancy. Patients with a serum creatinine greater than 1.5 mg/dL have significantly increased risk of deterioration of renal function during or after pregnancy. Preeclampsia occurs in over one-third of patients with lupus nephritis compared to less than 15% of patients without nephritis.

Table 37–1 CRITERIA FOR DIAGNOSIS OF SLE

1. **Malar rash**
   Fixed erythema, flat or raised, over the malar eminences, tending to spare the nasolabial folds
2. **Discoid rash**
3. **Photosensitivity**
   Skin rash as a result of unusual reaction to sunlight, by patient history or physician observation
4. **Oral ulcers**
   Oral or nasopharyngeal ulceration, usually painless, observed by a physician
5. **Arthritis**
   Non-erosive arthritis involving two or more peripheral joints and characterized by tenderness, swelling, or effusion
6. **Serositis**
   Pleuritis—convincing history of pleuritic pain or rub heard by a physician or evidence of pleural effusion

   or

   Pericarditis—documented by electrocardiogram or rub or by evidence of pericardial effusion
7. **Renal disorder**
   Persistent proteinuria > 0.5 g/d or > 3+ if quantitation not performed

   or

   Cellular casts—may be red cell, hemoglobin, granular, tubular, or mixed
8. **Neurologic disorder**
   Seizures in the absence of offending drugs or known metabolic derangements, eg, uremia, ketoacidosis, or electrolyte imbalance

   or

   Psychosis in the absence of offending drugs or known metabolic derangements, eg, uremia, ketoacidosis, or electrolyte imbalance
9. **Hematologic disorder**
   Hemolytic anemia with reticulocytosis

   or

   Leukopenia < 4000/mm^3 total on two or more occasions

   or

   Lymphopenia < 1500/mm^3 on two or more occasions

   or

   Thrombocytopenia < 100,000/mm^3 in the absence of offending drugs
10. **Immunologic disorder**
    Positive tests for antiphospholipid antibodies

    or

    Anti-DNA: antibody to native DNA in abnormal titer

    or

    Anti-Sm: presence of antibody to Sm nuclear antigen

    or

    False-positive serologic test for syphilis known to be positive for at least 6 mo and confirmed by *Treponema pallidum* immobilization or fluorescent treponemal antibody absorption test
11. **Antinuclear antibodies**
    An abnormal titer of antinuclear antibody by immunofluorescence or an equivalent assay at any point and in the absence of drugs known to be associated with "drug-induced **lupus**" syndrome

Table 37–2 CLINICAL MANIFESTATIONS OF SLE

FEATURE OF SLE	% FREQUENCY AT ANY TIME
Arthralgia/myalgia	95
Fatigue	90
Arthritis	90
Hematologic changes	90
Fever	80
Alopecia	71
Weight loss	60
Photosensitivity	58
Butterfly rash	50
Clinical lupus nephritis	50
Lymphadenopathy	50
Pleurisy	50+
Anemia	50+
aPL antibodies	25
Neuropsychiatric disorder	20

Table 37–3 LUPUS-INDUCING DRUGS

DEFINITE	POSSIBLE
Hydralazine	Phenytoin
	Aldomet
	Sulfonamides
	PTU
	Nitrofurantoin
	Atenolol
	Metoprolol
	Captopril

Other complications of pregnancy associated with SLE include intrauterine growth restriction (IUGR) (12%-32%), preterm birth (50%, typically due to preeclampsia, IUGR, or abnormal FHR testing), and neonatal lupus from autoantibodies that cross the placenta causing skin lesions, thrombocytopenia, anemia, and hepatitis. Women with anti-Ro and anti-La antibodies from Sjögren syndrome (anti-SSA and anti-SSB) also have a risk of congenital heart block in the fetus.

Preconception counseling should include renal function evaluation with a 24-hour urine collection for total protein and creatinine clearance, serum creatinine, urinalysis, CBC and platelet count, liver function tests, complement levels, ds-DNA levels, and anti-SSA and SSB antibodies, and the patient should be tested for lupus anticoagulant and anticardiolipin antibodies (ACA). Patients considering pregnancy should be apprised of the risks to themselves and the fetus from SLE, and the need to discontinue NSAIDs and cytotoxic drugs such as methotrexate prior to pregnancy. It is also recommended that they delay conception until at least 6 months after remission of any SLE flare.

Antenatal care should include visits every 2 weeks in the first and second trimesters and then weekly in the third to observe for hypertension, fundal height abnormalities, proteinuria, and symptoms of a lupus flare. Baseline labs should include a completion of their preconception labs if not recently obtained including 24-hour urine, CBC, and early dating ultrasound as well as a repeat of the lupus anticoagulant and anticardiolipin antibodies if previously negative. Serial ultrasounds for growth should be considered every 3 to 4 weeks after 20 weeks and biweekly non-stress tests (NSTs) or other fetal monitoring should commence by 32 weeks (earlier if IUGR is suspected).

With the exception of methotrexate, most anti-lupus medications may be continued during pregnancy. Commonly used medications and potential side effects are listed in Table 37–4.

Table 37–4 MEDICATIONS FOR SLE

NSAIDs
- Aspirin, NSAIDs should be discontinued.

Antimalarials
- Hydroxychloroquine (Plaquenil): stopping in pregnancy associated with lupus flare; may be first-line therapy.

Immunosuppressive agents
- Cyclosporine appears safe in humans.
- Azathioprine (Imuran) appears safe in humans; associated with IUGR.
- Cyclophosphamide (Cytoxan) should be avoided (cleft lip, skeletal abnormalities).
- Methotrexate should be avoided (embryolethal, associated with multiple congenital anomalies).

Glucocorticoids
- Avoid fluorinated glucocorticoids (cross placenta).
- Prednisone, prednisolone, methylprednisolone preferred.

If a lupus flare is suspected, it is critical to distinguish it from preeclampsia. Decreased levels of complement, the presence of urinary casts, and increased levels of ds-DNA antibodies may be present in lupus and are rarely seen in preeclampsia, which is more likely to evidence an increased level of uric acid. If the flare is mild-moderate (such as skin or joint pain), prednisone may be given at 15 to 20 mg/d or increase a prior dose to at least 20 to 30 mg/d. In severe flares without renal or CNS manifestation, a rheumatology consult as an outpatient is preferred. Glucocorticoids at 1.0 to 1.5 mg/kg per day should result in clinical improvement in 5 to 10 days. Steroids should be tapered when clinical improvement is noted; if symptoms recur during or after tapering, consider cyclosporine, hydroxychloroquine (Plaquenil), or azathioprine (Imuran) therapy. A severe flare with CNS or renal involvement requires hospitalization, a rheumatology consult, and IV glucocorticoids such as 10 to 30 mg/kg/d of methylprednisolone for 3 to 6 days.

While most patients with lupus fare well during pregnancy, a subset has the additional risk of antiphospholipid syndrome (aPL syndrome) and its increasingly complicated course. The criteria for the aPL syndrome are listed in Table 37–5. It is advisable to test for both lupus anticoagulant and anticardiolipin antibodies (IgG and IgM), since a patient may have lupus anticoagulant or ACA alone or in combination. Clinically significant values include positive lupus anticoagulant, medium- or high-positive IgG, and probably isolated IgM positivity as well.

Table 37–5 CRITERIA FOR DIAGNOSIS OF aPL SYNDROME[a]

Clinical Criteria
- **Pregnancy Loss**
- Recurrent spontaneous abortion[b]
- Unexplained fetal death
- **Thrombosis**
- Venous thrombosis
- Arterial thrombosis, stroke
- **Autoimmune thrombocytopenia**
- **Other disorders**
- Autoimmune hemolytic anemia
- Transient ischemic attacks
- Amaurosis fugax
- Chorea gravidarum
- Livedo reticularis

Laboratory Criteria
- **Lupus anticoagulant**
- **Anticardiolipin antibodies > 15-20 IgG binding units**

[a]At least one clinical and one lab criteria required for diagnosis of aPL syndrome.
[b]Three or more spontaneous abortions with no more than one live birth.

Obstetric complications of aPL syndrome include pregnancy loss rates as high as 90% which may occur as second- or third-trimester IUFD. Recurrent spontaneous abortion is also associated with aPL syndrome as is early preeclampsia, IUGR and placental insufficiency, preterm birth, autoimmune thrombocytopenia, and venous or arterial thrombosis. The three goals of aPL treatment during pregnancy therefore include suppression of the immune system, prevention of thrombosis, and improvement of placental blood flow by decreasing the thromboxane-to-prostacyclin ratio.

Early trials of aPL therapy in pregnancy reported successful pregnancies using high-dose (≥ 40 mg/d) prednisone and low-dose aspirin, but more recent reports demonstrate **comparable efficacy and fewer complications with heparin and low-dose aspirin.** Initiation of heparin therapy should begin as soon as pregnancy is confirmed using 10,000 to 20,000 U/d in two doses of unfractionated heparin (UFH) if no prior thrombosis (increasing to the higher dose in the third trimester), or full anticoagulation with UFH if prior thrombosis. Low-molecular-weight heparin may be used instead of UFH, and low-dose aspirin should be included with any heparin therapy. IVIg has been used as an adjunct to heparin and aspirin with high cost and uncertain benefits.

Surveillance of the patient with aPL syndrome in pregnancy is similar to other connective tissue diseases, and includes intensive monitoring for preeclampsia, IUGR, placental insufficiency, and thrombosis. Thromboprophylaxis or full anticoagulation should continue for 6 weeks postpartum and the patient should be counseled about the lifetime risk of thrombosis. Oral contraceptives are contraindicated with aPL syndrome in patients not on anticoagulation.

The pregnant patient with SLE who enters pregnancy with no recent flare or nephritis has an excellent chance of a successful outcome. Recent flares, nephritis, an elevated serum creatinine, or concurrent aPL syndrome markedly increases risk to both mother and fetus and should trigger additional monitoring and usually consultation with maternal-fetal medicine and rheumatology specialists.

Comprehension Questions

37.1   A 29-year-old patient is seen for a preconceptional visit. She has a history of lupus. Which of the following characteristics place her health at greatest risk?

A. Current BP of 120/80 mm Hg.

B. Serum creatinine of 1.8 mg/dL.

C. Most recent lupus flare 8 months ago.

D. Current medications include prednisone and azathioprine.

37.2 For optimal pregnancy outcome, patients should be advised to wait at least 6 months before attempting conception with which of the following conditions?
A. Lupus nephritis
B. Positive antinuclear antibody titer
C. Discontinuing methotrexate
D. Resolution of rash of discoid lupus

37.3 A lupus flare may be distinguished from preeclampsia using which of the following?
A. Level of proteinuria
B. Presence of thrombocytopenia
C. Urinary casts
D. Severe hypertension
E. IUGR

37.4 A patient with lupus and aPL syndrome will have the best outcome with fewest complications when administered which of the following therapies?
A. Baby aspirin alone
B. Heparin plus baby aspirin
C. Prednisone plus baby aspirin
D. Prednisone alone

ANSWERS

37.1 **B.** Patients with lupus and a serum creatinine greater than 1.5 mg/dL who become pregnant have a high risk of renal deterioration during or after pregnancy.

37.2 **A.** Patients who conceive while experiencing lupus nephritis have a greater than 50% risk of lupus flare during pregnancy and a 7% chance of permanent renal insufficiency after pregnancy.

37.3 **C.** A lupus flare during pregnancy may be difficult to distinguish from superimposed preeclampsia. Measuring complement levels which are decreased and observing for the presence of urinary casts (which should not be seen in preeclampsia) may help determine the presence of a lupus flare.

37.4 **B.** When the aPL syndrome occurs with lupus, surveillance and therapy should be intensified for fetal and maternal complications. Therapy including prophylactic levels of heparin (with no history of thrombosis) or therapeutic anticoagulation (with a thrombosis history) plus low-dose aspirin offers the best efficacy with the lowest risk of side effects.

Clinical Pearls

See US Preventive Services Task Force Study Quality levels of evidence in Case 1

➤ Pregnancy should be postponed at least for 6 months after lupus nephritis (Level II-3).

➤ Patients with a serum creatinine greater than 1.5 mg/dL have an increased risk of deterioration of renal function during pregnancy (Level II-2).

➤ Other than methotrexate, most medications used to treat lupus are reasonable options during pregnancy (Level III).

➤ Antenatal evaluation of the lupus patient includes complement levels and renal function tests as well as determination of the presence of the lupus anticoagulant and anticardiolipin antibodies, if not previously detected (Level III).

➤ Pregnant women with lupus should undergo additional monitoring including serial sonograms for fetal growth and regular fetal monitoring until delivery (Level III).

➤ Patients with lupus and aPL syndrome are at additional maternal and fetal risk and should receive heparin and low-dose aspirin for optimal pregnancy outcome (Level I).

➤ Pregnant women with aPL syndrome should receive postpartum thromboprophylaxis (Level III).

REFERENCES

1. Burkett G. Lupus nephropathy and pregnancy. *Clin Obstet Gynecol.* 1985;28:310-323.
2. Georgiou PE, Politi EN, Katsimbri P, Sakka V, Drosos AA. Outcome of lupus pregnancy: a controlled study. *Rheumatology.* 2000;39:1014-1019.
3. Khamashta M. Systemic lupus erythematosus and pregnancy. *Best Prac Res Clin Rheumatol.* 2006;20:685-694.
4. Lockshin M. Lupus pregnancies and neonatal lupus. *Springer Semin Immunopathol.* 1994;16:247-259.
5. Molad Y. Systemic lupus erythematosus and pregnancy. *Curr Opin Obstet Gynecol.* 18:613-617.
6. Petri M. Prospective study of systemic lupus erythematosus pregnancies. *Lupus.* 2004;13:688-689.
7. Petri M, Magder L. Classification criteria for systemic lupus erythematosus: a review. *Lupus.* 2004:13;829-837.
8. Tincani A, Bazzani C, Zingarelli S, Lojacono A. Lupus and the antiphospholipid syndrome in pregnancy and obstetrics: clinical characteristics, diagnosis, pathogenesis, and treatment. *Semin Thromb Hemost.* 2008;34:267-273.
9. Warren JB, Silver RM. Autoimmune disease in pregnancy: systemic lupus erythematosus and antiphospholipid syndrome. *Obstet Gynecol Clin N Am.* 2004;31:345-372. *This is an all encompassing review of SLE and aPL syndrome with an extensive review of etiology including genetics, epidemiology, and evaluation and management.*
10. Witter FR. Management of the high-risk lupus pregnant patient. *Rheum Dis Clin N Am.* 2007;33:253-265.

Case 38

A 27-year-old G1P0 Caucasian woman at 35 weeks' gestation comes into the obstetrical triage unit complaining of increasing shortness of breath, fatigue, and swelling of her legs and feet. She states that these symptoms have begun abruptly over the last 2 days, and seem to be worsening. She denies cough, history of asthma, or fever. She states that she sleeps on three pillows to be comfortable. Her prenatal course has been unremarkable. On examination, her BP is 110/80 mm Hg, HR 120 beats/min (bpm), RR 40 breaths/min and labored, and oxygen saturation 89%. The lung examination reveals rales in the bilateral lung fields, without wheezes. The heart has a rapid heart rate. The abdomen is soft and nontender. The uterus is nontender with a fundal height of 35 cm. The fetal heart tones are in the 170 bpm range. There is 3+ pitting edema of bilateral lower extremities up to the knees. A stat chest radiograph is performed revealing cardiomegaly and bilateral pulmonary infiltrates.

➤ What is the most likely diagnosis?

➤ What is your next therapeutic step?

➤ What would be your diagnostic approach?

ANSWERS TO CASE 38:
Peripartum Cardiomyopathy

Summary: This is a 27-year-old woman G1P0 at 35 weeks' gestation who presents with dyspnea, orthopnea, and fatigue. She has tachycardia, tachypnea with labored breathing, and hypoxemia. She is not hypertensive. There are no wheezes on chest examination. The chest x-ray reveals marked cardiomegaly and bilateral pulmonary infiltrates.

➤ **Most likely diagnosis:** Congestive heart failure/possible peripartum cardiomyopathy.

➤ **Next therapeutic step:** Since the patient is alert on arrival to the hospital and the airway is not obviously compromised the priority at this time is to decrease the work of breathing, the improvement of oxygenation, and maintenance of circulatory status. The first therapeutic interventions would be to provide oxygen by mask with the patient in a Fowler position, obtain IV access, and administration of a diuretic such as furosemide.

➤ **Diagnostic approach:** CBC, urinalysis, comprehensive metabolic panel, arterial blood gas, ECG, and echocardiogram.

ANALYSIS

Objectives

1. Be able to describe the clinical presentation of peripartum cardiomyopathy (PPCM).
2. Be able to describe the diagnostic approach and differential diagnosis of peripartum cardiomyopathy.
3. Be able to list the treatment of peripartum cardiomyopathy.
4. Be able to describe the counseling of patients including the recurrence of PPCM.

Considerations

Peripartum cardiomyopathy is an infrequent but potentially life-threatening condition of unknown cause that occurs in previously healthy women during the peripartum period. The National Hospital Discharge Survey (1990-2002) estimated that it occurs in 1 in every 2289 live births in the United States.[1]

It is characterized by left ventricular dysfunction and symptoms of heart failure that can arise in the last trimester of pregnancy or up to 5 months after delivery. Although the diagnosis can be suspected clinically by the exclusion of other causes of heart failure, it is echocardiographic and a cardiac ultrasound needs to be obtained. As with the patient described in this case, oxygenation and diuresis are important while approaching the diagnostic plan.

APPROACH TO
Peripartum Cardiomyopathy

Clinical Presentation

The diagnosis of PPCM should be considered whenever women present with heart failure during the peripartum period.[2]

Symptoms of heart failure such as dyspnea, dizziness, pedal edema, and orthopnea can occur even in normal pregnancies, but they always need to be evaluated. Therefore, a pregnant woman in whom peripartum cardiomyopathy is developing may consider her symptoms to be normal. If swelling and other heart failure symptoms develop suddenly in an otherwise normal pregnancy, this should prompt further investigation.[3]

Symptoms and signs that should raise the suspicion of heart failure include paroxysmal nocturnal dyspnea, chest pain, nocturnal cough, new regurgitant murmurs, pulmonary crackles, elevated jugular venous pressure, and hepatomegaly.[2]

Pulmonary edema was a presenting symptom in all 106 patients with PPCM in a study conducted in China in 2007.[4] The clinical presentation was similar to that of congestive heart failure but was highly variable; 17% of cases were diagnosed antepartum and 83% postpartum. The mean age at diagnosis was 28 ± 6 years.[4]

Delayed diagnosis may be associated with higher rates of illness and death; therefore physicians should consider peripartum cardiomyopathy in any peripartum patient with unexplained cardiopulmonary symptoms. Although the symptoms of heart failure can be difficult to differentiate from those of late pregnancy, a heightened suspicion can help.[5]

Diagnostic Approach

The differential diagnosis of PPCM relies on a high index of suspicion in conjunction with timing of symptoms (in respect to pregnancy) and echocardiographic identification of new left ventricular systolic dysfunction.

The diagnostic criteria include (1) development of CHF secondary to deceased left ventricular systolic function in the last month of pregnancy or within 5 months after delivery; (2) absence of preexisting cardiac dysfunction; (3) absence of determinable cause of cardiomyopathy; and (4) left ventricular systolic dysfunction demonstrated by classic echocardiographic criteria: ejection fraction less than 45%, or M-mode fractional shortening less than 30%, or both, and end-diastolic dimension more than 2.7 cm/m^2 (Table 38–1).[5]

Table 38–1 DIAGNOSTIC CRITERIA FOR PERIPARTUM CARDIOMYOPATHY
• Cardiac failure occurring in the last month of pregnancy or within 5 mo of delivery
• Absence of identifiable cause for the cardiac failure
• Absence of heart disease prior to the last month of pregnancy
• LV systolic dysfunction by echocardiographic criteria:
• LVEF < 45 % and/or
• Fractional shortening < 30 %
• End-diastolic dimension > 2.7 cm/m^2

Data from Pearson GD, Veille JC, Rahimtoola S, et al. Peripartum cardiomyopathy: National Heart, Lung, and Blood Institute and Office of Rare Diseases (National Institutes of Health) workshop recommendations and review. *JAMA*. 2000;283:1183-1188; and Demakis JG, Rahimtoola SH, Sutton GC, et al. Natural course of peripartum cardiomyopathy. *Circulation*. 1971;44:1053-1061.

The electrocardiogram is nonspecific and may demonstrate normal sinus rhythm or a sinus tachycardia; dysrhythmias may also be present. Left ventricular hypertrophy, inverted T waves, Q waves, and nonspecific ST-segment changes have also been reported.[3]

The chest x-ray will likely demonstrate pulmonary edema, cephalization of pulmonary flow, cardiomegaly, and occasionally pleural effusions but these changes are nonspecific.

The aims during the diagnosis are to exclude other causes of cardiomyopathy and to confirm left ventricular systolic dysfunction by echocardiography. An endomyocardial biopsy is not routinely necessary for the diagnosis.

The etiology of this disease remains uncertain, but a number of possible causes of PPCM have been proposed, including myocarditis, abnormal immune response to pregnancy, maladaptive response to the hemodynamic stresses of pregnancy, stress activated cytokines, viral infection, and prolonged tocolysis. In addition, there have been a few reports of familial PPCM, raising the possibility that some cases of PPCM are actually familial dilated cardiomyopathy unmasked by pregnancy.[2] Risk factors for PPCM are listed in Table 38–2.

Differential Diagnosis

See Table 38–3. In the differential diagnoses of PPCM other causes of acute cardiopulmonary decompensation during pregnancy need to be considered. Such conditions include pulmonary embolism and complications of late pregnancy itself (eg, preeclampsia or amniotic fluid embolism). Other possible causes of decompensation include accelerated hypertension, diastolic dysfunction, systemic infection, and non-cardiogenic pulmonary edema. The history and physical examination and the echocardiogram would be helpful in differentiating among these conditions.

Table 38–2 PPCM RISK FACTORS AND ASSOCIATIONS

- African American ethnic background
- Age > 30 years
- Multiparity
- Twin pregnancy
- Preeclampsia
- Others:
  - Familial
  - Malnutrition (selenium and zinc deficiencies)
  - Long-term tocolytic Rx
  - Cocaine ingestion
  - Chlamydia infection
  - Living in tropical or subtropical region
  - Anemia
  - Infection
  - Cesarean delivery

Preeclampsia is by far the most common of these complications and should be excluded on the basis of history and physical examination.

The incidence of pulmonary thromboembolism which is also increased during pregnancy can be a presenting feature of PPCM.

Table 38–3 DIFFERENTIAL DIAGNOSIS OF PERIPARTUM CARDIOMYOPATHY

Preeclampsia
Noncardiogenic pulmonary edema
Pulmonary thromboembolism
Amniotic fluid embolism
Malignant hypertension
Aortic stenosis
Mitral stenosis
Ischemic heart disease
Cardiomyopathy:
  Alcoholic
  Cocaine
  Diabetic
  Dilated
Hypertrophic
Restrictive
Pulmonary disease

Treatment

During pregnancy   When considering tests or treatments in pregnancy, the welfare of the fetus is always considered along with that of the mother. Coordinated management with consultants (an obstetrician, maternal-fetal medicine, internal medicine, or cardiology) is essential.

- Digoxin, beta-blockers, loop diuretics, and drugs that reduce afterload such as hydralazine and nitrates have been proven to be safe and are the mainstays of medical therapy of heart failure during pregnancy.[5,6]
- Beta-blockers have strong evidence of efficacy in patients with heart failure and patients taking these agents prior to diagnosis can continue to use them safely.[6,7]
- Angiotensin-converting enzyme (ACE) inhibitors and angiotensin receptor blockers (ARBs) are contraindicated in pregnancy because they can cause birth defects, although they are the main treatments for postpartum women with heart failure. The teratogenic effects occur particularly in the second and third trimester, with fetopathy characterized by fetal hypotension, oligohydramnios, anuria, and renal tubular dysplasia. However, a recent study suggested a risk of malformations even after first-trimester exposure to ACE inhibitors.[8]

After delivery   After delivery, the treatment is identical to that for nonpregnant women with dilated cardiomyopathy.

- ACE inhibitors and ARBs. The target dose is one-half the maximum antihypertensive dose.[6]
- **Diuretics** are given for symptom relief. Spironolactone or digoxin is used in patients who have New York Heart Association class III or IV symptoms (see Table 38–4). The goal with spironolactone is 25 mg/d after the dosing of other drugs is maximized. The goal with digoxin is the lowest daily dose to obtain a detectable serum digoxin level, which should be kept at less than

Table 38–4 NEW YORK HEART FUNCTIONAL ASSOCIATION

CLASS	CLINICAL IMPLICATIONS	LIMITATION OF ACTIVITIES
I	Good tolerance of exercise without symptoms (chest pain, angina, dyspnea, palpitations, fatigue)	None
II	Symptomatic with moderate exercise	With ordinary activities
III	Symptomatic with light exercise or ordinary activities	With less than ordinary activities
IV	Symptomatic at rest	Unable to perform any physical activities

1.0 ng/mL. In the Digitalis Investigation Group trial,[10] serum digoxin levels of 0.5 to 0.8 ng/mL (0.6-1.0 nmol/L) were most beneficial, and levels of 1.1 to 1.5 ng/mL (1.4-1.9 nmol/L) were associated with an increase in deaths related to heart failure.[9]

- **Beta-blockers** are recommended for peripartum cardiomyopathy, as they improve symptoms, ejection fraction, and survival.[5] Nonselective beta-blockers such as carvedilol and selective ones such as metoprolol succinate have shown benefit. The goal dosage is carvedilol 25 mg twice a day (50 mg twice a day for larger patients) or metoprolol succinate 100 mg once a day.[6]

- **Anticoagulation treatment.** The natural history of PPCM includes a high incidence of thromboembolism. These observations were noted before initiation of mandatory bed rest, which was the standard of care in the past. Cases of arterial, venous, and cardiac thrombosis have been reported in women with peripartum cardiomyopathy, and the risk may be related to the degree of chamber enlargement, systolic dysfunction, and the presence of atrial fibrillation.[7] Anticoagulation with subcutaneous heparin (ie, 5000 U heparin subcutaneously twice daily) should be strongly considered in this population. Coumadin, on the other hand, should be avoided during first trimester because it can cause birth defects.[2]

- **Cardiac transplantation.** Patients with severe heart failure despite maximal drug therapy need cardiac transplantation to survive and to improve their quality of life. However, fewer than 3000 hearts are available for transplantation worldwide per year. Therefore, ventricular assist devices are indicated as a bridge to transplantation.[6]

- Patients with symptomatic ventricular arrhythmias should be considered for defibrillator implantation.[6]

- Other therapies include pentoxifylline (may improve outcomes, left ventricular function, and symptoms when added to conventional therapy), intravenous immunoglobulin (may improve the ejection fraction in several studies and reduce the levels of inflammatory cytokines), immunosuppressive therapy (could be considered in patients with proven myocarditis), calcium channel blockers, statins, monoclonal antibodies, interferon beta, immunoadsorption, therapeutic apheresis, bromocriptine, and cardiomyoplasty.[6]

How Long to Treat?

Patients with peripartum cardiomyopathy who recover normal left ventricular function at rest or with low-dose dobutamine can be allowed to taper and then discontinue heart failure treatment in 6 to 12 months under the supervision of a cardiologist or internist.[6]

Counseling

Even after full recovery of left ventricular function, subsequent pregnancies carry a risk of relapse of peripartum cardiomyopathy. A study in Haiti followed

99 patients, 15 of whom became pregnant again. Eight of the women (53%) who became pregnant again experienced worsening heart failure and long-term systolic dysfunction.[10]

A South African study reported that of six functional class I women (see Table 38-4) who became pregnant after an initial episode of PPCM, two died within 8 weeks of delivery, and the other four continued to have heart failure symptoms.[9] In the United States, Elkayam and colleagues[11] reported the subsequent outcomes of 44 women with history of PPCM. Of these, 28 had recovered systolic function, with ejection fractions of 50% or higher before becoming pregnant again, and 16 had not. The ejection fraction fell in both groups during pregnancy, but in the first group it fell by more than 20% in only 6 (21%), and none died. In contrast, in the group without recovery it fell by more than 20% in 5 (31%), and 3 (19%) died.[11]

Patients who recover normal left ventricular function and have normal left ventricular contractile reserve after dobutamine challenge may undertake another pregnancy safely, but they should be warned of the risk of recurrence even with fully recovered left ventricular function.[11] Dorbala et al[12] performed dobutamine stress echocardiography to measure maximal inotropic contractile reserve in six women presenting with peripartum cardiomyopathy, and it correlated accurately with subsequent recovery of left ventricular function.[13]

Based on these data, recommendations for further pregnancies are the following:

- If left ventricular function has recovered fully, subsequent pregnancy is not contraindicated, but the patient should be told that, although the recurrence risk is low, it is not absent.
- If left ventricular function has recovered partially, perform dobutamine stress echocardiography. If the left ventricular inotropic response to dobutamine is normal, then patients can be counseled as above; if the left ventricular inotropic response to dobutamine is abnormal, then the risk is moderate and pregnancy is not recommended.
- If left ventricular function has not recovered at all, the risk is high, and subsequent pregnancy is not recommended.[6,12]

Comprehension Questions

38.1   The diagnosis of PPCM is based on parameters obtained by which of the following?
  A. ECG
  B. Echocardiogram
  C. Arterial blood gas showing hypoxemia and respiratory alkalosis
  D. Chest x-ray demonstrating pulmonary edema and cardiomegaly

38.2   The most common cause of pulmonary edema during pregnancy is which of the following?
   A. Cocaine induced
   B. Arrhythmia
   C. Peripartum cardiomyopathy
   D. Preeclampsia

38.3   Angiotensin receptor blockers are not used during pregnancy because of which of the following reasons?
   A. They are not effective.
   B. Their half-life is decreased during pregnancy.
   C. They can cause oliguria and occasionally fetal death.
   D. They can cause arrhythmias during pregnancy.

ANSWERS

38.1   **B.** The diagnosis of cardiomyopathy is mainly echocardiographic.

38.2   **D.** Although the differential diagnosis of all cases of pulmonary edema should include pulmonary edema, during pregnancy the most common cause of pulmonary edema is preeclampsia.

38.3   **C.** Angiotensin receptor blockers can cause oliguria, anuria, and occasionally fetal death and are contraindicated during pregnancy.

Clinical Pearls

See US Preventive Services Task Force Study Quality levels of evidence in Case 1

➤ Suspect peripartum cardiomyopathy in any peripartum patient with unexplained symptoms of heart failure (Level III).

➤ Heightened suspicion is important when a pregnant woman presents with signs of heart failure, because early diagnosis allows proven treatment to be started (Level III).

➤ Pregnant women should not receive angiotensin-converting enzyme inhibitors, angiotensin receptor blockers, or warfarin because of potential teratogenic effects (Level II-2).

➤ An initial left ventricular end-systolic dimension less than 5.5 cm, a left ventricular ejection fraction greater than 30%, and a low cardiac troponin level may predict a better outcome (Level II-3).

➤ Subsequent pregnancies carry a high risk of relapse, even in women who have fully recovered left ventricular function (Level II-3).

REFERENCES

1. Mielniczuk LM, Williams K, Davis DR, et al. Frequency of peripartum cardiomyopathy. *Am J Cardiol.* 2006;97:1765-1768.
2. Abboud J, Murad Y, Chen-Scarabelli C, et al. Peripartum cardiomyopathy: a comprehensive review. *Int J Cardiol.* 2007;118:295-303.
3. Brown CS, Bertolet BD. Peripartum cardiomyopathy: a comprehensive review. *Am J Obstet Gynecol.* 1998;178:409-414.
4. Hu CL, Li YB, Zou YG, et al. Troponin T measurement can predict persistent peripartum cardiomyopathy left ventricular dysfunction in peripartum cardiomyopathy. *Heart.* 2007;93:488-490.
5. Pearson GD, Veille JC, Rahimtoola S, et al. Peripartum cardiomyopathy: National Heart, Lung, and Blood Institute and Office of Rare Diseases (National Institutes of Health) workshop recommendations and review. *JAMA.* 2000;283:1183-1188.
6. Ramaraj R, Sorrell V. Peripartum cardiomyopathy: causes, diagnosis, and treatment. *Cleve Clin J Med.* 2009 May;76(5):289-296.
7. Sliwa K, Forster O, Zhanje F, et al. Outcome of subsequent pregnancy in patients with documented peripartum cardiomyopathy. *Am J Cardiol.* 2004;93:1441-1443, A10.
8. Cooper WO, Hernandez-Diaz S, Arbogast PG, et al. Major congenital malformations after first-trimester exposure to ACE inhibitors. *N Engl J Med.* 2006; 354:2443-2451.
9. Rathore SS, Curtis JP, Wang Y, et al. Association of serum digoxin concentration and outcomes in patients with heart failure. *JAMA.* 2003;289:871-888.
10. Fett JD, Christie LG, Murphy JG. Brief communication: outcomes of subsequent pregnancy after peripartum cardiomyopathy: a case series from Haiti. *Ann Intern Med.* 2006;145:30-34.
11. Elkayam U, Tummala PP, Rao K, et al. Maternal and fetal outcomes of subsequent pregnancies in women with peripartum cardiomyopathy. *N Engl J Med.* 2001;344:1567-1571.
12. Dorbala S, Brozena S, Zeb S, et al. Risk stratification of women with peripartum cardiomyopathy at initial presentation: a dobutamine stress echocardiography study. *J Am Soc Echocardiogr.* 2005;18:45-48.
13. Demakis JG, Rahimtoola SH, Sutton GC, et al. Natural course of peripartum cardiomyopathy. *Circulation.* 1971;44:1053-1061.

Case 39

A 22-year-old G1 P0 with a monochorionic diamniotic twin gestation is seen in your office at 24 weeks for follow-up sonogram. The patient notes fetal activity daily and occasional uterine contractions. Her vital signs are normal and she has gained 4 lb since her last visit at 20 weeks, when ultrasound revealed appropriate and concordant growth with normal amniotic fluid volume. Fundal height today is 30 cm.

On ultrasound, twin A appears normal and has grown appropriately since the last ultrasound, although the amniotic fluid volume appears moderately increased. Twin B's estimated fetal weight (EFW) is equivalent to 22 weeks' gestational age (GA). The bladder is difficult to visualize, and amniotic fluid volume is markedly decreased. No fetal movement of twin B is noted, although the fetal heart rate is 140 bpm.

➤ What is the most likely diagnosis?

➤ What is your next step?

➤ What are potential complications of the patient's disorder?

ANSWERS TO CASE 39:
Twin-Twin Transfusion

Summary: This is a 22-year-old G1P0 woman with monozygotic twins at 24 weeks' gestation with discordant growth and polyhydramnios in one sac and oligohydramnios in the other.

> **Most likely diagnosis:** Twin-twin transfusion syndrome (TTTS).

> **Next step:** Evaluate fetal well-being and the potential utility of various treatment modalities.

> **Potential complications:** Fetal polycythemia/fetal anemia; hydrops; intrauterine demise; preterm birth; preeclampsia.

ANALYSIS

Objectives

1. List risk factors for twin-twin transfusion syndrome.
2. Identify ultrasound findings that confirm the diagnosis of TTTS.
3. Explain a management scheme for TTTS.
4. Discuss situations in which laser ablation of placental vessels should be considered.

Considerations

This is a 22-year-old primigravida with a monochorionic, diamniotic twin gestation with a significant fluid discrepancy between the fetuses. One fetus has polyhydramnios and the other has oligohydramnios. Additionally, there is weight discordance between the two fetuses. This is highly suspicious for twin-twin transfusion syndrome (TTTS). Approximately 30% of all twin pregnancies are monochorionic, and the incidence of TTTS in monochorionic, diamniotic gestations is approximately 10% to 20%. Early identification is important due to the high perinatal mortality and the possible need for intervention. Because monochorionic twins have a higher perinatal morbidity, its identification is important, such as in the first trimester. This can be achieved by sonographic assessment of the dividing membrane.

APPROACH TO
Twin-Twin Transfusion

The **diagnosis** of TTTS is based on the presence of a monochorionic placenta and amniotic fluid discrepancy. Monochorionicity is diagnosed by the following sonographic findings:

- Same-sex twins
- A thin intertwin membrane
- The absence of a "twin peak" (also known as the "lambda") sign
- The presence of a "T-sign," in which the membranes diverge from the placental surface at a 90 degree angle
- A fused placenta
- Only two membranes between fetuses (if the ultrasound is done early enough and the membranes can be counted)

After monochorionicity is established, the remainder of the evaluation is based on fetal hemodynamics and growth. One fetus, the **recipient**, is volume overloaded, sometimes with signs of cardiac failure, and has polyhydramnios (maximum vertical pocket of over 8 cm). The recipient may be large for gestational age (LGA) or appropriate for gestational age (AGA). The other fetus, the **donor**, is dehydrated and has oligohydramnios (maximum vertical pocket of less than 2 cm). The donor may be SGA or AGA.

Growth discrepancy is many times a sign of chronic TTTS; however, in some cases the underlying etiology of growth discrepancy may be placental insufficiency or an abnormal placental cord insertion.

Once TTTS is suspected, Doppler analysis of the umbilical artery, middle cerebral artery, and of the ductus venosus, as well as echocardiograms of both fetuses are performed. The purpose of the echocardiogram is to evaluate cardiac function and signs of cardiac failure or valvular insufficiency.

Quintero et al[1] designed a staging system for TTTS which consists of the following:

Stage I: Polyhydramnios in the recipient, severe oligohydramnios in donor but urine visible within the bladder of the donor.

Stage II: Polyhydramnios in the recipient; the appearance of a "stuck" donor fetus, urine not visible within the donor's bladder and oligohydramnios.

Stage III: Polyhydramnios and oligohydramnios as well as critically abnormal Dopplers (at least one abnormal Doppler finding: absent or reverse end-diastolic flow in the umbilical artery, reverse flow in the ductus venosus or pulsatile umbilical venous flow) with or without urine visualized within the donor's bladder.

Stage IV: Presence of ascites or hydrops (fluid collection in two or more cavities) in either donor or recipient.

Stage V: Demise of either fetus.

Other investigators have modified the Quintero staging system by further subdividing stage III based on **cardiac function**. There is a wide range of severity across the many patients who present in stage III. The cardiac function profile can be used to better define the severity of TTTS within this group. Signs of valvular incompetence, ventricular wall thickening, and cardiac dysfunction (as determined by the Tei index) are used to assess cardiac function and subdivide stage III into stage III a, b, c.

Pathophysiology

Sometimes in several combinations, 95% of monochorionic twin placentas contain inter-fetal vascular connections of some kind. These connections may be vein-to-vein, artery-to-vein, vein-to-artery, and artery-to-artery within a placental cotyledon. Depending on the number and type of vascular connections, the blood flow between the twins may be balanced or unbalanced. "Unbalanced" denotes net flow away from one fetus and toward another (see Figure 39–1).

There is increasing evidence that the pathophysiology of TTTS may also include the renin and angiotensin system. The donor fetus—dehydrated and volume depleted—will produce angiotensin as a protective mechanism to maintain volume. However, because of the vascular shunting which underlies TTTS, the recipient is also exposed to the donor-produced angiotensin, further complicating the volume-overloaded recipient twin.

CLINICAL APPROACH

Once TTTS is diagnosed and the stage is determined, then the treatment approach is made. The treatment modalities can include:

- Microseptostomy
- Amnioreduction
- Laser ablation of the intertwin fetal vessels
- Selective fetal reduction

The treatment choice will depend on the gestational age at which TTTS presents as well as the severity. Prior to deciding upon a treatment plan, fetal evaluation should include the following:

- Ultrasound for growth
- Tests of fetal well-being—biophysical profile, umbilical artery Doppler, middle cerebral artery Doppler
- Assessment of the amniotic fluid volume
- Fetal echocardiogram for cardiac function and performance index

Treatment

Septostomy is performed in attempt to equalize the fluid dynamics between the fetuses. A small hole is created in the intertwin membrane to restore amniotic fluid in the donor fetus' sac. This can be problematic if the defect

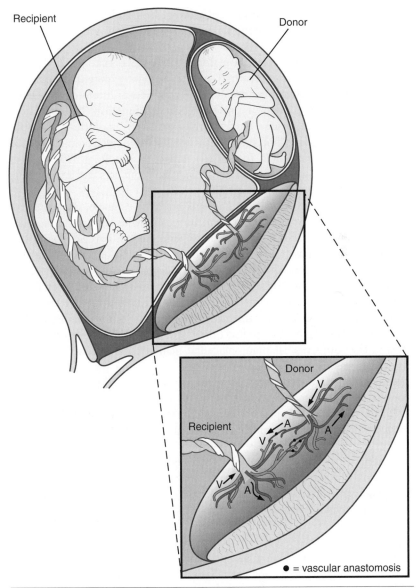

Figure 39–1. Twin-twin transfusion syndrome with the donor twin being smaller and with oligohydramnios and the recipient twin being larger and with hydramnios. Note the numerous arterial (donor) to venous (recipient) anatomoses which allows for the TTTS.

expands, as the large septostomy creates a functional monoamniotic gestation, which carries inherent risks of cord entanglement. Because of this risk, a fetoscopic approach to septostomy has been proposed. In this case, a laser is used to create a **microseptostomy**; use of the laser creates very small holes and cautery of the edges is felt to prevent tearing. In a multicenter prospective trial, Saade et al[2] compared amnioreduction to septostomy and found the survival in each arm was 65%.

Amnioreduction was initially performed to relieve maternal abdominal discomfort and shortness of breath. It was also thought to potentially decrease the risk of preterm delivery as a result of the uterine overdistension. It is likely that amnioreduction also improves placental function by decreasing intrauterine pressure created by the large amount of amniotic fluid in the recipient sac. The survival in one series with aggressive serial amnioreduction (reduction of amniotic fluid to normal) ranged widely, from 37% to 83%. However, this retrospective series contained small numbers and a wide range of gestational age and severity of TTTS.

The earlier in pregnancy the diagnosis of TTTS is made, the worse the prognosis. The majority of patients who are treated with amnioreduction will require serial amnioreductions, sometimes performed on a weekly basis. This treatment approach addresses the problematic symptoms of TTTS. The benefit to amnioreduction is that it is easily available and less invasive for the mother, but it does not fully address the underlying pathophysiology of TTTS.

Cases presenting early in pregnancy may benefit from definitive treatment by **fetoscopic laser ablation** of the placental intertwin fetal vessels. Laser ablation aims to eliminate the unidirectional shunting of blood from the donor fetus to the recipient, balancing placental hemodynamics. Laser ablation is considered definitive treatment, since the underlying pathophysiology is directly addressed; a second procedure is rarely necessary. However, laser ablation is significantly more invasive for the patient.

When compared to serial amnioreduction, the **overall** survival is similar and was not statistically significantly different (61% vs 51% for laser ablation and serial amnioreductions, respectively) in one nonrandomized comparison of patients at two different centers (one performed laser ablation and the other serial amnioreduction). However, in this same study, the survival of **at least one twin** with laser ablation was 79%—survival of at least one twin with serial amnioreduction was 60%.

The Eurofetus trial is the only prospective, randomized trial to compare the efficacy of laser therapy with serial amnioreduction. Patients were eligible if they had stage I TTTS with a gestational age between 16 and 26 weeks. The study was stopped when an analysis revealed that the survival at 28 days of life and 6 months of life was significantly higher in the laser group when compared to serial amnioreduction (76% vs 56% and 76% vs 51%, respectively). Of note, the amnioreduction group had a survival of 38%, significantly lower than previously reported. In the Eurofetus trial, fewer fetuses in the laser group had neurologic abnormalities on neuroimaging studies when compared to the amnioreduction group (52% vs 31%). It must be noted, however, that this does not necessarily correlate with neurologic developmental delay or cerebral palsy.

Fetoscopic umbilical cord cauterization is reserved for end-stage TTTS, in which one fetus is so compromised that death is imminent. In this procedure, the umbilical cord of the severely compromised fetus is cauterized to protect the healthier fetus from death or neurologic damage as a result of co-twin death.

There is a small subset of patients who will respond to a single amnioreduction and do not require serial procedures. Since this is a less invasive approach to management of these pregnancies, an amnioreduction is recommended first before more aggressive and invasive therapies are chosen. If a single amnioreduction does not lead to lasting normalization of the amniotic fluid indices, more definitive therapy is recommended, particularly in early gestations.

Screening

The best time to determine chorionicity is **early in the pregnancy**. When the gestation is evaluated in the first or early second trimester, the positive predictive value for properly assigning chorionicity using sonographic findings (placental location[s], the lambda and T signs, and/or fetal gender) is as high as 98%. By the mid-second trimester the same ultrasound findings have a positive predictive value of only 88%.

All monochorionic pregnancies should be evaluated frequently for the onset of TTTS. It is not possible to accurately predict which pregnancies will go on to develop TTTS. It is especially important to watch carefully for TTTS in the earlier stages of pregnancy, since the more definitive and invasive treatment options may be preferable earlier in the pregnancy and become unavailable as the gestation advances. Screening monochorionic pregnancies every 2 weeks by evaluating growth and amniotic fluid volume is one method with which to aggressively monitor for TTTS.

Comprehension Questions

39.1   A 34-year-old G2P1001 woman at 32 weeks' gestation is noted to have a twin gestation. The patient has been researching on the internet about different complications and asks about TTTS. The obstetrician reviews the records and specifically counsels the patient that she is not likely to develop TTTS. Which of the following is likely to be present in this patient?

A. Monochorionic diamniotic twin gestation
B. Polyhydramnios in the recipient sac
C. Oligohydramnios in the donor sac
D. Dichorionic twins with abnormal umbilical artery Dopplers
E. Growth restriction in one fetus of a monochorionic pair

39.2   A 29-year-old G1P0 woman at 30 weeks' gestation with a diagnosis of
        TTTS. The obstetrician has counseled the patient about various ther-
        apy options that are available. Which of the following is LEAST likely
        to be a treatment of TTTS?
        A. Microseptostomy
        B. Laser ablation of the intertwin surface placental vessels
        C. Amnioreduction with microseptostomy
        D. Selective fetal reduction
        E. Focused ultrasonic energy of the shared fetal vessels

39.3 to 39.5 Matching. Please match the following clinical vignette with the
              stage of the TTTS.
        A. Stage I
        B. Stage II
        C. Stage III
        D. Stage IV
        E. Stage V

39.3   A 41-year-old G3P2002 woman at 25 weeks' gestation is diagnosed
        with TTTS based on one fetus with oligohydramnios and the other
        with polyhydramnios. One fetus is noted to have loss of end-diastolic
        flow of the umbilical artery.

39.4   A 27-year-old G1P0 woman at 28 weeks' gestation with TTTS, and
        one fetus with fetal ascites.

39.5   A 35-year-old G3P2011 woman at 23 weeks' gestation with one fetus
        having oligohydramnios and the other with polyhydramnios, and car-
        diac dysfunction on echocardiogram.

39.6   A 32-year-old G4P2012 woman is at 25 weeks' gestation. She had been
        diagnosed as having monochorionic twins based on a first-trimester
        ultrasound showing the "T sign" of the dividing membrane. Which of
        the following is most accurate regarding this patient?
        A. Fetal gender is useful in determining zygosity.
        B. Number of placentas is useful in determining zygosity.
        C. The T sign is better visualized in the second trimester rather than
           the first trimester.
        D. Once the pregnancy has progressed beyond 24 weeks' gestational
           age and has not developed TTTS, then the patient is at low risk
           and can be followed monthly.
        E. A family history of twins is useful in determining zygosity.

ANSWERS

39.1   **D.** Dichorionic placentation is not associated with TTTS since there are two separate placentas, one for each fetus and the hemodynamic shifts between the fetuses is not present as it can be in monochorionic placentas. 95% of monochorionic placentas have vascular connections and the risk of TTTS in monochorionic pregnancies is 10% to 20%. The diagnosis is made by finding a monochorionic gestation with oligohydramnios in one sac and polyhydramnios in the other. If the problem is chronic then a growth discrepancy can be appreciated.

39.2   **E.** Ultrasound energy to the fetal vessels is not a therapy. All of the other treatment modalities (A-D) are reasonable and can be done in sequence or in combination. A patient will often have an amnioreduction first to see if the pregnancy responds before proceeding with more invasive therapy. During the fetoscopic laser ablation procedure an amnioreduction is performed so that the final maximum vertical pocket is less than 5 cm. A microseptostomy is also done at the time of the fetoscopy at some centers. The selective fetal reduction is reserved for severe, terminal cases in which one fetus has a very poor prognosis and is expected to die.

39.3   **C.** Oligohydramnios and polyhydramnios in the face of critically abnormal Doppler flow studies such as absent or reverse end-diastolic flow is indicative of stage III TTTS.

39.4   **D.** Ascites or hydrops in either the recipient or donor twin is consistent with stage IV disease, and implies serious fetal compromise.

39.5   **C.** Oligohydramnios and polyhydramnios by themselves are consistent with stage I disease, but the presence of cardiac dysfunction upstages the severity to stage III. Thus, in general, every patient with TTTS in stage I to III should have cardiac echocardiography to assess for further severity. The use of echocardiogram is to stage all TTTS, and can help to subcategorize those in stage III, since this category is fairly broad. Based on cardiac dysfunction an initial assessment of stage I or II can be increased to stage III after the echocardiogram. All patients with TTTS should have an echocardiogram as part of staging.

39.6   **A.** Monozygotic twins are at greater risk for complications. Different fetal genders are highly suggestive of dizygotic gestations. The number of placentas is not helpful, as often the placentas will fuse. The fetal membranes are better seen in the first trimester rather than later in the pregnancy. Even after 24 weeks' gestation TTTS can develop. It is difficult to predict which pregnancies will go on to develop TTTS and which will not. Sometimes TTTS can evolve very rapidly; therefore, it is recommended that the pregnancy be followed closely until delivery.

Clinical Pearls

See US Preventive Services Task Force Study Quality levels of evidence in Case 1

➤ The neonatal survival at 28 days of life and 6 months of life was significantly higher in the laser group when compared to serial amnioreduction (76% vs 56% and 76% and 51%, respectively) in the Eurofetus trial (Level I).

➤ Early ultrasound is useful in determining chorionicity and amnionicity in multifetal gestations (Level III).

➤ There is a wide range of severity across the many patients who present in stage III. The cardiac function profile can be used to better define the severity of TTTS within this group (Level III).

REFERENCES

1. Quintero RA, Morales WJ, Allen MH, et al. Staging of twin-twin transfusion syndrome. *J Perinatol.* 1999;19:550-555.
2. Saade GR, Belfort MA, Berry DL, et al. Amniotic septostomy for the treatment of twin oligohydramnios-polyhydramnios sequence. *Fetal Diagn Ther.* 1998;13:86-93.
3. Barrea C, Alkazaleh F, Ryan G, et al. Prenatal cardiovascular manifestations in the twin-to-twin transfusion syndrome recipients and the impact of therapeutic amnioreduction. *Am J Obstet Gynecol.* 2005;192:892-902.
4. Elliott JP, Urig MA, Clewell WH. Aggressive therapeutic amniocentesis for treatment of twin-twin transfusion syndrome. *Obstet Gynecol.* 1991;77:537-540.
5. Lee YM, Cleary-Goldman J, Thaker HM, Simpson LL. Antenatal sonographic prediction of twin chorionicity. *Am J Obstet Gynecol.* 2006;195:863.
6. Machin GA. Why is it important to diagnose chorionicity and how do we do it? *Best Pract Res Clin Obstet Gynaecol.* 2004 Aug;18(4):515-530.
7. Mahieu-Caputo D, Dommergues M, Delezoide AL, et al. Twin-to-twin transfusion syndrome: role of the fetal renin-angiotensin system. *Am J Pathol.* 2000;156:629-636.
8. Mahony BS, Petty CN, Nyberg DA, et al. The "stuck twin" phenomenon: ultrasonographic findings, pregnancy outcome, and management with serial amniocenteses. *Am J Obstet Gynecol.* 1990;163:1513-1521.
9. Michelfelder E, Gottliebson W, Border W, et al. Early manifestations and spectrum of recipient twin cardiomyopathy in twin-twin transfusion syndrome: relation to Quintero stage. *Ultrasound Obstet Gynecol.* 2007 Dec;30(7):965-971.
10. Pinette MG, Pan Y, Pinette SG, et al. Treatment of twin-twin transfusion syndrome. *Obstet Gynecol.* 1993;82:841-846.
11. Reisner DP, Mahony BS, Petty CH, et al. Stuck twin syndrome: outcome in 37 consecutive cases. *Am J Obstet Gynecol.* 1993;169:991-995.
12. Rodestal A, Thomassen PA. Acute polyhydramnios in twin pregnancy. A retrospective study with special reference to therapeutic amniocentesis. *Acta Obstet Gynecol Scand.* 1990;69:297-300.
13. Saade GR, Olson G, Belfort MA, et al. Amniotomy: a new approach to the "stuck twin" syndrome. *Am J Obstet Gynecol.* 1995;172:429-434.
14. Urig MA, Clewell WH, Elliott J. Twin-twin transfusion syndrome. *Am J Obstet Gynecol.* 1990;163:1522-1526.

Case 40

A 32-year-old G3P0202 married African American woman at 31 weeks' gestation arrives in the labor and delivery suite complaining of recurrent intermittent abdominal pain. She describes an increase in back pain yesterday and some mucous-like discharge today. She has noted no bleeding or leaking of fluid, but says she feels as if she is "starting her period." In reviewing her prenatal record, you note that her first pregnancy resulted in a 28-week vaginal delivery of a 1200 g female, who is currently 7 years old and doing well. Her second baby, a male, is a healthy 3 years old, although he was delivered at 33 weeks' gestation.

On examination, she is afebrile, her BP is 120/80 mm Hg, pulse is 80 bpm and regular, and RR is 16 breaths/min. She appears to be in mild distress and holds her abdomen and moans every 3 to 5 minutes. Her abdomen is gravid with a fundal height of 32 cm, and soft, although you note two contractions by palpation during your 10-minute examination with her. Sterile speculum examination is negative for nitrazine and ferning, and no blood is noted. Membranes are visualized through the cervix. On digital examination, her cervix is dilated 3 cm, effacement is 80%, and station of the fetal vertex is at −1. The electronic fetal monitor shows a reassuring fetal heart rate of 140 bpm with mild contractions every 3 to 4 minutes.

➤ What is the most likely diagnosis?

➤ What is your next step?

➤ What are potential complications of the patient's disorder?

ANSWERS TO CASE 40:

Idiopathic Preterm Labor

Summary: This is a 32-year-old G3P0202 woman with two prior preterm deliveries who is in preterm labor at 31 weeks. Because of the risk of imminent preterm birth, she should receive tocolytics in an attempt to delay delivery for at least 48 hours in order to administer antibiotics to reduce the risk of group B *Streptococcus* and corticosteroids to reduce the risk of respiratory distress syndrome.

➤ **Most likely diagnosis:** Idiopathic preterm labor.

➤ **Next step:** Begin hydration, administer tocolytics, corticosteroids, and antibiotics.

➤ **Potential complications:** Preterm birth with neonatal complications of respiratory distress syndrome (RDS), necrotizing enterocolitis (NEC), patent ductus arteriosus (PDA), and neonatal death.

ANALYSIS

Objectives

1. Understand the epidemiology of preterm birth.
2. Recognize risk factors that predispose to preterm delivery.
3. Understand methods of preventing or delaying preterm delivery.

Considerations

This is a 32-year-old G3P0202 patient with two prior preterm births presenting at 31 weeks with contractions and cervical dilation. She is at high risk for recurrent preterm birth because of the prior pregnancies. If there are no signs of infection, placental separation, or fetal stress, she is a candidate for tocolytics in an attempt to delay delivery for at least 48 hours in order to administer corticosteroids to obtain maximum effect to the fetus. Antibiotics effective against group B *Streptococcus* are customarily administered until her GBS status is known. Although in most circumstances, the etiology of preterm labor is unknown, a diligent search should be undertaken for a possible cause. Her clinical situation and the potential for neonatal damage underscore the importance of preterm birth in the United States today.

APPROACH TO

Idiopathic Preterm Labor

Epidemiology of Preterm Birth

Preterm birth, or delivery at less than 37 weeks' gestational age, is a leading health problem in the United States, with annual costs exceeding $20 billion. Since 1999, prematurity exceeded congenital anomalies as the leading cause of neonatal mortality in this country for all racial and ethnic groups. The preterm birth rate has risen in most industrialized countries, with the US rate increasing from 9.5% in 1981 to 12.7% in 2005. A dramatic recent epidemiologic change is the shift in just one decade (1992-2002) from 40 to 39 weeks as the most common length of gestation for singleton births in the United States. The obstetric precursors leading to preterm birth are: (1) delivery for maternal or fetal indications (30%-35%); (2) spontaneous preterm labor with intact membranes (40%-45%); and (3) preterm premature rupture of the membranes (PPROM, 25%-30%). Spontaneous preterm birth is most commonly caused by preterm labor in white women, but by PPROM in black women. Preterm births can also be grouped according to gestational age, since about 5% of preterm births occur at less than 28 weeks, about 15% at 28 to 31 weeks, about 20% at 32 to 33 weeks, and 60% to 70% at 34 to 36 weeks. Rather than having a specific etiology in most cases, preterm labor is now thought to be a syndrome initiated by multiple mechanisms, including infection or inflammation, uteroplacental ischemia or hemorrhage, uterine overdistension, stress, and other immunologically mediated processes.

Risk Factors for Preterm Birth

The lowest gestational age for which an increased risk of preterm birth is seen in subsequent pregnancies is 18 weeks' gestation. Previous births before 17 weeks' gestation do not appear to confer an increased risk of recurrent preterm delivery. In the United States and the United Kingdom, women classified as black, African American, and Afro-Caribbean are consistently reported to be at higher risk of preterm delivery: preterm birth rates are in the range of 16% to 18% for black women compared with 5% to 9% for white women. Some investigators have speculated on mechanisms. Black women in both the United States and the United Kingdom are three times more likely to have bacterial vaginosis than are white women, and this difference could explain half of the excess preterm births in black women. East Asian and Hispanic women typically have low preterm birth rates. In many immigrant groups, the greater the length of time spent living in the United States, the higher the rate of preterm birth. A low prepregnancy BMI is associated with an increased risk of spontaneous preterm birth, whereas obesity can be protective. Women with low serum concentrations of iron, folate, or zinc have more preterm births than those with measurements within the normal range.

Microbiologic studies suggest that intrauterine infection might account for 25% to 40% of preterm births. By studying microbial "footprints" in the amniotic cavity (such as PCR detection of *Ureaplasma urealyticum*) in addition to traditional culture methods, this number may be an underestimate. At 21 to 24 weeks' gestation, most spontaneous births are associated with histological chorioamnionitis compared to about 10% at 35 to 36 weeks. Trichomoniasis seems to be associated with preterm birth with a relative risk (RR) of about 1.3. Chlamydia does not appear to be associated with preterm birth. Syphilis and gonorrhea are probably associated with preterm birth with a RR of about 2.0. Vaginal group B *Streptococcus*, *U urealyticum*, and *Mycoplasma hominis* colonizations are not associated with an increased risk of preterm birth. Several nongenital tract infections, such as pyelonephritis and asymptomatic bacteriuria, pneumonia, and appendicitis, are associated with, and probably predispose to, preterm birth. Periodontal disease may also be a risk factor. On the other hand, viral DNA material in amniotic fluid has not been linked to preterm birth.

Both digital and ultrasound examinations of the cervix have shown that cervical shortening is a risk factor for preterm delivery. Ultrasound has been shown to be useful in identifying women at increased risk for preterm birth in asymptomatic low-risk women with cervical length of less than 25 mm at 24 weeks' gestation. Women with preterm contractions, on the other hand, with a cervical length of over 30 mm, have about a 1% chance of delivering within the next week. Fetal fibronectin, a marker of chorio-decidual disruption, is typically absent from cervico-vaginal secretions from 24 weeks' gestation until near term; however, 3% to 4% of women undergoing routine screening at 24 to 26 weeks are positive, and are at substantially increased risk of preterm delivery. In questionable cases of preterm labor, only about 1% of women with a negative test deliver in the next week. Genetic association studies have been used to identify single-nucleotide polymorphisms in several genes associated with preterm labor and PPROM. While maternal carriage of a polymorphism in the *IL6* gene did not result in an increased risk of spontaneous preterm birth for white or black women, black women who were carriers of the *IL6* allele and who had bacterial vaginosis had a twofold greater risk of preterm birth than did those who carried the variant but did not have such infection.

Methods to Reduce PTB

Work in a standing position compared with that in a sitting position and work at night compared to work during the day have been associated with an increased rate of preterm birth (PTB). A Cochrane review reported that smoking cessation programs in pregnancy successfully reduce the incidence of preterm birth. Although genital-tract infection and colonization are consistently associated with an increased risk of preterm birth, antibiotic treatment does not reliably reduce this risk. Screening for and treatment of U urealyticum, group B Streptococcus, bacterial vaginosis (BV), and Trichomonas vaginalis does not reduce the rate of preterm birth, and, in the case of trichomonas and metronidazole, can actually increase the risk of prematurity.

Dietary supplementation with omega-3 polyunsaturated fatty acids has been associated with reduced production of inflammatory mediators, and a randomized trial of omega-3 supplements undertaken in women at risk of preterm birth showed a reduction in the preterm birth rate as did a randomized trial of supplemental fish oil. The risk of preterm birth was reduced by about a third in two trials of progesterone supplementation, given as intramuscular injections of 250 mg per week of 17α-hydroxyprogesterone caproate and as daily vaginal progesterone, although two systematic reviews noted that studies of progesterone have not been sufficiently powered to detect an effect on neonatal or infant outcomes. Progesterone has not been uniformly beneficial in all populations at risk, including patients with twins.

In a meta-analysis of data from four trials, the risk of birth before 35 weeks' gestation was reduced with cerclage in women with previous preterm birth and a short cervix (defined as less than 25 mm) in the present pregnancy. Cerclage in women with short cervices who did not have previous preterm births showed no advantage. In women with twins, cerclage for short cervix was associated with an increased risk of preterm birth.

Pharmacologic Therapy for Women in Preterm Labor

Treatment to arrest preterm labor established by progressive cervical dilation and effacement or membrane rupture does not prolong pregnancy sufficiently to allow further intrauterine growth and maturation. Treatment can, however, defer preterm birth long enough to allow for interventions that reduce neonatal morbidity and mortality. Antibiotic treatment of all women with threatened preterm labor to prevent neonatal infection with group B Streptococcus is recommended because preterm infants have an increased risk of this infection. Antenatal administration of corticosteroids to the mother reduces neonatal morbidity and mortality from respiratory distress, intraventricular hemorrhage, necrotizing enterocolitis, and patent ductus arteriosus. A single course consists either of two doses of 12 mg betamethasone given intramuscularly, 24 hours apart, or four doses of 6 mg dexamethasone given intramuscularly every 12 hours. The duration of fetal benefit after a course of glucocorticoids is uncertain. Data suggest that a repeat course might confer modest additional neonatal benefit, whereas multiple courses can reduce fetal growth. The earliest gestational age at which corticosteroids are administered is either 23 or 24 weeks.

Tocolytic drugs are used to prolong pregnancy in women with acute risk of preterm birth caused mainly by active preterm labor and, less commonly, by ruptured membranes. The main rationale for use of these drugs is a 48-hour delayed delivery that allows transfer to a specialist unit and the administration of corticosteroids. No studies have shown that any tocolytic drug can reduce the rate of preterm birth. The Cochrane database meta-analyses suggest that calcium-channel blockers and an oxytocin antagonist (atosiban) can delay delivery by 2 to 7 days with an optimum risk-benefit ratio. The Cochrane analysts concluded that β_2-agonist drugs, such as ritodrine and terbutaline, can delay delivery by 48 hours, but carry greater side-effects than other agents, and that magnesium sulfate is ineffective. Magnesium, however, is currently the subject of intense review after studies have shown that intrapartum administration may reduce the risk of cerebral palsy. Although the cyclooxygenase inhibitor indomethacin reduced the occurrence of preterm birth when compared with placebo and other tocolytic agents in some controlled trials, the Cochrane analysts reported that the volume of evidence did not allow firm conclusions about efficacy. In light of this information, it is interesting that a recent survey noted that almost all maternal–fetal medicine specialists in this country recommend tocolysis in the setting of acute preterm labor. Magnesium and nifedipine are the most commonly prescribed first-line tocolytics, according to the survey.

Continued suppression of contractions after acute tocolysis does not reduce the rate of preterm birth. Posthospitalization surveillance with outpatient monitoring of uterine contractions also has no effect on the rate of preterm birth or low birth weight, or gestational age at delivery.

Summary

It is clear that spontaneous preterm birth causes a tremendous health care burden for the individual patient as well as society overall. Our current understanding of the etiologies, detection, and intervention is insufficient to make a dramatic impact of this important disease. Associated conditions and risk factors have not uniformly led to successful intervention in randomized controlled trials. More research is critically important for gains to be made in unlocking the mechanisms and making meaningful strides in preterm birth.

Comprehension Questions

40.1   The most common length of gestation for singleton births in the United States is which of the following?
A.   37 weeks
B.   38 weeks
C.   39 weeks
D.   40 weeks

40.2   The lowest gestational age at delivery associated with an increased risk of preterm birth in subsequent pregnancy is which of the following?
A. 16 weeks
B. 18 weeks
C. 20 weeks
D. 22 weeks

40.3   At 24 weeks' gestation, the threshold cervical length below which the risk of preterm birth increases is which of the following?
A. 2.0 cm
B. 2.5 cm
C. 3.0 cm
D. 3.5 cm

40.4   Cerclage has been shown to reduce preterm birth when a patient has a history of prior preterm delivery in which of the following circumstances?
A. Positive fetal fibronectin (fFN)
B. Cervical length less than 2.5 cm
C. Positive fern test
D. Twin gestation

ANSWERS

40.1   **C.** Due to the increased number of preterm births in this country, the most common gestational age at delivery since 2002 is 39 weeks.

40.2   **B.** Women with a previous delivery prior to 37 weeks' gestation remain at increased risk for subsequent preterm birth unless the delivery occurred before 18 weeks gestation. No increase in subsequent preterm birth has been seen when a pregnancy ends prior to 18 weeks.

40.3   **B.** Cervical length at 24 weeks should be over 2.5 cm. When it is noted by ultrasound to be less than 2.5 cm, the patient should be considered to be at increased risk for preterm birth.

40.4   **B.** Cerclage has been shown to reduce the rate of PTB if placed in a patient with a history of a prior preterm birth and cervical length of less than 2.5 cm. Patients with either of those risk factors alone, or with the risk factor of twins, have not been shown to benefit by placement of a cerclage.

Clinical Pearls

See US Preventive Services Task Force Study Quality levels of evidence in Case 1

▶ The obstetric precursors leading to preterm birth are indicated preterm birth (30%-35%), spontaneous preterm labor (40%-45%), and preterm premature rupture of the membranes (25%-30%) (Level II-2).

▶ Rather than having one specific etiology, preterm labor is now thought to be a syndrome initiated by multiple mechanisms, including infection or inflammation, uteroplacental ischemia or hemorrhage, uterine overdistension, stress, and other immunologically mediated processes (Level III).

▶ Microbiologic studies suggest that intrauterine infection might account for 25% to 40% of preterm births, although with sophisticated measurement of microbial "footprints" in amniotic fluid, the number is likely higher (Level II-3).

▶ Women with cervical length less than 2.5 cm who are over 20 weeks gestation are at increased risk for preterm birth, while those with uterine contractions and cervical length greater than 3.0 cm have around a 1% chance of delivering within the next week (Level II-2).

▶ No studies have shown that any tocolytic drug can reduce the rate of preterm birth (Level I).

REFERENCES

1. Damus K. Prevention of preterm birth: a renewed national priority. *Curr Opin Obstet Gynecol.* 2008;20:590-596.
2. Fox NS, Gelber SE, Kalish RB, Chasen SE. Contemporary practice patterns and beliefs regarding tocolysis among U.S. maternal–fetal medicine specialists. *Obstet Gynecol.* 2008;112:42-47.
3. Goldenberg RL, Culhane JF, Iams JD, Romero R. Epidemiology and causes of preterm birth. *Lancet.* 2008;371:75-84.
4. Huddleston JF, Sanchez-Ramox L, Huddleston KW. Acute management of preterm labor. *Clin Perinatol.* 2003;30:803-824.
   This review outlines our understanding of the mechanism of labor and how tocolytics may intervene to delay or prevent preterm birth.
5. Iams JD, Romero R, Culhane JF, Goldenberg RL. Primary, secondary, and tertiary interventions to reduce the morbidity and mortality of preterm birth. *Lancet.* 2008;371:164-175.
6. Smith V, Devane D, Begley CM, Clarke M, Higgins S. A systematic review and quality assessment of systematic reviews of randomised trials of interventions for preventing and treating preterm birth. *Eur J Obstet Gynecol.* 2008;doi:10.1016/j.ejogrb.2008.09.008.
   This paper reports on the quality of reviews of techniques for preventing and treating preterm birth.

Case 41

A 32-year-old G2P0010 African American woman at 28 weeks' gestation comes into the obstetrical triage unit complaining of leakage of fluid per vagina approximately 4 hours previously. She denied uterine contractions or vaginal bleeding. Her prenatal course has been unremarkable. She had a miscarriage at 8 weeks' gestation previously. On examination, her BP is 100/78 mm Hg, HR 82 beats per minute, RR 18 breaths/min, and temperature 98.3°F. Her heart and lung examinations are normal. The abdomen is soft and nontender. The uterus is nontender with a fundal height of 27 cm. The fetal heart tones are in the 140 bpm range. A speculum examination reveals gross pooling of fluid in the vagina, and the cervix appears to be visually closed.

➤ What is the most likely diagnosis?

➤ What are your next steps?

➤ How would you manage the patient if she went into labor?

ANSWERS TO CASE 41:
Preterm Premature Rupture of Membranes (PPROM)

Summary: A 32-year-old G2P0010 African American woman at 28 weeks' gestation has symptoms of vaginal leakage of fluid 4 hours previously. She is afebrile. The fetal heart tones are in the 140 bpm range. A speculum examination reveals gross pooling of fluid in the vagina, and the cervix appears to be visually closed.

➤ **Most likely diagnosis:** Preterm premature rupture of membranes (PPROM).

➤ **Next steps:**

1. Confirm the diagnosis: ferning test; pH testing (nitrazine paper) on vaginal fluid.
2. Baseline assessment of maternal and fetal well-being:
   a. CBC, urinalysis, comprehensive metabolic panel
   b. GBS culture. Consider an assay for gonorrhea and chlamydia
   c. Consider a urine drug screen
   d. Obstetric ultrasound
   e. Electronic fetal monitoring (if fetus is viable) and monitoring for contractions
3. Broad-spectrum antibiotics.
4. Corticosteroids for fetal lung maturation.
5. Consider pros and cons of expectant management.
6. Stabilization and transfer to a perinatal center where the fetus can be managed (if appropriate).

➤ **Managing the patient if she went into labor:**
   ➤ Assessment of maternal vital signs.
   ➤ Sterile speculum examination before digital examination.
   ➤ Assessment of the presentation and residual amniotic fluid volume by ultrasound.
   ➤ Penicillin for GBS prophylaxis (unless a recent GBS culture [within 5 weeks] is available with negative results).
   ➤ Intrapartum fetal heart rate monitoring.
   ➤ Consider the placement of an intrauterine pressure catheter for amnioinfusion if a vaginal delivery is an option and decelerations are noted.
   ➤ Consider intravenous magnesium sulfate for neuroprotection.

ANALYSIS

Objectives

1. Be able to describe the risk factors of PPROM.
2. Be able to describe the management of PPROM.
3. Be able to describe the complications of PPROM including early second-trimester PPROM.

Considerations

This is a 32-year-old G2P0010 African American woman at 28 weeks' gestation that presented with PPROM. Any pregnant patient that presents to a labor and delivery unit with complaints of leaking fluid requires prompt and thorough evaluation to rule in or out the possibility of PPROM. Maternal evaluation for signs of infection or sepsis (clinical assessment, vitals and labs) is important as infection is clinically evident in 13% to 60% of PPROM patients. Fetal assessment is initiated with external fetal monitors to evaluate fetal heart tones and uterine activity. PPROM is ruled in or out primarily on sterile speculum examination (positive nitrazine, pooling on Valsalva maneuver, and visualized ferning on microscopy). False positives may result from intravaginal semen, cervical mucus, blood, *Trichomonas*, and some antiseptics. Additionally, the patients described loss of fluid may be related to the intermittent loss of urine. During a speculum examination, cultures must be obtained for evaluation of infectious etiology (gonorrhea/Chlamydia probe, wet mount) and GBS carrier status (with culture and sensitivities for penicillin-sensitive patients). Cervical dilation is assessed visually and digital manipulation is avoided as it has been shown to increase infection rates. Intrauterine evaluation is continued with ultrasound to assess for the gestational age, fetal weight, presentation, placental location, and amniotic fluid index. Laboratory investigation includes CBC, type and screen, comprehensive metabolic panel (CMP), and urinalysis. If there is concern for illegal drug use it is reasonable to obtain urine toxicology. The treatment plan is then determined once fetal and maternal status, gestational age, and labor status have been appropriately assessed.

APPROACH TO

Preterm Premature Rupture of Membranes (PPROM)

Premature rupture of membranes (PROM) is defined as the ROM prior to the onset of labor. Preterm PROM (PPROM) is the ROM that occurs prior to $37^0/_7$ weeks. Approximately 3% of all pregnancies are complicated by PPROM and is the underlying etiology of one-third of preterm births.[1] Normal fetal membranes are biologically very strong in preterm pregnancies. The weakening mechanism is likely multifactorial. Studies have shown PPROM to be associated with intrinsic (intrauterine stretch/strain from polyhydramnios and multifetal pregnancies, cervical incompetence) and extrinsic factors (ascending bacterial infections that release proteases and metalloproteinase).[2] There is evidence demonstrating an association between ascending infection from the lower genital tract and PPROM. In women with PPROM about one-third of pregnancies have positive amniotic fluid cultures[3,4] and studies have shown that bacteria have the ability to cross intact membranes.[5,6] Other risk factors include smoking, placental abruption, prior PPROM, cocaine, previous cervical lacerations/surgeries, short cervical length (< 25 mm), trauma, and positive fetal fibronectin (see Table 41–1). A study by Lee et al showed a recurrence rate of 16.7% in patients with prior pregnancy complicated by PPROM.[7]

PPROM is associated with significant maternal and fetal morbidity and mortality. The time from rupture of membranes to delivery is known as "latency." The latency period is inversely proportional to the gestational age at PPROM. Latency period of 1 week or less is present in 50% to 60% of PPROM patients.[8] During this period amnionitis occurs in 13% to 60%, and abruptio placentae occurs in 4% to 12%.[8] Maternal and fetal complications decrease with increasing gestational age at the time of PPROM. Multiple complications have been associated with PPROM (see Table 41–2).

The primary maternal morbidity is chorioamnionitis. Incidence varies with population and gestational age at PPROM, with reported frequency from 15% to 40%.[2] Women with intrauterine infection deliver earlier than noninfected women.[9] Chorioamnionitis typically precedes fetal infection but this is not always the case, and therefore close clinical monitoring is required. Fetal morbidity and mortality varies with gestational age, the treatment rendered and the presence of comorbidities, particularly infection. The most common complication is respiratory distress syndrome (RDS). Other serious fetal complications include necrotizing enterocolitis, intraventricular hemorrhage, and

Table 41–1 RISK FACTORS FOR PPROM

MATERNAL	FETAL
Collagen disease	Polyhydramnios
Cervical insufficiency	Congenital anomalies
Smoking	Multiple gestations
Cocaine use	
Cervical infections (gonorrhea; chlamydia)	
COPD	

Table 41–2 COMPLICATIONS OF PPROM	
MATERNAL	**FETAL**
Chorioamnionitis	Prematurity
Endometritis	Pulmonary hypoplasia
Sepsis	Deformities/contractures
Postpartum hemorrhage	Neonatal sepsis
	IVH
	NEC

sepsis. The three causes of neonatal death associated with PPROM are prematurity, sepsis, and pulmonary hypoplasia. Preterm infants born with sepsis have a mortality rate four times higher than those without sepsis.[9]

Making the Diagnosis

Management of PPROM starts with initial evaluation and diagnosis of rupture of membranes. The patient typically complains of a "gush" of fluid but some patients will report persistent leakage of fluid. This patient history of rupture of membranes is accurate in 90% of cases.[10] Diagnosis is established on sterile speculum evaluation. Confirmatory findings include pooling of amniotic fluid in posterior fornix and/or leakage of fluid on Valsalva; positive nitrazine test of fluid (vaginal pH 4.5-6.0, amniotic fluid pH 7.1-7.3, nitrazine turns dark blue above 6.0-6.5); amniotic fluid *ferning* on microscopy. Friedman and McElin found that two positive findings had an accuracy of 93.1%.[10] More recently, other tests have been evaluated in the diagnosis of ruptured membranes and fetal fibronectin and elevated insulin-like growth factor binding protein-1 in cervico-vaginal secretions have reported sensitivities of 94% and 75% and specificities of 97%, respectively.[11,12]

Should the initial tests be ambiguous or negative, in the face of continued clinical suspicion other diagnostic modalities can be utilized. The ultrasound finding of oligohydramnios is usually confirmatory. Occasionally for cases when the history of PROM is suspicious and other physical tests are negative, the transabdominal intraamniotic injection of indigo-carmine (1-2 mL in 4-9 mL sterile saline) needs to be considered. In these cases the presence of blue dye on a vaginal pad after ambulation would confirm the leaking of amniotic fluid.

At the time of the initial evaluation, the patient's cervical os should be visually assessed for dilatation and possible prolapse of umbilical cord or fetal limb. Brown et al found visual estimation of cervical dilation had a positive predictive value of 86.5% and negative predictive value of 100%.[13] Digital evaluation of cervix should be avoided; Lewis et al found that in PPROM patients gestational ages 24 to 35 weeks, who underwent digital vaginal examination, had a significantly decreased mean latency period (2.1 vs 11.3 days).[14] Ultrasound evaluation of the gestational age, fetal weight, fetal presentation, placental location, and assessment of amniotic fluid index (AFI) are vital for treatment planning. A low AFI (< 5.0 cm) and low maximum vertical fluid pocket (< 2.0 cm) at the time of initial assessment is associated with shorter latency, increased RDS, and increased composite morbidity (death or RDS, early sepsis, stage 2-3 necrotizing enterocolitis, and/or grade III-IV intraventricular hemorrhage).[15]

Management

Patients diagnosed with PPROM would benefit from an admission to the hospital in all likelihood until delivery.

Once PPROM is verified, the treatment plan must balance the maternal, fetal, neonatal risks/benefits of prolonged pregnancy or expeditious delivery and possible inclusion of medical intervention. Many studies have demonstrated benefits in conservative management for gestations of less than 34 weeks, whereas the management of pregnancies complicated by PPROM between 34 and 37 weeks of gestation continues to be controversial.[16]

A retrospective series examining neonatal outcome following cases with PPROM between 32 weeks and 36 weeks showed that the specific gestation for reduced morbidity was 34 weeks.[17] The incidence of respiratory distress syndrome and the length of hospital stay were reduced in infants delivered after 34 weeks of gestation. The incidence of RDS was 22.5% and 5.8% at 33 and 34 weeks, respectively. Although the incidence beyond 34 weeks was relatively low, the condition affected infants into the 36th week, with incidences of 10.4% to 1.5% at 35 and 36 weeks, respectively.

- **PPROM at $34^{0}/_{7}$ to $36^{6}/_{7}$ weeks:**
  Naef et al showed that conservative management at this gestational age range lead to increased risk of maternal amnionitis (16% vs 2%), prolonged maternal length of stay (5.2 vs 2.6 days), and lower mean cord pH (7.25 vs 7.35).[16] Additionally, there is increase of umbilical cord compression/prolapse and placental abruption. In addition the risk of severe morbidity and mortality to the fetus in this age range is low. Thus, expeditious delivery in this gestational age range is most reasonable. If GBS status is not verifiable or a patient has risk factors, GBS prophylaxis should be given. In this gestational age range, there is no significant data to support corticosteroids for fetal lung maturity.

- **PPROM at $32^{0}/_{7}$ to $33^{6}/_{7}$ weeks:**
  In this gestational age range there remains a significant risk for RDS, approximately 35%. Therefore, an attempt to determine fetal lung maturity (FLM) can be considered. FLM can be determined from vaginal pooling sample to assess phosphatidylglycerol (PG) levels. In most cases the risk-benefit ratio does not justify an amniocentesis in this clinical setting.

- **PPROM under 32 weeks:**
  In the absence of clinical signs of labor, abruption, or maternal or fetal signs of infection most patients in this gestational age will benefit from an expectant management with daily assessment of the maternal and fetal well-being.
1. Antenatal assessment:
   a. Maternal: The criteria for the diagnosis of clinical chorioamnionitis include maternal pyrexia, tachycardia, leukocytosis, uterine tenderness, malodorous vaginal discharge, and fetal tachycardia. During inpatient observation, the woman should be regularly examined for such signs of intrauterine infection and an abnormal parameter or a combination of them may indicate intrauterine infection. The frequency of maternal and fetal assessments (temperature, pulse, and fetal heart rate auscultation) should be between 4 and 8 hours.[18,19,20]

   Maternal fever (above 38.0°C) in the absence of other sources of infection, offensive vaginal discharge, and fetal tachycardia (rate above 160 bpm) indicate clinical chorioamnionitis. There is a variation in the literature regarding the accuracy of the laboratory tests of leukocytosis and raised C-reactive protein in the prediction of chorioamnionitis. The sensitivities and false-positive rates for leukocytosis in the detection of clinical chorioamnionitis range from 29% to 47% and 5% to 18%, respectively.[18,20] The specificity of C-reactive protein is 38% to 55%.[18,20,21] The presence of leukocytosis may be useful clinically in cases where there is doubt about the diagnosis of chorioamnionitis.

   b. Fetal: Electronic fetal heart rate tracing is useful because fetal tachycardia may represent a sign of fetal infection and is frequently used in the clinical definition of chorioamnionitis in some studies. Fetal tachycardia predicts 20% to 40% of cases of intrauterine infection with a false-positive rate of about 3%.[18,22,23] There are no randomized controlled trials to support the use of frequent biophysical or Doppler assessment. The disparity in the literature evaluating these tests of fetal well-being suggests that, although some studies have shown benefit, overall the tests are of limited value in differentiating between fetuses with and without infection.[24]

2. Use of corticosteroids: A meta-analysis of 15 randomized controlled trials involving more than 1400 women with preterm rupture of the membranes demonstrated that antenatal corticosteroids reduced the risks of respiratory distress syndrome (RR 0.56; 95% confidence interval [CI] 0.46-0.70), intraventricular hemorrhage (RR 0.47; 95% CI 0.31-0.70), and necrotizing enterocolitis (RR 0.21; 95% CI 0.05-0.82).[25] They do not appear to increase the risk of infection in either mother (RR 0.86; 95% CI 0.61-1.20) or baby (RR 1.05; 95% CI 0.66-1.68).[25]

3. Use of antibiotics: Twenty-two trials involving over 6000 women with PPROM before 37 weeks were included in a meta-analysis.[26] The use of antibiotics following PPROM was associated with a statistically significant

reduction in chorioamnionitis (RR 0.57; 95% CI 0.37-0.86). There was a significant reduction in the numbers of babies born within 48 hours (RR 0.71; 95% CI 0.58-0.87) and 7 days (RR 0.80; 95% CI 0.71-0.90). Neonatal infection was significantly reduced in the babies whose mothers received antibiotics (RR 0.68; 95% CI 0.53-0.87). There was also a significant reduction in the number of babies with an abnormal cerebral ultrasound scan prior to discharge from hospital (RR 0.82; 95% CI 0.68-0.98).[26]

4. Use of tocolytics: Prophylactic tocolysis in women with PPROM without uterine activity is not recommended. Women with PPROM and uterine activity who require intrauterine transfer or antenatal corticosteroids should be considered for tocolysis. Three randomized studies of a total of 235 women with PPROM reported that the proportion of women remaining undelivered 10 days after membrane rupture was not significantly higher in those receiving tocolysis compared with those receiving none.[27-29] A recent retrospective case–control study showed that tocolysis after PPROM did not increase the interval between membrane rupture and delivery or reduce neonatal morbidity.[30]

- **PPROM under 23 weeks:**
  There are insufficient data to make recommendations in the setting of PPROM under 23 to 24 weeks including the possibility of home, daycare, and outpatient monitoring. It would be considered reasonable to maintain the woman in hospital for at least 48 hours before a decision is made to allow her to go home.[24] The management of these cases should be individualized and outpatient monitoring restricted to certain groups of women after careful consideration of other risk factors and the access to the hospital.

Delivery

1. Timing: If the diagnosis of chorioamnionitis is made, regardless of the gestational age of the fetus it is in the best interest for the mother and the fetus to be separated and to begin the process of delivery, if it has not started on its own by then. Parents need to be counseled at that point of the fetal chances for survival and the associated morbidities. Arrangements need to be made to provide the fetus with the best possible facilities if time allows it.
   Other indications for delivery include spontaneous labor, death of the fetus, cord prolapse, abruption of the placenta, or demonstration of fetal lung maturity.

2. Interventions during delivery: If the patient is a candidate for a vaginal delivery and the fetal tracing exhibits recurrent variable decelerations (associated with oligohydramnios) the placement of an intrauterine pressure catheter and amnioinfusion might improve the tracing and increase the likelihood for a vaginal delivery. If a GBS culture is not available prior to delivery antibiotic prophylaxis is recommended. Neuroprophylaxis with magnesium sulfate can also be considered for fetuses under 34 weeks.

3. Route: The route of delivery in the setting of PPROM will depend on the urgency of the indication (eg, cord prolapse is more common in PPROM), the previous surgical history of the mother (cesarean sections in particular), presentation of the fetus, number of fetuses, and presence or absence of labor. The rates of cesarean section are increased among women with PPROM.

4. After delivery: Women who deliver as a result of PPROM need to be counseled to seek early prenatal care in future pregnancies and on the use of 17α-hydroxyprogesterone for the prevention of recurrent episodes of PPROM.[31] Cervical length monitoring may be beneficial in a subset of patients and needs to be considered in the evaluation of these patients in subsequent pregnancies.

Comprehension Questions

41.1   What is the contribution of PPROM to the rate of preterm labor?
        A. 15%
        B. 30%
        C. 66%
        D. 80%

41.2   A 33-year-old woman G1P0 at $36^0/_7$ weeks' gestation complains of leakage of clear fluid per vagina. Speculum examination is consistent with spontaneous preterm premature rupture of membranes. The patient would prefer nonintervention and for a natural labor course. Which of the following statements is the most accurate in counseling of this patient of expectant management versus induction of labor?
        A. Expectant management has been shown to lead to equal perinatal and maternal outcomes.
        B. Expectant management has an equal perinatal and maternal outcome in GBS-negative individuals.
        C. Intramuscular corticosteroids would be recommended if expectant management is entertained.
        D. Maternal infection and length of stay are increased with expectant management.

41.3   A 22-year-old G1P0 woman at 25 weeks' gestation is admitted to the hospital with a diagnosis of PPROM. Which of the following is the most accurate statement regarding the use of corticosteroids?
        A. Has been shown to reduce the risk of NEC.
        B. Has been shown to increase the risk of maternal infection.
        C. Has been shown to increase the risk of neonatal sepsis.
        D. Should not be administered until the patient reaches 28 weeks' gestation.

ANSWERS

41.1　**B.** PPROM contributes to approximately a third of the cases of preterm labor.

41.2　**D.** PPROM between 34 and 36 weeks' gestation is generally best treated by delivery. Expectant management in this gestational age window is associated with a higher likelihood of maternal infection, greater length of stay, and lower cord pH values.

41.3　**A.** Corticosteroid use has been associated with a reduction of NEC, intraventricular hemorrhage (IVH), and RDS, without increasing the risk of maternal or neonatal infection, provided that there is no overt infection evident.

Clinical Pearls

See US Preventive Services Task Force Study Quality levels of evidence in Case 1

➤ The diagnosis of spontaneous rupture of the membranes is best achieved by maternal history followed by a sterile speculum examination of the vagina and cervix (Level II).

➤ Ultrasound examination is useful in some cases to help confirm the diagnosis (Level III).

➤ Digital examination should be avoided when PPROM is suspected (Level III).

➤ Routine amniocentesis is not recommended for women with PPROM (Level II).

➤ Antenatal corticosteroids should be administered in women with PPROM (Level I).

➤ Prophylactic tocolysis in women with PPROM without uterine activity is not recommended (Level I).

➤ The use of antibiotics for up to 1 week after diagnosis prolongs the latency period and outcomes of PPROM (Level I).

➤ Delivery should be considered for all cases at 34 weeks of gestation (Level I).

➤ The recurrence of PPROM can be reduced in future pregnancies with the prophylactic administration of 17α-hydroxyprogesterone caproate (Level I).

REFERENCES

1. Hyagriv NS, Canavan TP. Preterm premature rupture of membranes: diagnosis, evaluation and management strategies. *BJOG.* 2005;1:32-37.
2. Creasy RK, Resnik R. Chapter 38: Premature rupture of the membranes. *Maternal-Fetal Medicine Principles and Practice*. 5th ed. Philadelphia, PA: WB Saunders; 2004; 723-739.
3. Carroll SG, Sebire NJ, Nicolaides KH. Pre-term pre-labour amniorrhexis. *Curr Opin Obstet Gynecol.* 1996;8:441-448.

4. Broekhuizen FF, Gilman M, Hamilton PR. Amniocentesis for Gram stain and culture in preterm premature rupture of the membranes. *Obstet Gynecol.* 1985;66:316-321.

5. Galask RP, Varner MW, Petzold CR, Wilbur SL. Bacterial attachment to the chorioamniotic membranes. *Am J Obstet Gynecol.* 1984;148:915-928.

6. Gyr TN, Malek A, Mathez–Loic, et al. Permeation of human chorioamniotic membranes by Escherichia coli in vitro. *Am J Obstet Gynecol.* 1994;170:223-227.

7. Lee T, Carpenter MW, Heber WW, Silver HM. Preterm premature rupture of membranes: risks of recurrent complications in the next pregnancy among a population-based sample of gravid women. *Am J Obstet Gynecol.* 2003;188:209-213.

8. Mercer BM. Preterm premature rupture of the membranes. *Obstet Gynecol.* 2003; 101:178-193.

9. Cotton DB, Hill LM, Strassner HT, Platt LD, Ledger WJ. Use of amniocentesis in preterm gestation with ruptured membranes. *Obstet Gynecol.* 1984;63:38-48.

10. Friedman ML, McElin TW. Diagnosis of ruptured fetal membranes. Clinical study and review of the literature. *Am J Obstet Gynecol.* 1969;104:544-550.

11. Gaucherand P, Guibaud S, Awada A, et al. Comparative study of three amniotic fluid markers in premature rupture of membranes: fetal fibronectin, alpha-fetoprotein, diaminooxidase. *Acta Obstet Gynecol Scand.* 1995;74:118-121.

12. Rutanen EM, Pekonen F, Karkkainen T. Measurement of insulin-like growth factor binding protein-1 in cervical/vaginal secretions: comparison with the ROM-check membrane immunoassay in the diagnosis of ruptured fetal membranes. *Clin Chim Acta.* 1993;214:73-81.

13. Brown CL, Ludwiczak, MH, Blanco J, Hirsch CE. Cervical dilation: accuracy of visual and digital examinations. *Obstet Gynecol.* 1993;81:215-216.

14. Lewis DF, Major CA, Towers, CV, Asrat T, Harding JA, Garite TJ. Effects of digital vaginal examinations on latency period in preterm premature rupture of membranes. *Obstet Gynecol.* 1992;80:630-634.

15. Mercer BM, Rabello YA, Thurnau GR, et al. The NICHD-MFMU antibiotic treatment of preterm PROM study: impact of initial amniotic fluid volume on pregnancy outcome. *Am J Obstet Gynecol.* 2006;194:438-445.

16. Naef RW 3rd, Albert JR, Ross EL, Weber BM, Martin RW, Morrison JC. Premature rupture of membranes at 34 to 37 weeks' gestation: aggressive versus conservative management. *Am J Obstet Gynecol.* 1998;178:126-130.

17. Neerhof MG, Cravello C, Haney EI, Silver RK. Timing of labor induction after premature rupture of membranes between 32 and 36 weeks' gestation. *Am J Obstet Gynecol.* 1999;180:349-352.

18. Ismail A, Zinaman MJ, Lowensohn RI, Moawad AH. The significance of C-reactive protein levels in women with premature rupture of membranes. *Am J Obstet Gynecol.* 1985;151:541-544.

19. Carlan SJ, O'Brien WF, Parsons MT, Lense JJ. Preterm premature rupture of membranes: a randomised study of home versus hospital management. *Obstet Gynecol.* 1993;81:61-64.

20. Romem Y, Artal R. C-reactive protein as a predictor for chorioamnionitis in cases of premature rupture of the membranes. *Am J Obstet Gynecol.* 1984;150:546-550.

21. Kurki T, Teramo K, Ylikorkala O, Paavonen J. C-reactive protein in preterm premature rupture of the membranes. *Arch Gynecol Obstet.* 1990;247:31-37.

22. Carroll SG, Papiaoannou S, Nicolaides KH. Assessment of fetal activity and amniotic fluid volume in the prediction of intrauterine infection in preterm prelabour amniorrhexis. *Am J Obstet Gynecol.* 1995;172:1427-1435.
23. Ferguson MG, Rhodes PG, Morrison JC, Puckett CM. Clinical amniotic fluid infection and its effect on the neonate. *Am J Obstet Gynecol.* 1985;151:1058-1061.
24. Royal College of Obstetricians and Gynaecologists. Preterm prelabour rupture of membranes. RCOG Guideline No. 44. London: RCOG, November 2006.
25. Harding JE, Pang J, Knight DB, Liggins GC. Do antenatal corticosteroids help in the setting of preterm rupture of membranes. *Am J Obstet Gynecol.* 2001;184:131-139.
26. Kenyon S, Boulvain M, Neilson J. Antibiotics for preterm rupture of membranes. *Cochrane Database Syst Rev* 2003;2:CD001058.
27. How HY, Cook CR, Cook VD, Miles DE, Spinnato JA. Preterm premature rupture of membranes: aggressive tocolysis versus expectant management. *J Matern Fetal Med.* 1998;7:8-12.
28. Levy D, Warsof SL. Oral ritodrine and preterm premature rupture of membranes. *Obstet Gynecol.* 1985;66:621-633.
29. Dunlop PDM, Crowley PA, Lamont RF, Hawkins DF. Preterm ruptured membranes, no contractions. *J Obstet Gynecol.*1986;7:92-96.
30. Combs CA, McCune M, Clark R, Fishman A. Aggressive tocolysis does not prolong pregnancy or reduce neonatal morbidity after preterm premature rupture of the membranes. *Am J Obstet Gynecol.* 2004;190:28-31.
31. Meis PJ, Klebanoff M, Thom E, et al. Prevention of recurrent preterm delivery by 17 alpha-hydroxyprogesterone caproate. *N Engl J Med.* 2003 Jun 12;348(24): 2379-2385.
32. ACOG Committee Opinion 455. Magnesium sulfate before anticipated preterm birth for neuroprotection. *Obstet Gynecol.* 2010;115:669-671.

Case 42

A 28-year-old woman, G2P1001, presented for prenatal care at 16 weeks' gestation. Her only complaint was excessive weight gain of 25 lb to this point in pregnancy. The patient had no other medical problems other than allergic rhinitis. Her obstetrical history was significant for a prior term vaginal delivery without complications.

On physical examination her vitals were as follows: BP 98/65 mm Hg, HR 95 bpm, BMI = 28 kg/mm^2. The only finding on examination was that the maternal abdomen was distended with a positive fluid wave and the uterus was difficult to palpate abdominally. There were no other significant findings. Given this examination finding, you question the patient further and she denies early satiety, bloating, nausea, vomiting, and fever/chills.

An ultrasound in the office showed a 16 weeks, 2 days intrauterine pregnancy. The maternal abdominal cavity showed a large amount of ascites. Ovaries could not be visualized. Magnetic resonance imaging (MRI) of the abdomen and pelvis was ordered and it revealed a large cystic mass extending from the pelvis to the abdominal cavity measuring 30 × 15 cm likely arising from the left ovary. The cyst was without wall thickening, septations, or projections. There was no apparent adenopathy or free fluid. The right ovary appeared normal. You call the patient to discuss the results of her MRI.

➤ What is your next step in the management?

➤ What is in your differential diagnosis of an adnexal mass in pregnancy?

ANSWERS TO CASE 42:
Adnexal Masses in Pregnancy

Summary: A 28-year-old G2P1001 at $16^2/_7$ weeks' gestation with an incidental finding of a large pelvic mass and ascites.

➤ **Next step:** The patient should be counseled that although most adnexal masses during pregnancy are benign and resolve, this particular mass is more concerning due its large size and the presence of ascites. Surgical management is the best option in this particular situation.

➤ **Differential diagnosis:** Common etiologies of adnexal masses in pregnancy include functional cysts (corpus luteum, hemorrhagic, simple) as well as dermoids, endometriomas, and paraovarian cysts. Borderline tumors or malignancy are less likely in general but are strong considerations in this case.

ANALYSIS

Objectives

1. Describe the characteristics of adnexal masses that are physiologic versus neoplasms.
2. Describe the diagnostic strategy for adnexal masses in pregnancy.
3. Describe the treatment of adnexal masses in pregnancy.

Considerations

There are several factors that must be considered when recommending surgery versus expectant management in a gravid patient with an adnexal mass. Sonographic characteristics, size, symptoms, persistence, and gestational age are all important considerations.

In general, adnexal masses with size > 5 cm, complex consistency (cystic and solid), presence of excrescences, mural nodules, septations, wall thickness, and ascites raise the concern for malignancy. With few exceptions, these masses should be excised regardless of concurrent pregnancy. Waiting until the fetus is term would generally not be considered appropriate with a lesion of this size because a potentially malignant lesion would have time to spread, thereby affecting the mother's overall survival. In general, the risk of malignancy of persistent masses in pregnancy is low. If surgical intervention is being considered, it should be planned for after 16 weeks' of gestation for two reasons. First, most adnexal masses are functional cysts and resolve by 16 weeks' gestation. Secondly, most spontaneous abortions occur in the first trimester and therefore waiting until later in pregnancy may help to avoid unnecessary surgery during pregnancy.

The first step in management is to evaluate the mass via imaging studies starting with gynecological sonogram and proceeding to a computed tomography scan (CT-scan) or an MRI. The most appropriate management for this particular patient given the size of the mass would be an exploratory laparotomy with an attempt to preserve the ovary. Additionally, the patient should be counseled that a staging procedure by a gynecologic oncologist may also be indicated based on intraoperative findings. Had the mass been smaller, perhaps a laparoscopic approach could have been initiated. The timing of the procedure would ideally occur at 16 to 18 weeks of gestation when most functional cysts have already resolved. Whether observation or antepartum surgical intervention is chosen, the patient should be properly counseled regarding the risks, benefits, and alternatives of the proposed management.

With expectant management, one of the more common complications in pregnant patients with adnexal masses is pain especially in those with larger masses. Pain can also be due to torsion which has a variable reported rate of less than 1% to 22% of cases. Rupture of adnexal masses in pregnancy is less common, occurring in less than 9% of cases. Another potential complication of adnexal masses in pregnancy is obstruction of labor which may occur in 2% to 17% of cases[1] (Level III). Much lower antepartum complication rates (< 2%) have been reported with expectant management in other studies[2,3,4] (Level II-2, Level III). Even with emergent surgery due to torsion or other acute complications, adverse pregnancy outcome is significantly low[4] (Level III).

The risks of surgery during pregnancy include miscarriage and preterm birth, however, these risks are minimized if surgery is performed in the second trimester. Both laparoscopy and laparotomy, when performed by skilled operators, have been shown to have similar pregnancy outcomes[5] (Level III). That being said, the risks of observation need to be balanced against the risks of surgical intervention. In this particular patient, the concern is twofold—the presence of a large adnexal mass and ascites, both of which are concerning for an ovarian neoplasm or malignancy.

APPROACH TO
Adnexal Masses in Pregnancy

The finding of an incidental adnexal mass in pregnancy has become more common with the routine use of ultrasound in prenatal care. For this reason, many incidental masses will be detected by ultrasound in the first or second trimester of pregnancy. Approximately 1% to 4% of pregnant women are diagnosed with an adnexal mass[2,6] (Level II-2). The majority of these masses are corpus luteum or other functional cysts that usually resolve by 16 weeks of gestation. Some adnexal masses persist and 1% to 8% of these masses represent malignant tumors[7,8,9-11] (Level II-3, Level II-2, Level III). Size is the best indicator of whether the mass requires surgical intervention. Slightly less than 100% of masses smaller than 5 cm in diameter will resolve spontaneously. Larger cysts have increased risk of torsion, rupture, and labor obstruction, therefore close monitoring and often surgery are necessary[12] (Level III).

Common adnexal lesions associated with pregnancy include simple cysts, hemorrhagic cysts, and hyperstimulated ovaries in patients who have undergone assisted fertility. Uncommon adnexal lesions specific to pregnancy include heterotopic pregnancy, hyperreactio luteinalis, theca lutein cysts with moles, and luteinomas. Some adnexal entities are found incidentally, such as teratomas, endometriomas, leiomyomas, hydrosalpinx, cystadenomas, and cystadenocarcinomas (see Table 42–1 for differential diagnosis).

Improvements in ultrasound technology have increased the ability to better characterize adnexal masses. The use of color Doppler imaging has been shown to significantly improve the ability to distinguish benign from malignant masses[13] (Level III). The sensitivity of ultrasound in distinguishing

Table 42–1 DIFFERENTIAL DIAGNOSIS OF ADNEXAL MASSES IN PREGNANCY

Functional
- Simple cysts
- Corpus luteum
- Hemorrhagic cysts

Nonfunctional
- Endometriomas
- Leiomyomas

Paraovarian
- Paraovarian cysts
- Hydrosalpinx
- Tubo-ovarian abscess

Unique to pregnancy
- Hyperstimulated ovaries
- Hyperreactio luteinalis
- Theca lutein cysts
- Luteomas
- Heterotopic pregnancy

Benign/malignant
- Teratomas
- Cystadenomas
- Cystadenocarcinomas

Nongynecologic
- Acute appendicitis
- Irritable bowel disease
- Adhesive disease

benign from malignant disease is 96.8% with specificity of 77%. Although the diagnosis of most adnexal pathologic conditions can be made on the basis of sonographic appearance alone, MRI may help when the sonographic appearance is not specific or the mass is unable to be adequately imaged. Familiarity with these clinicopathologic and imaging features is important for diagnosis and treatment[12] (Level III).

Most adnexal masses detected by sonography during pregnancy are simple cysts or hemorrhagic corpus luteum cysts. **Simple cysts** are unilocular and anechoic and have a smooth, thin wall. The prevalence of simple cysts at 8 to 10 weeks is 5.3% dropping to 1.5% by 14 weeks gestation. **Follicular cysts** are simple cysts that develop in response to monthly cyclical hormonal change and are less than 2 cm in size[5] (Level III). **Corpus luteum cysts** support pregnancy by maintaining progesterone levels. These cysts enlarge during the first trimester, regress by the 12th week of gestation, and disappear later on in the pregnancy[12] (Level III). Sonographic appearance varies from simple to complex with internal debris and thick walls. The corpus luteum is typically surrounded by a circumferential rim of color Doppler flow with a low-resistance Doppler pattern often referred to as the "*ring of fire.*" These cysts are prone to rupture and hemorrhage.

Hemorrhagic cysts can have a variety of sonographic appearances due to the changing appearance of the blood clot[12] (Level III). Hemorrhagic cysts appear as predominantly anechoic masses that contain hypoechoic material within them[12] (Level III). Acutely hemorrhagic cysts can appear as echogenic masses with internal echoes more hyperechoic than surrounding normal ovarian parenchyma in a "*fishnet*" or reticular pattern. The appearance over time may evolve to include a solid component representing a retracting blood clot with low-level echoes. Color Doppler interrogation will show no vascularity within the solid component.

The mature cystic *teratoma is the most common benign ovarian neoplasm to* be diagnosed in pregnancy. **Teratomas** show a complex echo pattern on ultrasound due to the presence of fat, solid components, and calcified material[12] (Level III). Sonographic appearances include the presence of a hyperechoic nodules, acoustic shadowing due to dense calcifications and multiple interdigitating lines representing hair floating in sebum[12] (Level III). Teratomas my be pedunculated and are prone to undergoing torsion and rupture, leading to peritonitis[12] (Level III). The most common sonographic appearance of **endometriomas** is that of diffuse homogenous low-level internal echoes although the appearance may vary from a cystic lesion to a solid mass depending on the stage of degradation of blood products[5] (Level III).

Lesions specific to pregnancy include hyperstimulated ovaries. **Ovarian hyperstimulation syndrome** appears as markedly enlarged ovaries (> 5 cm) containing multiple, large, peripherally located, thin-walled cysts that sometimes exude fluid from hemorrhage or ascites. They usually regress later in pregnancy or after delivery[12] (Level III). **Hyperreactio luteinalis** are similar in appearance to hyperstimulated ovaries but are seen in patients who have not undergone ovulation induction. They are thought to result from hypersensitivity of the ovary to circulating human chorionic gonadotropin (hCG) which may or may not be high[12] (Level III). These can commonly be mistaken for an ovarian neoplasm, however, MRI can be useful in distinguishing it from, or decreasing the likelihood of, a neoplasm[12] (Level III). **Theca lutein cysts** are reported with complete hydatiform moles 14% to 30% of the time which are stimulated by high levels of circulating hCG. They appear as anechoic, multiloculated, ovarian cysts[12] (Level III). The presence of a uterus filled with small cysts is the key to the diagnosis. Partial molar pregnancy is not likely to have theca lutein cysts. **Luteomas** are rare solid lesions that occur unique to pregnancy. Fewer than 200 cases of luteoma have been reported in the literature.[14]. Luteomas cause maternal virilization in 25% to 30% of cases and carry a 50% risk of virilizing a female fetus[12] (Level III). On sonography, they appear as heterogeneous solid masses, predominantly hypoechoic compared with normal ovarian tissue, with thick walls and irregular internal contours in an enlarged ovary[12] (Level III). They are often highly vascular and mimic ovarian neoplasms[12] (Level III). The appearance of virilizing symptoms in the pregnant patient leads to this diagnosis. When a luteoma is suspected, laparotomy can be avoided during pregnancy because the lesions regress after delivery[12] (Level III).

Paraovarian lesions are virtually always from a benign etiology and therefore do not require surgical intervention during pregnancy. Paraovarian cysts are common benign lesions usually 1 to 2 cm in size appearing as simple, anechoic structures. The sonographic appearance of a hydrosalpinx is characteristically an elongated tubular cystic structure with incomplete septations or nodules from thickened endosalpingeal folds[5] (Level III).

Leiomyomas are the most common solid adnexal masses found during pregnancy. Sonographic appearance is variable depending on whether the myoma has undergone degeneration, infarction, or necrosis. **Tubo-ovarian abscess** is another adnexal mass where the normal morphological pattern of the ovary is lost and replaced by a complex cystic structure. There are also **nongynecologic causes** of adnexal masses that need to be considered during pregnancy including acute appendicitis, irritable bowel disease, or adhesive disease from prior surgeries.

When an ovarian cyst is complex (and not hemorrhagic), the likelihood of neoplasm is increased. The *most common malignancies during pregnancy* are germ cell tumors, stromal or epithelial tumors of low malignant potential (LMP).[15] **Dysgerminoma** is a type of germ cell tumor accounting for less than 5% of ovarian cancers overall. It is the most common invasive malignant neoplasm in pregnancy (excluding epithelial tumors). Sonographic appearance of dysgerminomas is likely to be a solid mass with anechoic areas from hemorrhage or necrosis. Prognosis is very good as it is sensitive to chemotherapy and radiation. **Sex-cord stromal tumors** such as fibromas, thecomas, or granulose cell tumors, although uncommon overall, are potential malignancies detected during pregnancy.

Epithelial neoplasms include cystadenomas, cystadenocarcinomas, and tumors of low malignant potential (LMP). **Cystadenomas** may be simple cysts or have thin septations. *Serous* cystadenomas are the most common type with 20% being bilateral. They tend to be anechoic, whereas *mucinous* tumors have low-level internal echoes with multiple septations. Approximately 10% to 15% of cystadenomas are of LMP which have cytological features of malignancy without evidence of stromal invasion[5] (Level III). Irregular septations, mural nodules, and increased vascularity by color Doppler interrogation on ultrasound increase the likelihood of malignancy.

The management of asymptomatic adnexal masses that persist during pregnancy remains controversial. Traditionally, these patients are treated by exploratory laparotomy and tumor resection at 16 to 20 weeks of gestation despite the lack of supporting data[12] (Level III). Surgery is performed to rule out malignancy and prevent complications such as torsion, cyst rupture, and obstruction of labor. Abdominal surgery during pregnancy is associated with its own complications, including spontaneous miscarriage, rupture of membranes, preterm labor, and preterm birth[12] (Level III). Advances in ultrasonography have caused practitioners to question whether surgical intervention is warranted in all pregnant patients with adnexal masses.

Observation has therefore been proposed for select patients with an adnexal mass during pregnancy[8,13] (Level II-2, Level III). To our knowledge, no prospective studies randomizing between observation and surgery have been performed. Schmeler et al (2005) performed a retrospective study whereby they reviewed the records of women with adnexal masses greater than 5 cm during pregnancy (N = 59) and evaluated the circumstances of each case as well as final outcome. Seventeen (29%) of these women had surgery and 42 (71%) were observed during pregnancy then underwent cystectomy or oophorectomy at time of cesarean section. Two of the surgical cases were by laparoscopy and the rest via laparotomy. Five of 17 (29%) surgical cases were diagnosed with a malignancy on final pathologic analysis. None of those cases which were observed had a malignancy. All of the malignant masses had complex features on ultrasonography compared with 30% of benign cases[13] (Level III). The authors propose that in select cases, close observation is a reasonable alternative to antepartum surgery in patients with an adnexal mass during pregnancy.

Tumor Markers in Pregnancy

In general, CA-125 levels are not useful because CA-125 can be elevated in pregnancy, especially in the first trimester and again at time of delivery. During the second and third trimesters, serum levels were below 35 U/mL[16] (Level II-2). Although alpha-fetoprotein (AFP) screening is used to detect neural tube defects, markedly elevated AFP levels are seen with endodermal sinus tumors[17] (Level III). As for lactate dehydrogenase (LDH), it does not change in pregnancy and therefore can be assayed in pregnancy to follow the course of a dysgerminoma.

Comprehension Questions

42.1   A 31-year-old G1P0 woman presents to your office at 32 weeks of gestation with an adnexal mass which is described on sonogram as having a complex echo pattern and calcified material. There is no free fluid and the mass is 5 cm. What is the most likely diagnosis?

     A. Benign cystic teratoma

     B. Hemorrhagic corpus luteum cyst

     C. Ovarian hyperstimulation syndrome

     D. Theca lutein cyst

42.2   A 29-year-old G1P0 woman at 10 weeks of gestation presents with an adnexal mass of 4 cm in size that is thin walled without septations or projections. What is the best management for this patient?

     A. Perform immediate exploratory laparotomy and staging procedure.

     B. Perform a laparoscopic excision of mass during second trimester.

     C. Repeat ultrasound in the second trimester.

     D. Refer her to a gynecologic oncologist for the remainder of her pregnancy.

42.3   A 19-year-old G2P1001 woman at 15 weeks' gestation is noted to have a 9 cm adnexal mass. She complains of abdominal pain that is crampy in nature and associated with nausea and vomiting. Which of the following is the most likely diagnosis?

     A. Abruptio placenta

     B. Chorioamnionitis

     C. Ovarian torsion

     D. Rupture of membranes

ANSWERS

42.1   **A.** Teratomas are the most common benign ovarian neoplasm diagnosed in pregnancy and the mass described in this example is consistent with the sonographic features of a teratoma.

42.2   **C.** This adnexal mass is small (< 8 cm) and simple, and is most likely a physiologic cyst. Simple cysts that are less than 5 cm usually resolve by the second trimester and therefore observation is the best approach.

42.3   **C.** Ovarian torsion is a potential complication of an adnexal mass during pregnancy. This is a clinical diagnosis. Doppler flow studies of the ovarian vessels may or may not be helpful.

Clinical Pearls

See US Preventive Services Task Force Study Quality levels of evidence in Case 1

➤ Almost 100% of simple cysts smaller than 5 cm will resolve spontaneously by second trimester (Level III).

➤ Malignancy is most likely with thick-walled cyst, containing thick septations and internal projections. Increased flow by color Doppler in this setting is also suspicious (Level II-3).

➤ Adnexal masses greater than 5 cm are at risk for torsion, rupture, and sometimes labor obstruction in pregnancy (Level II-3).

➤ Risks of abdominal surgery during pregnancy include spontaneous miscarriage, rupture of membranes, preterm labor, and preterm birth (Level III).

➤ If surgical intervention can be planned and is necessary, performing it during the early second trimester is recommended (Level III).

REFERENCES

1. Leiserowitz GS. Managing ovarian masses in pregnancy. *Obstet Gynecol Surv.* 2006;61(7):463-470.
   A thorough review article on the management of adnexal masses during pregnancy including the use of diagnostic testing and options for treatment (Level III).

2. Bernard LM, et al. Predictors of persistence of adnexal masses in pregnancy. *Obstet Gynecol.* 1999;93:585-589 (Level II-2).

3. Zanetta G, Mariani E, Lissoni A, et al. A prospective study of the role of ultrasound in the management of adnexal masses in pregnancy. *BJOG.* 2003;110:578-583.
   A large prospective cohort study of pregnant women with adnexal masses of greater than 3 cm who underwent observation or surgery based on sonographic appearance. The authors conclude that expectant management is successful in majority of cases with low incidence of malignancy or antepartum complications (Level II-2).

4. Whitecar MP, Turner S, Higby MK. Adnexal masses in pregnancy: a review of 130 cases undergoing surgical management. *Am J Obstet Gynecol.* 1999;181:19-24.
   A review of 130 cases of adnexal masses in pregnancy which showed that emergent surgery does not increase the risk of adverse pregnancy outcome (Level III).

5. Glanc P. Adnexal masses in the pregnant patient: a diagnostic and management challenge. *Ultrasound Q.* 2008;24(4):225-240 (Level III).

6. Nelson MJ, Nelson MJ, Cavalieri R, Graham D, Sanders RC. Cysts in pregnancy discovered by sonography. *J Clin Ultrasound.* 1986;14:509-512 (Level II-3).

7. Fleischer AC, Boehm FH, James AE Jr. Sonography and radiology of pelvic masses and other maternal disorders. *Semin Roentgenol.* 1982;17:172-181 (Level II-3).

8. Thorton JG, and Phelps RL. Ovarian cysts in pregnancy: does ultrasound make traditional management inappropriate? *Obstet Gynecol.* 1987;69:717-720 (Level II-2).

9. Ghossain MA, Buy JN, Ruiz A, et al. Hyperreactio luteinalis in a normal pregnancy: sonographic and MRI findings. *J Magn Reson Imaging.* 1998;8:1203-1206 (Level III).

10. Baltarowich OH, Kurtz AB, Pasto ME, Rifkin MD, Needleman L, Goldberg BB. The spectrum of sonographic findings in hemorrhagic ovarian cysts. *AJR Am J Roentgenol.* 1987;148:901-905 (Level III).

11. Ritchi WGM. Ultrasound evaluation of normal and induced ovulation. In: Callen PW (ed). *Ultrasonography in Obstetrics and Gynecology.* 3rd ed. Philadelphia, PA: WB Saunders Co; 1994:582 (Level II-3).

12. Chiang G, and Levine D. Imaging of adnexal masses in pregnancy. *J Ultrasound Med.* 2004;23:805-819 (Level III).

13. Schmeler KM, Mayo-Smith WW, Peipert JF, Weitzen S, Manuel MD, Gordinier ME. Adnexal masses in pregnancy: surgery compared with observation. *Obstet Gynecol.* 2005;105(5):1098-1103.
    Between 1990 and 2003, 127,177 deliveries were performed at our institution. An adnexal mass 5 cm in diameter or greater was diagnosed in 63 (0.05%) patients. Antepartum surgery was performed in 17 patients (29%): 13 because of ultrasound findings that suggested malignancy and 4 secondary to ovarian torsion. The remaining patients were observed, with surgery performed in the postpartum period or at the time of cesarean delivery. The majority of masses were dermoid cysts (42%). Four patients were diagnosed with ovarian cancer (6.8% of masses, 0.0032% of deliveries), and one patient (1.7%) had a tumor of low malignant potential. Antepartum surgery due to ultrasound findings that caused concern was performed on all five women diagnosed with a malignancy or borderline tumor, compared with 12 (22%) of the patients with benign tumors (P < 0.01). The authors conclude that in select cases, close observation is a reasonable alternative to antepartum surgery in patients with an adnexal mass during pregnancy (Level III).

14. Choi JR, Levine D, Finberg H. Luteoma of pregnancy: sonographic finding in two cases. *J Ultrasound Med.* 2000;19(12):877-881.

15. ACOG Practice Bulletin. Management of adnexal masses. *Obstet Gynecol.* 2007 Jul;110(1):201-214.

16. Kobayashi F, Sagawa N, Nakamura K, et al. Mechanism and clinical significance of elevated CA-125 levels in sera of pregnant women. *Am J Obstet Gynecol.* 1989;160:563-566.
    CA-125 was found to peak at 10 weeks gestation and again at the time of delivery. During the second and third trimesters, serum levels were below 35 U/mL. CA-125 is very high in the amniotic fluid during the second trimester. These investigators conclude that elevated CA-125 levels in maternal sera are found at the time of chorionic invasion or placental separation (Level II-2).

17. Christman JE, Teng NN, Lebovic GS, Sikic BI. Delivery of a normal infant following cisplatin, vinblastine, and bleomycin (PVB) chemotherapy for malignant teratoma of the ovary during pregnancy. *Gynecol Oncol.* 1990;37:292-295 (Level III).

Case 43

A 36-year-old primigravida at 28 weeks' gestation is seen in your office for a routine prenatal visit. She has had an uncomplicated pregnancy to date including normal maternal serum screening at 16 weeks' gestation. Ultrasound at 18 weeks' gestation revealed an appropriately grown singleton infant with no obvious anatomic anomalies and normal amniotic fluid volume. She currently reports normal fetal activity and rare uterine contractions since her last visit in your office. She denies vaginal leaking or bleeding. She does feel that she has grown much larger over the past 4 weeks than in comparable 4-week intervals during this pregnancy, and says that when she is at work, many people think she is "due any day" because of her increasing abdominal girth.

On physical examination, she is alert and oriented, and states she feels well. Her blood pressure is 120/80 mm Hg and her weight is 138 lb, which is up 6 lb over the past month. Her fundal height is 36 cm. Ultrasound in your office reveals a vertex fetus with estimated fetal weight of 1500 g, normal head circumference/abdominal circumference ratio, and amniotic fluid index of 26 with single deepest vertical pocket of 10 cm.

➤ What is the most likely diagnosis?

➤ What is your next step?

➤ What are potential complications of the patient's disorder?

ANSWERS TO CASE 43:

Polyhydramnios

Summary: This is a 36-year-old at 28 weeks with a rapidly enlarging fundal height due to excessive amniotic fluid volume.

➤ **Most likely diagnosis:** Hydramnios (or polyhydramnios).

➤ **Next step:** Evaluate fetal anatomy, test for maternal diabetes, and monitor for preterm labor.

➤ **Potential complications:** Preterm labor, preterm PROM and abruptio placenta, fetal anomalies, maternal diabetes, abnormal fetal presentation, postpartum hemorrhage.

ANALYSIS

Objectives

1. Describe the production and regulation of amniotic fluid.
2. List risk factors for oligo- and polyhydramnios.
3. Explain fetal anatomic reasons for abnormal amniotic fluid volume measurements.
4. List maternal reasons for abnormal amniotic fluid volume measurements.
5. Discuss management of the pregnancy with excess or inadequate amniotic fluid volume.

Considerations

This patient represents a commonly seen issue in obstetrics—an unexplained increase in amniotic fluid in the third trimester. Although this patient's ultimate etiology may be as simple as maternal hyperglycemia, and may indicate little or no excessive fetal or maternal morbidity, half or more of cases of polyhydramnios remain idiopathic with no obvious cause discovered even after birth. This case should include maternal glucose screening, repeat ultrasound evaluation for anomalies that cause polyhydramnios and an estimation of fetal weight, and assessment for uterine contractions and prodromal preterm labor. If the workup is negative, follow-up ultrasound in 2 to 3 weeks would be the next step in her care.

APPROACH TO
Polyhydramnios

Normal Amniotic Fluid

Although term human fetuses vary in size, an average 3.5 kg fetus contains about 2500 mL of water, 350 mL of which is intravascular and 1000 mL of which is intracellular, the remainder being extracellular. The placenta contains about 500 mL of water, and 500 to 1200 mL of water is present in the amniotic fluid. Amniotic fluid functions include those of a physical nature to protect the fetus and cord, a functional nature to allow substrate for breathing, movement, and swallowing activities, and a homeostatic nature to protect against infection and regulate uterine activity.

Amniotic Fluid Dynamics

During the first trimester, amniotic fluid is isotonic with maternal or fetal plasma and represents a transudate of plasma, either from the fetus across nonkeratinized fetal skin or from the mother across the uterine decidua and/or placental surface. With advancing gestation, amniotic fluid composition diverges from that of plasma as the transudative process becomes negligible by 22 to 23 weeks' gestation. Amniotic fluid osmolality and sodium composition decrease, felt to be the result of dilute fetal urine. During the second half of pregnancy, in keeping with the increasing fetal urine production, amniotic fluid urea, creatinine, and uric acid increase resulting in amniotic fluid concentrations of urinary by-products two to three times higher than fetal plasma. At this time, amniotic fluid is formed primarily from fetal lung fluid (about 100 mL/d) and fetal urine (7-10 mL/kg/h) and is eliminated primarily by fetal swallowing (up to 1 L/d). Fetal lung fluid production is affected by a diversity of fetal physiologic and endocrine factors including AVP (amniotic vertical pocket), catecholamines, and cortisol (all of which decrease lung fluid production), effects that may explain the enhanced clearance of lung fluid in fetuses delivered after labor compared to elective cesarean section.

The amount of fluid swallowed by the fetus daily does not equal the amount of fluid produced by the sum of kidneys and lungs, and because the volume of amniotic fluid does not greatly increase during the last half of pregnancy, intramembranous transfer of fluid is suspected to maintain this equilibrium. The intramembranous pathway refers to the route of absorption from the amniotic cavity directly across the amnion into fetal vessels (as opposed to the transmembranous pathway which refers to absorption from amniotic fluid to maternal blood within the uterus). In sheep, the intramembranous pathway, combined with fetal swallowing, approximately equals the flow of urine and lung liquid under homeostatic conditions. In humans, indirect evidence supports the existence of a similar pathway. This intramembranous pathway may explain the observation that in upper GI tract obstruction in the human fetus with no fetal swallowing, only 40% develop polyhydramnios.

Amniotic Fluid Volume Measurements

In invasive studies using amniocentesis to instill dye with remeasuring after mixing, neither single maximum vertical pocket (MVP) nor the four quadrant amniotic fluid index (AFI) produce very accurate evaluation of actual volume. Since clinical correlations are established between these ultrasound estimates and clinical outcome, however, the absolute volume present is not a primary issue. Categorization of polyhydramnios by MVP is more closely associated with clinical outcome, and in management comparisons reported in the Cochrane database in 2008, neither MVP nor AFI was superior in preventing admission to the NICU, an umbilical artery pH less than 7.1, the presence of meconium, an APGAR score of less than 7 at 5 minutes, or cesarean delivery. However, the AFI was associated with significantly more diagnoses of oligohydramnios and more women had inductions of labor and cesarean sections for fetal stress. The authors concluded that the MVP was the preferred method to assess AFV during fetal assessment, since the AFI increased the diagnosis of oligohydramnios and intervention without improvement in peripartum outcomes.

Oligohydramnios

Reduced amniotic fluid has been linked with numerous adverse pregnancy outcomes, and thus its detection is critical. Subjective assessments of low amniotic fluid volume have been replaced by quantitative measures of either MVP (also referred to as single deepest pocket, or SDP) or amniotic fluid index (AFI). Both of these measurements were introduced in the literature in the 1980s, with the AFI initially being promoted as the more accurate method to assess fluid volume. In an attempt to confirm previously reported normative data with both techniques, however, Magann et al[1] reported that when using an AFI of ≤ 5 cm or SDP of less than 2 cm as criteria for oligohydramnios, 8% of normal gravidas were falsely labeled as having oligohydramnios compared to only 1% with the SDP. In reviewing randomized clinical trials comparing AFI to SDP, using the SDP to detect oligohydramnios was superior and resulted in fewer unnecessary interventions with similar fetal outcomes. The SDP is also the method of amniotic fluid assessment used in the biophysical profile (BPP). Thus, he and others recommend the SDP less than 2 cm as the most appropriate method to detect oligohydramnios.

Oligohydramnios prior to 20 weeks gestation is rare, and should prompt a careful search for renal agenesis, bladder outlet obstruction, another significant fetal anomaly, or rupture of the fetal membranes. After 20 weeks, additional reasons to be considered are inadequate prerenal volume (in situations such as IUGR, twin-twin transfusion syndrome, or unexplained markedly elevated MS-AFP which may indicate placental dysfunction and high perinatal mortality rates). Uterine and maternal etiologies should be sought, including intravascular dehydration or preeclampsia, and a careful search for PROM should occur as well in all cases of oligohydramnios after 20 weeks. When borderline oligohydramnios is suspected, maternal hydration should be considered, as improvements in AFI have been noted after IV or PO fluid administration in several studies.

Isolated oligohydramnios in the third trimester when other fetal testing is reassuring is an area of ongoing debate. In a recent national survey of perinatologists, 92% of respondents felt isolated oligohydramnios represented a potential precursor of adverse pregnancy outcome, but only 33% felt induction of labor could decrease adverse outcomes.

Polyhydramnios

Excessive amniotic fluid complicates up to 4% of pregnancies, usually being associated with a normal neonatal outcome. However, as Table 43–1 indicates, the greater the degree of excess fluid, the more likely an adverse outcome becomes. Over 50% of patients with polyhydramnios have no identifiable cause, and when detected in the third trimester or when associated with macrosomia, usually have a good outcome. When detected in the second trimester or when associated with low or normal birth weight, however, nearly 30% of infants will have an abnormality detected during or after the first year of life, and experts recommend in those cases, careful antenatal ultrasound evaluation of fetal movement (to exclude hypotonia), and the fetal face and heart as possible causes of the hydramnios.

When an antenatal cause is identified, it usually is the result of maternal diabetes, multiple gestation, GI tract obstruction, underlying neurologic disorders that prevent or reduce fetal swallowing, cardiac anomalies (structural, functional, or rhythm disturbances), or chromosomal or genetic disorders.

Table 43–1 DEGREE OF HYDRAMNIOS, FREQUENCY, PERINATAL MORTALITY, AND ANOMALY RATE					
DEGREE	SDP	AFI	FREQUENCY	PNM	ANOMALIES
Mild	> 8 cm	> 24 cm	68%	50/1000	≤ 6%
Moderate	> 11 cm	> 32 cm	19%	190/1000	Up to 45%
Severe	> 15 cm	> 44 cm	13%	540/1000	Up to 65%

Data from Harman CR. Amniotic fluid abnormalities. *Semin Perinatol.* 2008;32:288-294.

SDP = Single deepest vertical pocket; AFI = amniotic fluid index; PNM = perinatal mortality

Structural fetal anomalies associated with hydramnios have an associated 9% to 10% risk of aneuploidy, compared to the 1% risk of aneuploidy with isolated hydramnios, and patients should be counseled regarding amniocentesis accordingly. Rh isoimmunization, metabolic disorders, and fetal infections may also cause hydramnios and should be considered prior to categorizing the etiology as idiopathic.

Management of the patient with unexplained hydramnios includes evaluation for preterm labor, preterm rupture of membranes and abruptio placenta, abnormal presentation in labor, and postpartum hemorrhage. At delivery, the infant's pediatrician should be notified of the history of hydramnios so a thorough evaluation of the neonate can occur.

Comprehension Questions

43.1   Complete bladder outlet obstruction viewed sonographically at 16 weeks' gestation would be associated with which of the following?
A. Severe oligohydramnios
B. Normal amniotic fluid volume
C. Polyhydramnios
D. Unable to determine

43.2   Production of amniotic fluid includes which of the following organ systems?
A. lungs
B. liver
C. bone
D. CNS

43.3   Oligohydramnios is best detected clinically with few false positives using which of the following techniques?
A. AFI
B. SDP
C. Subjective assessment
D. Dye dilution techniques

43.4   Polyhydramnios, when idiopathic, is associated with neonatal abnormalities in which of the following ranges?
A. 10%
B. 20%
C. 30%
D. 40%

ANSWERS

43.1 **B.** Fetal skin keratinization occurs around mid-gestation, and at 16 weeks, complete bladder outlet obstruction would appear sonographically with normal amniotic fluid volume.

43.2 **A.** In addition to fetal urination, the fetal lungs produce up to 100 mL of amniotic fluid daily.

43.3 **B.** Diagnosing oligohydramnios using the single deepest pocket measurement is associated with fewer false positives, and similar perinatal outcomes to the AFI calculation.

43.4 **C.** Idiopathic polyhydramnios detected prior to the third trimester and not associated with macrosomia is associated with neonatal abnormalities in 28% or more of infants.

Clinical Pearls

See US Preventive Services Task Force Study Quality levels of evidence in Case 1

➤ Amniotic fluid is isotonic with fetal and maternal plasma prior to 22 weeks' gestation (Level II-3).
➤ In addition to fetal swallowing and lung and urinary production, the intramembranous pathway regulates amniotic fluid volume (Level II-2).
➤ The single deepest pocket (SDP) is superior to the amniotic fluid index (AFI) when evaluating for oligohydramnios, and results in fewer false-positive results (Level II-1).
➤ Idiopathic polyhydramnios has an up to 28% chance of neonatal abnormality, and should prompt a careful newborn examination (Level II-3).

REFERENCES

1. Magann EF, Chauhan SP, Doherty DA, Magann MI, Morrison JC. The evidence for abandoning the amniotic fluid index in favor of the single deepest pocket. *Am J Perinatol.* 2007;24:549-558.
2. Beall MH, van den Wijngaard JPHM, van Gemert MJC, Ross, MG. Amniotic fluid water dynamics. *Placenta.* 2007;28:816-823.
3. Dashe JS, McIntire DD, Ramus RM, Santos-Ramos R, Twickler DM. Hydramnios: anomaly prevalence and sonographic detection. *Obstet Gynecol.* 2002;100:134-139.
4. Dorleijn DMJ, Cohen-Overbeek TE, Groenendaal F, Bruinse HW, Stoutenbeek P. Idiopathic polyhydramnios and postnatal findings. *J Matern Fetal Neonatal Med.* 2008 Dec;13:1-6.
5. Harman CR. Amniotic fluid abnormalities. *Semin Perinatol.* 2008;32:288-294.

6. Nabhan AF, Abdelmoula YA. Amniotic fluid index versus single deepest vertical pocket as a screening test for preventing adverse pregnancy outcome. *Cochrane Database Syst Rev* 2008; 3. Art. No.:CD006593. doi: 10.1002/14651858.CD006593.pub2.

7. Schwartz N, Sweeting R, Young BK. Practice patterns in the management of isolated oligohydramnios: a survey of perinatologists. *J Matern Fetal Neonatal Med.* 2008 Dec;16:1-5.

Case 44

A 32-year-old G4P1113 woman presents for a routine prenatal visit at 22 weeks' gestation by a sure LMP consistent with an 8-week sonogram. She has no significant past medical or surgical history. Her obstetric history is significant for a full-term vaginal delivery followed by a twin vaginal delivery at 36 weeks. She also had a first-trimester miscarriage between the first and second pregnancies.

She is employed as a youth counselor at the local elementary school. Her children are in daycare 2 days per week. She denies use of alcohol and tobacco, and is a vegetarian. She reports having had "cold" symptoms 3 to 4 weeks ago when her children were all sick for 2 days.

On physical examination, her blood pressure is 108/62 mm Hg, pulse of 74 bpm, respiratory rate of 18 breaths/min. Her weight is 165 lb and the urine dipstick is negative for protein or glucose. The fundal height is 26 cm. She reports the sensation of fetal movement and denies contractions. The patient undergoes a fetal anatomical survey which is significant for a single intrauterine gestation. The fetal growth parameters are consistent with the established gestational age. There is polyhydramnios of 24 cm and bilateral pleural effusions are noted. There is a small rim of ascites at the level of the fetal abdominal circumference. There are no gross structural anomalies noted. The placenta is posterior and unremarkable.

➤ What is the most likely diagnosis?

➤ What is the next step in evaluating this patient?

➤ What are the potential maternal risks?

➤ What are the potential fetal risks?

ANSWERS TO CASE 44:
Nonimmune Hydrops

Summary: A multigravida at 22 weeks' gestation with increased fundal height and ultrasound findings of polyhydramnios, bilateral pleural effusions, and ascites.

➤ **Most likely diagnosis:** The diagnosis is fetal hydrops. Fetal hydrops can be immune or nonimmune. As the patient's blood type is Rh+ with a negative antibody screen, a nonimmune process is likely responsible for the fetal hydrops.

➤ **Next step:** The next step is to evaluate for causes of nonimmune hydrops fetalis (NIHF). In addition to fetal anomalies, placental abnormalities should be considered. Other common etiologies of NIH include genetic, infectious, and hematologic disorders and an evaluation of these should be performed.

➤ **Potential maternal risks:** It is important to be aware that maternal birth trauma from delivery of a large edematous fetus is possible. Mirror syndrome is a rare complication in which maternal pulmonary edema and preeclampsia develop. In addition, there is also an increased risk of cesarean delivery, postpartum hemorrhage, and retained placenta.

➤ **Potential fetal risks:** There is an increased risk of premature labor and/or premature rupture of membranes due to uterine overdistension. Dystocia at the time of delivery may also occur due to an edematous fetus. Pleural effusions may make resuscitation more difficult and may require drainage in the early neonatal period to improve the ability to ventilate. Lung hypoplasia due to the pleural effusions may make neonatal resuscitation impossible.

ANALYSIS

1. Describe the clinical presentation of hydrops fetalis.
2. Describe the causes of hydrops fetalis including immune and nonimmune causes.
3. Describe the diagnostic strategy of hydrops.

Considerations

The incidence of **nonimmune hydrops fetalis (NIHF)** ranges from 1/1500 to 1/3800 births[1-4,5] (Level III, Level II-2). This variation is likely due to differences in the definitions, populations studied, and the extent of the fetal evaluation when hydrops is noted. In addition, cases of fetal demise and pregnancy terminations are included in some studies and excluded in others.

Immune hydrops occurs in relation to red blood cell alloimmunization, most commonly to Rh(D) and Kell antibodies. In contrast, NIHF includes the causes of fetal hydrops that are not mediated by an immune mechanism. Prior to the widespread use of RhIg, red cell alloimmunization was the most common cause of fetal hydrops. However, nearly 90% of fetal hydrops cases are now related to nonimmune hydrops[1] (Level III).

Fetal hydrops is diagnosed by the presence of **excess fluid in two or more fetal compartments** including the pleural cavity (Figure 44-1), pericardial cavity, abdominal cavity (ascites; Figure 44-2), amniotic sac (polyhydramnios; Figure 44-3), and skin edema. Abnormalities within each organ system may lead to nonimmune hydrops fetalis. A brief list of some of the more common causes of NIHF will be presented as a comprehensive list of etiologies is beyond the scope of this chapter. Unfortunately, antenatal determination of the etiology of hydrops is only successful 50% to 85% of the time. An additional 5% of cases may have an underlying etiology that can be determined after delivery while the remainder will be classified as idiopathic. Some of the more common causes of NIHF include disorders of the systems shown in Table 44-1.

This patient's pregnancy has been relatively uncomplicated to date except for a cold approximately 1 month ago. The initial evaluation of a patient with nonimmune fetal hydrops includes a detailed anatomy ultrasound, evaluation for fetal anemia by measuring peak systolic velocity (PSV) of the middle cere-

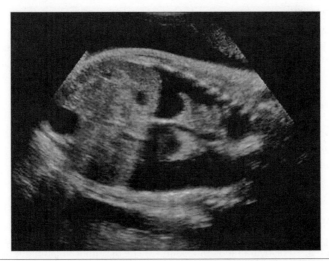

Figure 44–1. Bilateral pleural effusions. The fetal chest is filled with echolucent material, which represents pleural fluid. (*Reproduced, with permission, from Dr. Svena Julien.*)

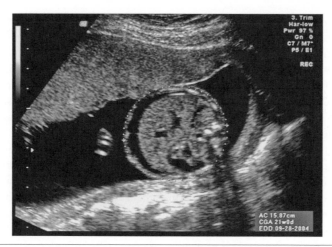

Figure 44–2.   Rim of ascites. Fetal abdomen has a moderately large echolucent border which constitutes ascites. (*Reproduced, with permission, from Dr. Svena Julien.*)

bral artery (MCA), and serologic testing for infection. Amniocentesis for fetal karyotype should also be offered to exclude a chromosomal abnormality. Prognosis depends on the underlying etiology and gestational age at which hydrops has occurred. In general, when nonimmune hydrops develops, the prognosis is uniformly poor.

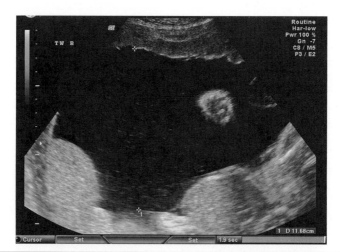

Figure 44–3.   Polyhydramnios. Ultrasound image of significant amniotic fluid. Note large amount of echolucent space from anterior uterine wall to posterior placenta (cursor at 11.7 cm). (*Reproduced, with permission, from Dr. Svena Julien.*)

Table 44–1 ETIOLOGIES OF FETAL HYDROPS

- **Genetic disorders (10%)**
  - Aneuploidy including monosomy X, trisomy 21, trisomy 18
  - Syndromes including skeletal dysplasias
  - Metabolic storage diseases including Hurler syndrome, Gaucher disease
- **Cardiovascular (40%)**
  - Structural lesions such as AVSD, hypoplastic left and right heart syndrome, cardiomyopathy
  - Arrhythmias including tachyarrhythmia and bradyarrhythmia
- **Pulmonary (10%)**
  - Pulmonary sequestration
  - Congenital cystic adenomatoid malformation of the lung
  - Diaphragmatic hernia
  - Pulmonary neoplasia and lymphangiectasia
  - Bronchogenic cysts
- **Infectious diseases (8%)**
  - Parvovirus
  - Cytomegalovirus
  - Syphilis
  - Coxsackie virus
  - Toxoplasmosis
  - Rubella virus
- **Gastrointestinal and renal**
  - Gut duplications and malrotation
  - Hepatobiliary vascular malformation and tumor
  - Congenital Finnish-type nephrosis
  - Posterior urethral valves
  - Prune belly syndrome
- **Hematologic (10%-27%)**
  - α Thalassemia
  - Aplastic anemia related to parvovirus infection
  - Other red cell aplasias
  - Fetal hemorrhage
- **Placental abnormalities** including AV fistulas, chorioangiomas, umbilical cord thrombosis, and aneurysms
- **Other**
  - Twin-to-twin transfusion sequence

APPROACH TO
Nonimmune Hydrops Fetalis

The diagnosis of nonimmune fetal hydrops is made by the ultrasound findings of abnormal fluid in two or more fetal compartments. **Pleural effusions** may be visualized as echolucent fluid outlining the lungs. They may be unilateral or bilateral, and may lead to compression of lung tissue giving the appearance of small lungs. Over time, effusions may restrict the growth of the fetal lungs and put the fetus at risk for pulmonary hypoplasia. This is more common when hydrops develops prior to 20 weeks of gestation and is a common cause of neonatal mortality in infants surviving to delivery. A number of authors have described ultrasound techniques to determine the severity of lung hypoplasia, but none are consistently reliable[6] (Level III).

Pericardial effusions can be seen in fetuses with fetal hydrops and are described when the rim of fluid within the pericardial sac is greater than 4 to 5 mm. It is important not to mistake physiologic pericardial fluid for an effusion as 2 mm of fluid is normal[7] (Level II-2).

Fetal ascites is noted when a rim of fluid outlines the abdominal cavity and often the intraabdominal organs. It is important to distinguish true ascites from pseudoascites. Pseudoascites is an echolucent rim around the abdomen that actually represents prominent abdominal wall muscles. As the amount of ascites increases, the bowel may appear compressed and echogenic[8,9] (Level III).

An amniotic fluid index of greater than 24 cm or a maximum vertical pocket greater than 8 cm is consistent with **polyhydramnios.**[10] It is present in 40% to 75% of pregnancies complicated by nonimmune hydrops. Size greater than dates related to polyhydramnios is often the initial indication for a growth sonogram evaluation of the pregnancy.

Pathologic **skin edema** is a late finding in hydrops fetalis. It is defined as a tissue thickness of the subcutaneous tissue greater than 5 mm.[10] However, during the sonographic evaluation, subcutaneous fat should not be included in the measurement of edema (Figure 44-4).

Placentomegaly may occur due to edema of the intervillous spaces and may be a manifestation of nonimmune hydrops. However, be aware that significant polyhydramnios may lead to a thinned or compressed appearing placenta. In general, a placental thickness of greater than 4 to 6 cm is considered abnormal and should prompt further investigation[11,12] (Level III).

Once fetal hydrops is confirmed, an extensive examination of the fetal anatomy and placenta should be done. A number of potential causes of hydrops can be excluded based upon the finding of normal fetal anatomy. In addition, a thorough maternal history including ethnicity, family history of inherited disorders, travel history, and infectious agent exposure should be done. Given the vast number of etiologic possibilities, several laboratory studies may need to be undertaken concomitantly.

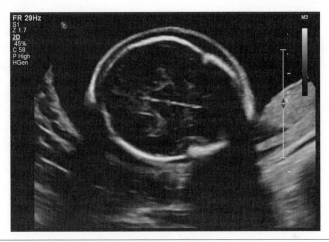

Figure 44–4. Scalp edema. Ultrasound image of significant scalp edema. (*Reproduced, with permission, from Dr. Svena Julien.*)

The initial evaluation includes the fetal anatomical survey. Following this examination, maternal blood type and antibody screen should be obtained. An amniocentesis for karyotype should be offered. Additional amniotic fluid should be obtained in order to test for viral pathogens using amniotic fluid PCR, and fluid may be frozen for analysis to exclude metabolic storage diseases in an at risk population. Additional sonographic evaluation can include a fetal echocardiogram to exclude a cardiac etiology of the hydrops, and interrogation of the fetal middle cerebral artery (MCA). The peak systolic velocity assessment of the MCA may be used to determine the presence of fetal anemia. If MCA Dopplers are found to be elevated, fetal blood sampling may be indicated. Other components of the evaluation include maternal CBC, serologic assessment for the TORCH pathogens including toxoplasmosis, CMV, HSV, rubella, as well as other viruses such as parvovirus B19, Coxsackie, and adenovirus.

Once the diagnosis has been established, the patient must be counseled regarding the prognosis for the pregnancy. The perinatal mortality rate remains greater than 50%, and may be as high as 100% according to some studies[13-16] (Level III). The overall prognosis is related to the underlying etiology of the hydrops. In addition, the gestational age at which the hydrops was noted impacts the prognosis. As noted earlier, hydrops with pleural effusions that develops prior to 20 weeks of gestation is associated with an increased risk of pulmonary hypoplasia and its associated morbidity. Aneuploid fetuses, as well as those with structural abnormalities are at greater risk of fetal demise[17,18] (Level III). Additional risks include preterm labor and premature rupture of membranes due to uterine overdistention. Premature delivery is independently associated with adverse outcomes, and these may be potentiated in a compromised fetus.

Given the poor prognosis associated with nonimmune hydrops, termination of the pregnancy may be considered. Management of an ongoing pregnancy should include therapeutic interventions specific to the etiology of the hydrops. For example, in cases of fetal anemia due to parvovirus infection, red blood cell transfusion should be considered. Antenatal surveillance should include serial fetal testing to assure overall fetal well-being. There is no established frequency for antenatal fetal testing, but several authors recommend weekly or twice weekly fetal surveillance. Delivery may be indicated depending upon the results of such testing, and should occur at a tertiary care center with neonatal staff available. A neonatal consultation and possibly pediatric subspecialty consultations should be obtained prior to delivery.

Maternal risks at the time of delivery include soft tissue trauma due to an edematous fetus, postpartum hemorrhage, and retained placenta. However, cesarean delivery should be reserved for the usual obstetric indications.

Comprehension Questions

44.1   In a fetus with new-onset hydrops related to parvovirus B19 infection at 29 weeks, what is the most appropriate screening test for fetal anemia?
A. Fetal blood sampling
B. Biophysical profile testing
C. Umbilical artery Doppler study
D. Middle cerebral artery Doppler study
E. Delivery and neonatal CBC

44.2   A 26-year-old G2P0 presents at 21 weeks with fetal hydrops. What is the initial workup for this patient following the anatomy ultrasound?
A. Fetal blood sampling
B. Fetal surveillance with BPP
C. Fetal karyotype
D. Fetal MRI

44.3   A 38-year-old G3P2 with Graves disease presents with size greater than dates at 23 weeks. She has two small children at home with a viral illness and nausea/vomiting. An ultrasound shows fetal hydrops. What is the most likely etiology of the hydrops?
A. Fetal cardiac anomaly
B. Acute parvovirus infection with fetal anemia
C. Listeria transplacental infection
D. Antibody mediated high-output cardiac failure
E. Feto-maternal hemorrhage

ANSWERS

44.1   **D.** Middle cerebral artery Doppler study has a high sensitivity for predicting fetal anemia.

44.2   **C.** Amniocentesis for fetal karyotype is the next step in the evaluation of fetal hydrops.

44.3   **A.** Fetal cardiac abnormality is the most likely underlying etiology for NIH accounting for approximately 40% of all cases.

Clinical Pearls

See US Preventive Services Task Force Study Quality levels of evidence in Case 1

➤ Hydrops fetalis is the sonographic finding of excess fluid in two or more fetal compartments (Level III).

➤ NIHF includes fetal hydrops not mediated by red cell antigens (Level III).

➤ The causes of NIHF are numerous and include infectious, genetic, metabolic, and structural organ system anomalies (Level II-3).

➤ Amniocentesis or CVS should be considered in all cases of NIHF (Level III).

➤ Infectious studies that should be obtained in NIHF include assays for toxoplasmodium, rubella, CMV, HSV, Coxsackie, adenovirus, parvovirus, and syphilis. These may be from maternal serology or amniotic fluid PCR studies (Level III).

➤ Coordination of care in continuing pregnancies should include consultation with neonatal staff and possibly pediatric subspecialists along with maternal-fetal medicine specialists (Level III).

REFERENCES

1. Sohan K, Carroll SG, De La Fuente S, et al. Analysis of outcome in hydrops fetalis in relation to gestational age at diagnosis, cause and treatment. *Acta Obstet Gynecol Scand.* 2001;80:726.
   Database review of fetal hydrops cases and survival rates. Prior to 24 weeks the most common association was fetal aneuploidy. After 24 weeks fetal cardiac arrhythmias, especially tachyarrhythmias and hydrothorax were the most common causes of hydrops. Though overall prognosis is still quite dismal, appropriate prenatal investigation and therapy may improve survival rates (Level III).
2. Carlson DE, Platt LD, Medearis AL, Horenstein J. Prognostic indicators of the resolution of nonimmune hydrops fetalis and survival of the fetus. *Am J Obstet Gynecol.* 1990;163:1785 (Level III).
3. Castillo RA, Devoe LD, Hadi HA, Martin S, Geist D. Nonimmune hydrops fetalis: clinical experience and factors related to a poor outcome. *Am J Obstet Gynecol.* 1986;155:812.

A review of the sonographic detection of 21 cases of fetal hydrops. The perinatal mortality rate was 95% and the most common cause was lung hypoplasia. Two factors that were consistently associated with poor perinatal outcomes were sonographically detected malformation and the presence of persistent pleural effusions (Level III).

4. Anandakumar C, Biswas A, Wong YC, et al. Management of non-immune hydrops: 8 years' experience. *Ultrasound Obstet Gynecol.* 1996;8:196.
   By sonography 100 fetuses with NIFH were identified. Ten percent were related to aneuploidy. Twenty-six fetuses were candidates for in-utero therapies including IUT, direct fetal drug therapy, and fetal pleuro-amniotic shunting. In carefully selected cases, in-utero therapy may lead to improvements in fetal and neonatal survival (Level III).

5. Moise KJ Jr, Carpenter RJ Jr, Hesketh DE. Do abnormal Starling forces cause fetal hydrops in red blood cell alloimmunization? *Am J Obstet Gynecol.* 1992;167:907 (Level II-2).

6. Dizon-Townson DS, Dildy GA, Clark SL. A prospective evaluation of fetal pericardial fluid in 506 second-trimester low-risk pregnancies. *Obstet Gynecol.* 1997;90:958 (Level III).

7. Di Salvo DN, Brown DL, Doubilet PM, et al. Clinical significance of isolated fetal pericardial effusion. *J Ultrasound Med.* 1994;13:291 (Level II-2).

8. Callen P. *Ultrasonography in Obstetrics and Gynecology.* 4th ed. Philadelphia, PA: WB Saunders; 2000.

9. Jones DC. Nonimmune fetal hydrops: diagnosis and obstetrical management. *Semin Perinatol.* 1995;19:447 (Level III).

10. Romero R, Pilu G, Jeanty P, Ghidini A, Hobbins J. *Prenatal Diagnosis of Congenital Anomalies.* Norwalk, CT: Appleton and Lange; 1988.

11. Arcasoy MO, Gallagher PG. Hematologic disorders and nonimmune hydrops fetalis. *Semin Perinatol.* 1995;19:502 (Level III).

12. Chitkara U, Wilkins I, Lynch L, et al. The role of sonography in assessing severity of fetal anemia in Rh- and Kell-isoimmunized pregnancies. *Obstet Gynecol.* 1988;71:393 (Level III).

13. Ismail KM, Martin WL, Ghosh S, et al. Etiology and outcome of hydrops fetalis. *J Matern Fetal Med.* 2001;10:175 (Level III).

14. Graves GR, Baskett TF. Nonimmune hydrops fetalis: antenatal diagnosis and management. *Am J Obstet Gynecol.* 1984;148:563 (Level III).

15. Heinonen S, Ryynanen M, Kirkinen P. Etiology and outcome of second trimester non-immunologic fetal hydrops. *Acta Obstet Gynecol Scand.* 2000;79:15 (Level III).

16. Wy CA, Sajous CH, Loberiza F, Weiss MG. Outcome of infants with a diagnosis of hydrops fetalis in the 1990s. *Am J Perinatol.* 1999;16:561 (Level III).

17. McCoy MC, Katz VL, Gould N, Kuller JA. Non-immune hydrops after 20 weeks' gestation: review of 10 years' experience with suggestions for management. *Obstet Gynecol.* 1995;85:578 (Level III).

18. Iskaros J, Jauniaux E, Rodeck C. Outcome of nonimmune hydrops fetalis diagnosed during the first half of pregnancy. *Obstet Gynecol.* 1997;90:321 (Level III).

Listing of Cases

Listing by Case Number

Listing by Disorder (Alphabetical)

Page numbers followed by *f* or *t* indicate figures or tables, respectively.